# The SAGES University M; Series

Editor-in-Chief, Brian P. Jacob

Ankit D. Patel • Dmitry Oleynikov
Editors

# The SAGES Manual of Robotic Surgery

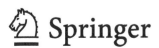 Springer

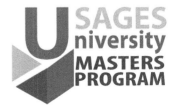

*Editors*
Ankit D. Patel
Department of General and Gastrointestinal
  Surgery
Emory Endosurgery
Emory University School of Medicine
Atlanta, GA, USA

Dmitry Oleynikov
Gastrointestinal, Minimally Invasive and
  Bariatric Surgery
The Center for Advanced Surgical
  Technology
University of Nebraska Medical Center
Omaha, NE, USA

Videos can also be accessed at http://link.springer.com/book/10.1007/978-3-319-51362-1

The SAGES University Masters Program Series
ISBN 978-3-319-51360-7       ISBN 978-3-319-51362-1    (eBook)
DOI 10.1007/978-3-319-51362-1

Library of Congress Control Number: 2017933834

Printed on acid-free paper

This Springer imprint is published by Springer Nature
The registered company is Springer International Publishing AG
The registered company address is: Gewerbestrasse 11, 6330 Cham, Switzerland

# Foreword

Several years ago I was asked to write a commentary on robotic surgery for a well-regarded surgical publication. At that time I was not a big fan of this new tool. I was impressed with the technological platform of robotic surgical systems and at that time I felt (as I still do today) that the platform held tremendous potential in the future. However, outcomes at that time were equivalent to standard laparoscopic surgery yet the one-time cost of the robot coupled with the ongoing costs of the service contract and the instruments used in each case were, in my view, exorbitant. I felt that given the relative lack of gold-standard evidence confirming that robotic surgery was associated with better patient outcomes when compared to current laparoscopic techniques and the cost which was associated with robotic surgical systems placed the new innovation in jeopardy. In short, I felt it was a little like using a Cadillac for a golf cart.

Spring forward several years; I must admit that I have developed a significantly different point of view. The robot does provide significant advantages in terms of ergonomics and enhanced minimally invasive surgical abilities for surgeons. In addition, it is a platform that can be further developed to facilitate smaller and smaller incisions. However, I still believe that it's important to point out that the robot is simply a tool—an expensive tool at that. In order to fully maximize the value of care provided to patients using this tool, surgeons must be efficient with setting up the device, have a clear understanding of the steps of an operation for which they are using the robot, minimize unnecessary use of expensive instruments during the conduct of an operation, and have equivalent outcomes to those reported for similar operations performed using laparoscopic or open techniques.

This manual provides a wealth of practical material regarding the application of robotics to common and complex minimally invasive surgery scenarios. Surgeons that actually do these operations using this tool wrote the chapters in this manual. The chapters give advice about room setup, patient positioning, proper robot positioning, as well as step-by-step descriptions of how each surgical procedure should be conducted. I am most impressed with the material compiled in this manual and I am convinced that the concepts outlined, if followed by the reader, will add to the value of care that we provide to our patients. Enjoy.

John F. Sweeney
Department of Surgery
Emory University School of Medicine
Atlanta, GA, USA

Emory Healthcare
Atlanta, GA, USA

# Preface

The number of robotic surgery procedures has significantly increased in the last few years, especially in general surgery and its subspecialties. Several advantages of the platform, such as three-dimensional visualization, articulating instruments, and improved ergonomics, have led to its adoption in minimally invasive procedures. As the techniques have evolved and been refined, it has allowed more surgeons access to a minimally invasive approach that they would have otherwise performed in a traditional open fashion, allowing potential benefits to the patient including less pain, less blood loss, and less wound-related complications. While laparoscopy continues to be the standard of care for cholecystectomy, robotics may be enabling in more complex gastrointestinal and hernia procedures.

This textbook is designed to present a comprehensive approach to the various applications of surgical techniques and procedures currently performed using a robotic surgical platform. The initial chapters address preliminary issues faced by surgeons and staff who may be initially undertaking these new techniques. These areas include training and credentialing, as well as instrumentation and platforms commonly used for these procedures. Subsequent chapters focus on specific disease processes and the robotic applications for those procedures, divided among the specialties. Written by unbiased experts in that field, each of these sections address issues such as patient selection, preoperative considerations, positioning and technical aspects of these operations, and how to avoid complications. Many have included their own experience and handy tips for a successful procedure.

The goal of the text is to embrace the robotic technology in its current form and what it holds in the future. Continuous technologic improvements will make the platform more versatile and improve access for surgeons and for patients. Inevitably other robotic and computer-aided technologies will follow in the future and may one day profoundly change how we perform surgery. We are grateful to these SAGES members for sharing their knowledge and we hope you will be able to utilize this in your new or current practice. We would also like to acknowledge Intuitive Surgical for allowing us to use their diagrams and pictures without any restrictions.

Atlanta, GA, USA                                    Ankit D. Patel
Omaha, NE, USA                                    Dmitry Oleynikov

# Contents

# Contributors

**Daniah Bu Ali, M.D.** Endocrine and Oncology Surgery Division, Department of Surgery, Tulane University School of Medicine, New Orleans, LA, USA

**Conrad Ballecer, M.D., F.A.C.S.** Center for Minimally Invasive and Robotic Surgery, Maricopa Integrated Health System, Phoenix, AZ, USA

**Daniel B. Jones, M.D.** Professor and Vice Chair, Department of Surgery, Harvard Medical School, Beth Israel Deaconess Medical Center, Boston, MA, USA

**Filip Bednar, M.D., Ph.D.** Department of Surgery, University of Michigan, Ann Arbor, MI, USA

**Partha Bhurtel, M.B.B.S.** Department of General Surgery, St. Elizabeth's Medical Center, Brighton, MA, USA

**James G. Bittner IV, M.D.** Virginia Commonwealth University, Medical College of Virginia, Richmond, VA, USA

**Alfredo M. Carbonell II, D.O., F.A.C.S., F.A.C.O.S.** Division of Minimal Access and Bariatric Surgery, Greenville Health System, University of South Carolina School of Medicine-Greenville, Greenville, SC, USA

**Aaron Carr, M.D.** Department of Surgery, University of California-Davis, Sacramento, CA, USA

**Robert Cerfolio, M.D., M.B.A.** Thoracic Surgery, Department of Surgery, University of Alabama Birmingham—Medical Center, Birmingham, AL, USA

**Julietta Chang, M.D.** Section of Surgical Endoscopy, Department of General Surgery, Digestive Disease Institute, Cleveland Clinic, Cleveland, OH, USA

**Ray K. Chihara, M.D., Ph.D.** Cardiothoracic Surgery, Emory University Hospital/ Emory University, The Emory Clinic, Atlanta, GA, USA

**Amareshewar Chiruvella, M.D.** Advanced Gastrointestinal/Minimally Invasive Surgery, University of Nebraska Medical Center, Omaha, NE, USA

**Christopher Crawford, M.D.** Advanced Gastrointestinal/Minimally Invasive Surgery, University of Nebraska Medical Center, Omaha, NE, USA

**Arturo Garcia, M.D.** Department of Surgery, University of California-Davis, Sacramento, CA, USA

**Angela A. Guzzetta, M.D.** Minimally Invasive and Bariatric Surgery, Department of Surgery, University of Texas Southwestern Medical Center, Dallas, TX, USA

**Michael E. Halkos, M.D., M.Sc.** Cardiothoracic Surgery, Emory University School of Medicine, Atlanta, GA, USA

**Cristina Harnsberger, M.D.** Department of Surgery, University of California, San Diego, Healthcare Systems, La Jolla, CA, USA

**Melissa E. Hogg, M.D., F.A.C.S.** Surgical Oncology, University of Pittsburgh Medical Center, Pittsburgh, PA, USA

**Dina S. Itum, M.D.** GI/Endocrine Division, Department of Surgery, UT Southwestern Medical Center, Dallas, TX, USA

Department of Surgery, Dallas VA Medical Center, Dallas, TX, USA

**Brian P. Jacob, M.D.** Associate Professor of Surgery, Department of Surgery, Icahn School of Medicine at Mount, Sinai, MY, USA

**D. Rohan Jeyarajah, M.D.** Surgical Oncology, Methodist Dallas Medical Center, Dallas, TX, USA

**Arinbjorn Jonsson, M.D.** Department of General & Gastrointestinal Surgery, Emory University School of Medicine, Atlanta, GA, USA

**Emad Kandil, M.D., M.B.A., F.A.C.S., F.A.C.E.** Endocrine and Oncology Surgery Division, Department of Surgery, Tulane University School of Medicine, New Orleans, LA, USA

**Sang-Wook Kang, M.D.** Department of Surgery, Yonsei University College of Medicine, Seoul, South Korea

**Jonathan C. King, M.D.** Department of Surgery, David Geffen School of Medicine at UCLA, Santa Monica, CA, USA

**Sam E. Kirkendall, M.D.** Department of Surgery, University of Texas Southwestern Medical Center, Dallas, TX, USA

**Crystal Krause, Ph.D.** Surgery, University of Nebraska Medical Center, Omaha, NE, USA

**Matthew Kroh, M.D.** Section of Surgical Endoscopy, Department of General Surgery, Digestive Disease Institute, Cleveland Clinic, Cleveland, OH, USA

Digestive Disease Institute, Cleveland Clinic, Abu Dhabi, UAE

**Omar Yusef Kudsi, M.D., M.B.A., F.A.C.S.** General Surgery, Tufts University School of Medicine, Brockton, MA, USA

**Sachin S. Kukreja, M.D.** Department of Surgery, University of Texas Southwestern Medical Center, Dallas, TX, USA

North Texas Veterans Affairs, Dallas, TX, USA

**Simone Langness, M.D.** Department of Surgery, University of California, San Diego, Healthcare Systems, La Jolla, CA, USA

**Edward Lin, D.O., F.A.C.S.** Emory Endosurgery Unit, Division of Gastrointestinal and General Surgery, Department of Surgery, Emory University School of Medicine, Atlanta, GA, USA

**Shanglei Liu, M.D.** Department of Surgery, University of California, San Diego, Healthcare Systems, La Jolla, CA, USA

**Nathaniel Lytle, M.D.** General Surgery, MIS/Bariatrics, Kaiser Permanente, Southeast Permanente Medical Group, Atlanta, GA, USA

**Emmanuel Moss, M.D., M.Sc., F.R.C.S.C.** Division of Cardiac Surgery, Jewish General Hospital/McGill University, Montreal, QC, Canada

**Dmitry Oleynikov, M.D., F.A.C.S.** Gastrointestinal, Minimally Invasive and Bariatric Surgery, The Center for Advanced Surgical Technology, University of Nebraska Medical Center, Omaha, NE, USA

**George Orthopoulos, M.D., Ph.D.** Department of General Surgery, St. Elizabeth's Medical Center, Brighton, MA, USA

**Sahil Parikh, D.O.** Department of Surgery, University of California-Davis, Sacramento, CA, USA

**Ankit D. Patel, M.D., F.A.C.S.** Department of General & Gastrointestinal Surgery, Emory Endosurgery, Emory University School of Medicine, Atlanta, GA, USA

**Lava Y. Patel, M.D.** Department of General & Gastrointestinal Surgery, Emory University School of Medicine, Atlanta, GA, USA

**Puraj P. Patel, D.O.** Division of Minimal Access and Bariatric Surgery, Greenville Health System, University of South Carolina School of Medicine-Greenville, Greenville, SC, USA

**Paul A.R. Del Prado, M.D.** Maricopa Integrated Health System, Pheonix, AZ, USA

**Brian E. Prebil, D.O.** Surgery, Arrowhead Hospital, Peoria, AZ, USA

**Sonia Ramamoorthy, M.D.** Department of Colorectal Surgery, University of California, San Diego, Healthcare Systems, La Jolla, CA, USA

**Seth Alan Rosen, M.D.** Department of Colorectal Surgery, Emory University, Johns Creek, GA, USA

**Manu S. Sancheti, M.D.** Cardiothoracic Surgery, Emory University Hospital/ Emory University, The Emory Clinic, Atlanta, GA, USA

**Neil D. Saunders, M.D.** Department of Surgery, Emory University School of Medicine, Atlanta, GA, USA

**Mihir M. Shah, M.D.** Emory Endosurgery Unit, Division of Gastrointestinal and General Surgery, Department of Surgery, Emory University School of Medicine, Atlanta, GA, USA

**Linda Schultz, M.D.** Society of American Gastrointestinal and Endoscopic Surgeons, Boston, MA, USA

**Jamil Luke Stetler, M.D.** General Surgery, Emory University Hospital, Atlanta, GA, USA

**Iswanto Sucandy, M.D.** Department of Surgery, University of Pittsburgh Medical Center, Pittsburgh, PA, USA

**Allan Tsung, M.D.** Research, Department of Surgery, University of Pittsburgh Medical Center, Pittsburgh, PA, USA

**Jarvis Walters, D.O.** Department of Surgery, Maricopa Integrated Health System, Phoenix, AZ, USA

**Jeffrey R. Watkins, M.D.** Methodist Dallas Medical Center, Dallas, TX, USA

**Benjamin Wei, M.D.** Cardiothoracic Surgery, Department of Surgery, University of Alabama Birmingham—Medical Center, Birmingham, AL, USA

**Martin R. Weiser, M.D.** Department of Surgery, Memorial Sloan Kettering Cancer Center, New York, NY, USA

**Herbert J. Zeh, M.D., F.A.C.S.** Surgical Oncology, University of Pittsburgh Medical Center, Pittsburgh, PA, USA

**Amer H. Zureikat, M.D., F.A.C.S.** UPMC Pancreatic Cancer Center, Surgical Oncology, University of Pittsburgh Medical Center, Pittsburgh, PA, USA

## Daniel B. Jones, Brian P. Jacob, and Linda Schultz

The SAGES MASTERS Program organizes educational materials along clinical pathways into discrete blocks of content which could be accessed by a surgeon attending the SAGES annual meeting or by logging into the online SAGES University (Fig. 1.1) [1]. The SAGES MASTERS program currently has eight pathways including: Acute Care, Biliary, Bariatrics, Colon, Foregut, Hernia, Flexible Endoscopy, and Robotic Surgery (Fig. 1.2). Each pathway is divided into three levels of targeted performance: Competency, Proficiency, and Mastery (Fig. 1.3). The levels originate from the Dreyfus model of skill acquisition [2], which has five stages: novice, advanced beginner, competency, proficiency, and expertise. The SAGES MASTERS Program is based on the three more advanced stages of skill acquisition: competency, proficiency, and expertise. *Competency* is defined as what a graduating general surgery chief resident or MIS fellow should be able to achieve; *Proficiency* is what a surgeon approximately 3 years out from training should be able to accomplish; and *Mastery* is what more experienced surgeons should be able to accomplish after seven

Adopted from Jones DB, Stefanidis D, Korndorffer JR, Dimick JB, Jacob BP, Schultz L, Scott DJ, SAGES University Masters Program: a structured curriculum for deliberate, lifelong learning. Surg Endoscopy, 2017, in press.

D.B. Jones, MD (✉)
Professor and Vice Chair, Department of Surgery, Harvard Medical School,
Beth Israel Deaconess Medical Center, Boston, MA 02215, USA
e-mail: djones1@bidmc.harvard.ed

B.P. Jacob, MD
Associate Professor of Surgery, Department of Surgery,
Icahn School of Medicine at Mount, Sinai, NY, USA
e-mail: bpjacob@gmail.com

L. Schultz
Society of American Gastrointestinal and Endoscopic Surgeons, Boston, MA, USA
e-mail: linda@sages.org

© Springer International Publishing AG 2018                                         3
A.D. Patel, D. Oleynikov (eds.), *The SAGES Manual of Robotic Surgery*,
The SAGES University Masters Program Series, DOI 10.1007/978-3-319-51362-1_1

**Fig. 1.1** MASTERS
Program logo

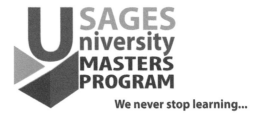

**Fig. 1.2** MASTER
Program clinical pathways

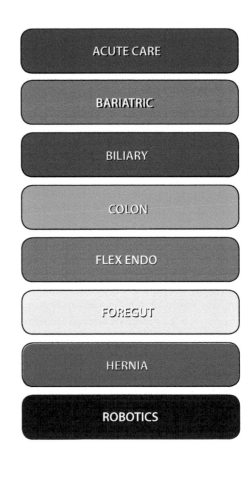

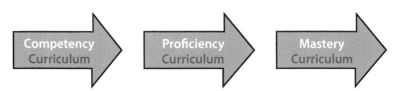

**Fig. 1.3** MASTERS Program progression

or more years in practice. Mastery is applicable to SAGES surgeons seeking in-depth knowledge in a pathway, including the following: Areas of controversy, outcomes, best practice, and ability to mentor colleagues. Over time, with the utilization of coaching and participation in SAGES courses, this level should be obtainable by the majority of SAGES members. This edition of the SAGES Manual—Robotic Surgery aligns with the current version of the new SAGES University MASTERS Program Robotic Surgery pathway (Table 1.1).

**Table 1.1** Robotic curriculum

| Curriculum elements | Competency |
|---|---|
| Anchoring procedure—Competency | 2 |
| CORE LECTURE | 1 |
| CORE MCE 70% | 1 |
| Annual meeting content | 8 |
| Guidelines | 1 |
| SA CME hours | 6 |
| Sentinel articles | 2 |
| Social media | 2 |
| Hands-on robotic proficiency verification | 12 |
| *Credits* | *35* |

| Curriculum elements | Proficiency |
|---|---|
| Anchoring procedure—Proficiency | 2 |
| CORE LECTURE | 1 |
| CORE MCE 70% | 1 |
| Annual meeting content | 5 |
| FUSE | 12 |
| Outcomes database enrollment | 2 |
| SA CME hours (ASMBS electives, SAGES or SAGES-endorsed) | 3 |
| Sentinel articles | 2 |
| Social media | 2 |
| *Credits* | *30* |

| Curriculum elements | Mastery |
|---|---|
| Anchoring procedure—Mastery | 2 |
| CORE LECTURE | 1 |
| CORE MCE 70% | 1 |
| Annual meeting content | 3 |
| Fundamentals of surgical coaching | 4 |
| Outcomes database reporting | 2 |
| SA CME credits (ASMBS electives, SAGES or SAGES-endorsed) | 5 |
| Sentinel articles | 2 |
| Serving as video assessment reviewer and providing feedback (FSC) | 4 |
| Social media | 6 |
| *Credits* | *30* |

## Robotic Surgery Curriculum

The Robotic Curriculum is a little different from the other SAGES MASTERS Program pathways. To complete the robotic pathway, a robotic surgeon should complete requirements in the corresponding pathway. For example, for successful completion of the Robotic Competency Curriculum for Hernia, the learner should be able to demonstrate a robotic ventral hernia for competency, a robotic inguinal hernia for proficiency, and a robotic complex abdominal wall reconstruction or a recurrent hernia repair to accomplish mastery. This recognizes the importance of understanding disease and also unique technical expertise of mastering the robot technology.

The key elements of the Robotic Surgery curriculum include core lectures for the pathway, which provides a 45-min general overview including basic anatomy, physiology, diagnostic workup, and surgical management. As of 2018, all lecture content of the annual SAGES meetings are labeled as follows: Basic (100), intermediate (200), and advanced (300). This allows attendees to choose lectures that best fit their educational needs. Coding the content additionally facilitates online retrieval of specific educational material, with varying degrees of surgical complexity, ranging from introductory to revisional surgery.

SAGES identified the need to develop targeted, complex content for its mastery level curriculum. The idea was that these 25-min lectures would be focused on specific topics. It assumes that the attendee already has a good understanding of diseases and management from attending/watching competency and proficiency level lectures. Ideally, in order to supplement a chosen topic, the mastery lectures would also identify key prerequisite articles from *Surgical Endoscopy* and other journals, in addition to SAGES University videos. Many of these lectures will be forthcoming at future SAGES annual meetings.

The MASTERS Program has a self-assessment, multiple-choice exam for each module to guide learner progression throughout the curriculum. Questions are submitted by core lecture speakers and SAGES annual meeting faculty. The goal of the questions is to use assessment for learning, with the assessment being criterion referenced with the percent correct set at 80%. Learners will be able to review incorrect answers, review educational content, and retake the examination until a passing score is obtained.

The MASTERS Program Robotic Surgery curriculum taps much of the of SAGES existing educational products including FLS, FES, FUSE, SMART, Top 21 videos and Pearls (Fig. 1.4). The Curriculum Task Force has placed the aforementioned modules along a continuum of the curriculum pathway. For example, FLS, in general, occurs during the Competency Curriculum, whereas the Fundamental Use of Surgical Energy (FUSE) is usually required during the Proficiency Curriculum. The Fundamentals of Laparoscopic Surgery (FLS) is a multiple-choice exam and a skills assessment conducted on a video box trainer. Tasks include peg transfer, cutting, intracorporeal and extracorporeal suturing, and knot tying. Since 2010, FLS has been required of all US general surgery residents seeking to sit for the American Board of Surgery qualifying examinations. The Fundamentals of Endoscopic Surgery (FES)

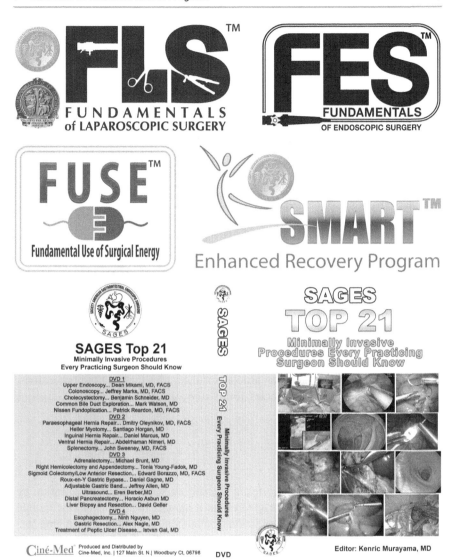

**Fig. 1.4** SAGES educational content: FLS, FUSE, FES, SMART, Top 21 video

assesses endoscopic knowledge and technical skills in a simulator. FUSE teaches about the safe use of energy devices in the operating room and is available at <u>FUSE. didactic.org</u>. After learners complete the self-paced modules, they may take the certifying examination.

The SAGES Surgical Multimodal Accelerated Recovery Trajectory (SMART) Initiative combines minimally invasive surgical techniques with enhanced recovery pathways (ERPs) for perioperative care, with the goal of improving outcomes and patient satisfaction. Educational materials include a website with best practices, sample pathways, patient literature, and other resources such as videos, FAQs, and an implementation timeline. The materials assist surgeons and their surgical team with implementation of an ERP.

Top 21 videos are edited videos of the most commonly performed MIS operations and basic endoscopy. Cases are straightforward with quality video and clear anatomy.

Pearls are step-by-step video clips of 10 operations. The authors show different variations for each step. The learner should have a fundamental understanding of the operation.

SAGES Guidelines provide evidence-based recommendations for surgeons and are developed by the SAGES Guidelines Committee following the Health and Medicine Division of the National Academies of Sciences, Engineering, and Medicine standards (formerly the Institute of Medicine) for guideline development [3]. Each clinical practice guideline has been systematically researched, reviewed, and revised by the SAGES Guidelines Committee and an appropriate multidisciplinary team. The strength of the provided recommendations is determined based on the quality of the available literature using the GRADE methodology [4]. SAGES Guidelines cover a wide range of topics relevant to the practice of SAGES surgeon members and are updated on a regular basis. Since the developed guidelines provide an appraisal of the available literature, their inclusion in the MASTERS Program was deemed necessary by the group.

The Curriculum Task Force identified the need to select required readings for the MASTERS Program based on key articles for the various curriculum procedures. Summaries of each of these articles follow the American College of Surgeons (ACS) Selected Readings format.

## Facebook™ Groups

While there are many great platforms available to permit online collaboration by user-generated content, Facebook (™) offers a unique, highly developed mobile platform that is ideal for global professional collaboration and daily continuing surgical education (Fig. 1.5). The Facebook groups allow for video assessment, feedback, and coaching as a tool to improve practice, and their use to enhance professional surgical education has been validated by Dr. Brian Jacob's International Hernia Collaboration closed Facebook group.

Based on the anchoring procedures determined via group consensus (Table 1.2) participants in the MASTERS Program will submit video clips on designated SAGES closed Facebook groups, with other participants and/or SAGES members providing qualitative feedback. Using crowdsourcing, other surgeons would comment and provide feedback.

Eight, unique vetted membership-only closed Facebook groups were created for the MASTERS Program, including a group for bariatrics, hernia, colorectal, biliary, acute care, flexible endoscopy, robotics, and foregut. The SAGES Robotic Surgery group is independent of the other groups already in existence and will be populated

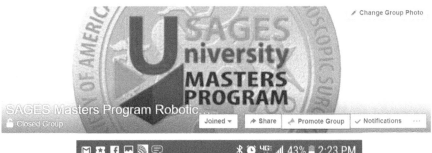

Change Group Photo

SAGES Masters Program Robotic...
Closed Group

Joined ▾ | ↗ Share | ⚹ Promote Group | ✓ Notifications | ⋯

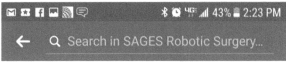

☒ ✉ ⨳ ☐ 🗺 ▧ 🗩  ≉ 🕐 ⁴ᴳ ⫴ 43% ▰ 2:23 PM

← 🔍 Search in SAGES Robotic Surgery...

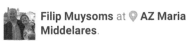

**Filip Muysoms** at 📍 **AZ Maria Middelares**.
Apr 2 at 3:51 AM • Gent, Belgium • ▣

At SAGES in Houston there was some discussion on the cost-effectivity of rTAPP groin repair. I my situation (Belgium) doing an rTAPP with only two instruments will keep the material cost for a case within the € package the hospital gets for such a case. I show a video doing as such: rTAPP with a needle driver and a hotshears only. Anyone strongly f...
Continue Reading

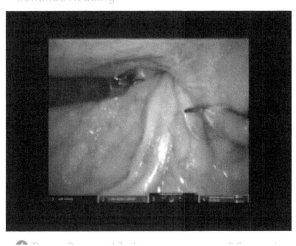

**Fig. 1.5** Robotic Surgery Facebook Group

**Table 1.2** Anchoring procedures for Robotic Surgery pathway

| Robotic Surgery anchoring procedure by pathway | Level |
|---|---|
| *Biliary* | |
| Multi-port cholecystectomy | Competency |
| Cholecystectomy with IOC or for uncomplicated acute cholecystitis | Proficiency |
| Cholecystectomy for difficult/severe acute cholecystitis or common bile duct exploration (CBDE) | Mastery |
| *Foregut* | |
| Nissen fundoplication | Competency |
| Paraesophageal Hernia Repair or Heller Myotomy | Proficiency |
| Redo fundoplication | Mastery |
| *Hernia* | |
| Primary ventral hernia repair | Competency |
| Primary inguinal hernia repair | Proficiency |
| Redo hernia or complex hernia (transversus abdominis release) | Mastery |
| *Bariatric* | |
| Sleeve gastrectomy or lap band | Competency |
| Roux-en-Y gastric bypass | Proficiency |
| Revisional bariatric surgery | Mastery |
| *Colorectal* | |
| Right colectomy | Competency |
| Left colectomy | Proficiency |
| Left colectomy with splenic flexure release, colectomy for complex inflammatory disease or advanced cancer | Mastery |

only by physicians, mostly surgeons or surgeons in training interested in a wide range of robotic surgery applications.

The group provides an international platform for surgeons and healthcare providers interested in optimizing outcomes in a surgical specialty to collaborate; share; discuss; and post photos, videos and anything related to a chosen specialty. By embracing social media as a collaborative forum, we can more effectively and transparently obtain immediate global feedback that potentially can improve patient outcomes, as well as the quality of care we provide, all while transforming the way a society's members interact.

For the first two levels of the MASTERS Program, Competency and Proficiency, participants will be required to post videos of the anchoring procedures and will receive qualitative feedback from other participants. However, for the mastery level, participants will submit a video to be evaluated by an expert panel. A standardized video assessment tool, depending on the specific procedure, will be used. A benchmark will also be utilized to determine when the participant has achieved the mastery level for that procedure.

Once the participant has achieved mastery level, he will participate as a coach by providing feedback to participants in the first two levels. MASTERS program participants will therefore need to learn the fundamental principles of surgical coaching. The key activities of coaching include goal setting, active listening, powerful inquiry, and constructive feedback [5, 6]. Importantly, peer coaching is much different than traditional education, where there is an expert and a learner. Peer coaching is a "co-learning" model where the coach is facilitating the development of the coached by using inquiry (i.e., open-ended questions) in a non-competitive manner.

Surgical coaching skills are a crucial part of the MASTERS curriculum. At the 2017 SAGES Annual Meeting, a postgraduate course on coaching skills was developed and video recorded. The goal is to develop a "coaching culture" within the SAGES MASTERS Program, wherein both participants and coaches are committed to lifelong learning and development.

The need for a more structured approach to the education of practicing surgeons as accomplished by the SAGES MASTERS program is well recognized [7]. Since performance feedback usually stops after training completion and current approaches to MOC are suboptimal, the need for peer coaching has recently received increased attention in surgery [5, 6]. SAGES has recognized this need and its MASTERS Program embraces social media for surgical education to help provide a free, mobile, and easy-to-use platform to surgeons globally. Access to the MASTERS Program groups enables surgeons at all levels to partake in the MASTERS Program curriculum and obtain feedback from peers, mentors, and experts. By creating surgeon-only private groups dedicated to this project, SAGES can now offer surgeons posting in these groups the ability to discuss preoperative, intraoperative, and postoperative issues with other SAGES colleagues and mentors. In addition, the platform permits transparent and responsive dialogue about technique, continuing the theme of deliberate, lifelong learning.

To accommodate the needs of this program, SAGES University is upgrading its web-based features. A new learning management system (LMS) will track progression and make access to SAGES University simple. Features of the new IT infrastructure will provide the ability to access a video or lecture on-demand in relation to content, level of difficulty, and author. Once enrolled in the MASTERS Program, the LMS will track lectures, educational products, MCE, and other completed requirements. Participants will be able to see where they stand in relation to module completion and SAGES will alert learners to relevant content they may be interested in pursuing. Until such time that the new LMS is up and running, it is hoped that the SAGES Manual will help guide learners through the MASTERS Program Curriculum.

## Conclusions

The SAGES MASTERS Program ROBOTIC SURGERY PATHWAY facilitates deliberate, focused postgraduate teaching and learning. The MASTERS Program certifies completion of the curriculum but is NOT meant to certify competency, proficiency, or mastery of surgeons. The MASTERS Program embraces the concept of lifelong learning after fellowship and its curriculum is organized from basic principles to more complex content. The MASTERS Program is an innovative, voluntary curriculum that supports MOC and deliberate, lifelong learning.

# References

1. Jones DB, Stefanidis D, Korndorffer JR, Dimick JB, Jacob BP, Schultz L, Scott DJ. SAGES University Masters program: a structured curriculum for deliberate, lifelong learning. Surg Endosc. 2017;31(8):3061–71.
2. Dreyfus SE. The five-stage model of adult skill acquisition. Bull Sci Technol Soc. 2004;24:177–81.
3. Graham R, Mancher M, Miller Woman D, Greenfield S, Steinberg E. Institute of Medicine (US) committee on standards for developing trustworthy clinical practice guidelines. In: Graham R, Mancher M, Wolman DM, Greenfield S, Steinberg E, editors. Clinical practice guidelines we can trust. Washington, DC: National Academies Press (US); 2011.
4. Guyatt GH, Oxman AD, Vist GE, Kunz R, Falck-Ytter Y, Alonso-Coello P, Schünemann HJ, GRADE Working Group. GRADE: an emerging consensus on rating quality of evidence and strength of recommendations. BMJ. 2008;336:924–6.
5. Greenberg CC, Ghousseini HN, Pavuluri Quamme SR, Beasley HL, Wiegmann DA. Surgical coaching for individual performance improvement. Ann Surg. 2015;261:32–4.
6. Greenberg CC, Dombrowski J, Dimick JB. Video-based surgical coaching: an emerging approach to performance improvement. JAMA Surg. 2016;151:282–3.
7. Sachdeva AK. Acquiring skills in new procedures and technology: the challenge and the opportunity. Arch Surg. 2005;140:387–9.

Sahil Parikh and Aaron Carr

## Introduction

Surgical management of gallbladder disease changed drastically with the advent of laparoscopic techniques in the 1990s. Initially, laparoscopic techniques were cumbersome due to the new orientation and lack of direct contact with tissues [1, 2]. This technology rapidly evolved with improved instrumentation and optics to become the standard approach for cholecystectomy [3, 4]. The course of robotic surgery began with the implementation of a camera steadying system to assist laparoscopic surgery. The field continued to advance with improved instrumentation to include fully wristed instruments with seven degrees of motion, 3D vision, fluorescently enhanced optics, and even remote access [5].

Multi-Port Robotic Cholecystectomy (MPRC) has been shown to be as safe as the laparoscopic approach with similar operative times and hospital lengths of stay [6, 7]. Breitenstein et al. compared laparoscopic cholecystectomies (LC) to MPRC and found similar outcomes between the two approaches [7]. Another study showed a decrease in robotic docking time from 12.1 to 4.9 min after the initial learning curve [8]. If studies with more than 50 cases are analyzed the average docking times for MPRC ranged from 4.3 to 17 min and average total operative time was 52.4–95.7 min [6–10] (Table 2.1). MPRC offers improved visualization and fully wristed instruments, but has not been widely adopted, likely due to the need for larger ports, robotic availability, and robotic docking time. In our experience, MPRC may still have an advantage in re-operative fields, obese patients, and when no surgical assistant is available.

MPRC also allows a safe and reliable method of training future surgeons and the learning curve is shorter than traditional laparoscopic surgery [8, 9]. This chapter

S. Parikh, D.O. • A. Carr, M.D. (✉)
Department of Surgery, University of California-Davis,
2221 Stockton Blvd, Sacramento, CA 95817, USA
e-mail: acarr@ucdavis.edu

© Springer International Publishing AG 2018
A.D. Patel, D. Oleynikov (eds.), *The SAGES Manual of Robotic Surgery*,
The SAGES University Masters Program Series, DOI 10.1007/978-3-319-51362-1_2

**Table 2.1** Multi-port robotic cholecystectomy outcomes

| | $N$ | Robotic docking time (min) | Console time (min) | Total time (min) | Major complication (bile leak, bleeding) |
|---|---|---|---|---|---|
| Vidovszky et al. (2006)[a] | | | | | |
| MPRC | 51 | 4.9 | 32.5 | 68.2 | None |
| Breitenstein et al. (2008) | | | | | |
| LC | 50 | – | – | 50.2 | 2% |
| MPRC | 50 | 17 | 30 | 54.6 | 2% |
| Kim et al. (2013) | | | | | |
| MPRC | 178 | 4.3 | 15.1 | 52.4 | 0.6% |
| Ayloo et al. (2014) | | | | | |
| LC | 147 | NA | NA | 89.6 | 2.0% |
| MPRC | 179 | NA | NA | 95.7 | 1.7% |

Data from PubMed search for SIRC with greater than 50 patients
*SIRC* single incision robotic cholecystectomy, *LC* conventional laparoscopic cholecystectomy, *MPRC* multi-port robotic cholecystectomy, *NA* not available
[a]After the initial learning curve

focuses on the safe application of robotic technology to biliary disease. The most commonly used robotic system is the da Vinci Si Surgical System (Intuitive Surgical Inc. Sunnyvale, CA). Although other platforms exist in various stages of development, our chapter will focus on the use of the da Vinci Si system. Many of the concepts will be broadly applicable to other systems.

## Indications

The indications for MPRC are similar to those of traditional laparoscopic cholecystectomy. These include symptomatic cholelithiasis, cholecystitis, acalculous cholecystitis, symptomatic gallbladder polyps or polyps greater than 10 mm, porcelain gallbladder, and biliary dyskinesia [11].

## Equipment and Operating Room Team Development

The three components of the da Vinci Surgical System are the Surgeon Console (SC), Vision Cart (VC) and Patient-side Cart (PSC). The SC is positioned away from the operative field and controls the instrumentation and visualization of the operative field. The VC is also positioned away from the operative field and contains supporting hardware and software, such as the optical light source, electrosurgical unit, and optical integration. The PSC is the only component docked within the operative field and is covered with sterile drapes. It has four articulated mechanical arms that control the instruments that are docked to the ports.

The efficient use of any system requires the coordination of all personnel involved. At our institution, we have achieved very efficient robotic docking times with organization and training of operating room personnel. Our structure consists of a robotic nurse manager, equipment specialist, circulating nurse, and scrub nurse. This structure is not limited to robotic cases but applies to any specialty cases. The robotic nursing supervisor specifically overseas all robotic cases to ensure the appropriate personnel and equipment are assigned to the room several days in advance. The equipment specialists are responsible for setup and troubleshooting of all laparoscopic and robotic equipment across multiple rooms. In our robotic rooms, they are responsible for the location of all robotic components and positioning of robotic equipment during the operation. The circulating nurse is responsible for additional equipment used during the operation. The scrub nurse is responsible for instrument exchange at the patient's bedside. Using this system, we achieved an average docking time of 5 min [8, 12].

## Patient Positioning and Peritoneal Entry

The patient is placed supine on the operating room table. After intubation, the elbows should be properly padded and secured in the adducted position. The bed is angled 45° with the head moving to the patient's right. The right arm is tucked, so the PSC can eventually be positioned over the patient's right shoulder. The scrub nurse and sterile instrument table are generally positioned near the foot of the bed. The SC is placed away from the operating room table. The VC can be positioned to the left or right, away from the sterile field (Fig. 2.1).

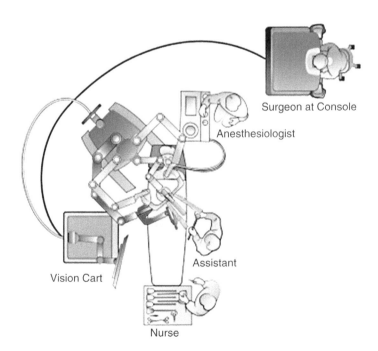

**Fig. 2.1**   Robotic equipment position during multi-port cholecystectomy

Access can be gained with a periumbilical incision to maintain at least a 15 cm distance from the camera to the operative field in the right upper quadrant. If there are no previous incisions in the area, we elevate the fascia and use either an open technique or veress needle in order to obtain pneumoperitoneum, followed by a 12 mm optical entry port. After peritoneal access is gained, the abdominal cavity is inspected through the periumbilical port. It can be helpful to use an extra-long 12 mm port because this allows adequate length for robotic docking independent of the patient's body habitus. Next, two separate 8 mm robotic ports are placed in the right upper quadrant, 8–10 cm away from one another. These robotic ports are best placed in line with one another and slightly cephalad to the camera port, positioning one along the mid-clavicular line and one along the anterior axillary line. Finally, an 8 mm robotic port is placed in the left upper abdomen. This is ideally placed in the midclavicular line and slightly more cephalad than the right sided abdominal ports (Fig. 2.2).

## Technical Pearls

- Placing the endotracheal tube to the left can avoid collision with the robotic arms.
- A footboard should be used to avoid inadvertent movement of the patient intra-operatively. Padding and taping of the ankles helps to avoid rolling of the foot during positioning.
- Care should be taken to place the left upper quadrant port so that a line between the port and gallbladder does not bisect the falciform ligament.
- In patients with prior abdominal incisions, we prefer a direct-access Hasson technique for abdominal access or left upper quadrant optical entry.
- In patients with a large distance between the umbilicus and right subcostal margin, a supraumbilical incision may be of greater benefit.

**Fig. 2.2** Port placement for multi-port robotic cholecystectomy (1): 8 mm robotic port for hook electrocautery. (2): 8 mm robotic port for infundibular grasper. (3): 8 mm robotic port for fundal grasper. Camera port: 12 mm extra-long port. Assistant: optional port placement

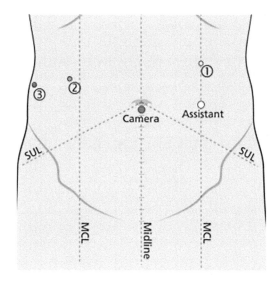

## Robotic Dissection

The patient is next placed in a reverse Trendelenburg position with a slight left lateral rotation. The sterile covered PSC subsystem is positioned over the right humeral area of the patient. The middle boom should be in line with the gallbladder and camera port.

The camera is initially docked. A 30° downward facing scope allows for excellent visualization after proper downward calibration and white-balancing. Following this, the 8 mm ports are docked. The ports should be docked to avoid collision with one another, with special care given to ensure that the camera arm is at its "sweet-spot," indicated by the blue line, once docked.

Under direct visualization, we place two graspers in the right upper abdominal ports and a hook cautery into the left upper quadrant port. The gallbladder is grasped in a manner similar to the laparoscopic approach. The lateral port is used for cephalad retraction on the fundus, while the medial port manipulates the infundibulum. We begin our dissection using the hook cautery on the gallbladder near the area of the cystic artery. The artery is traced down to open the peritoneum over the cystic duct/gallbladder junction. Next, the peritoneum is separated both lateral and medial to the gallbladder. We will carefully dissect within Calot's triangle until a critical view is obtained (Fig. 2.3).

We place medium sized hemo-o-lok clips on either side of the cystic duct and cystic artery prior to transection with robotic shears. Finally, the gallbladder is dissected off the liver with hook cautery. A 5 mm assistant port can be placed in either the right upper quadrant or between the camera port and left sided abdominal port if additional assistance is needed.

The lateral grasper is removed, and a laparoscopic grasper is inserted and placed on the gallbladder infundibulum. All remaining instruments and the camera are removed. The PSC is undocked and removed from the operative field, and the patient is placed in the level position. If the 10 mm camera was used, then a 5 mm laparoscopic camera is inserted into the remaining 8 mm right upper quadrant port. Under direct visualization, a laparoscopic retrieval bag is used through the 12 mm

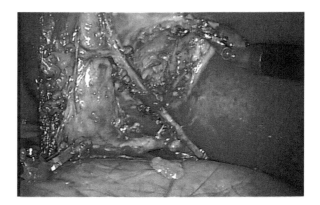

**Fig. 2.3** Critical view of a Calot's triangle (picture from the University of California, Davis Department of Surgery archive)

port to secure the gallbladder and remove it. If an 8 mm robotic camera was used, then it can be controlled manually through the 8 mm port. It is unnecessary to have the standard laparoscopic camera. The fascia of the 12 mm port is approximated and pneumoperitoneum is released. All sites are closed with absorbable suture and sterile dressing.

## Technical Pearls

- A 30° downward facing scope may offer more visual advantages when dissecting the cystic duct and artery. The robotic camera must be calibrated for upward or downward direction. We recommend always calibrating for both directions.
- Use of an 8 mm robotic camera obviates the need for standard laparoscopic instruments.
- Avoiding collision of robotic arms is paramount intra-operatively. This can be accomplished by adjusting the right lateral port to swing as wide as possible. The remaining ports should have a minimum of 8 cm between all joints.
- A higher grasping strength instrument may be better for retracting the fundus.
- Visual haptics are important with right lower quadrant retraction of the infundibulum because excessive retraction may cause injuries.
- If a cholangiogram needs to be performed, the table can remain in position. The C-arm can be brought into position from the left side after undocking and repositioning the PSC.

## Conclusion

Studies on MPRC have demonstrated its safety for treatment of a variety of gallbladder diseases. MPRC provides a safe and reliable method for cholecystectomy. The advantages of wristed instruments and improved visualization over standard laparoscopy have yet to be determined, but will likely have the most significant advantage in reoperative fields, obese patients, and when a surgical assistant is unavailable. It also allows for an optimal teaching platform of basic and advanced minimally invasive technique. The most important aspect of the application of new technology is strict adherence to the standard principles of good surgical technique.

## References

1. Soper NJ, Stockmann PT, Dunnegan DL, Ashley SW. Laparoscopic cholecystectomy. The new 'gold standard'? Arch Surg 1992;127(8):917–921; discussion 921–3.
2. Kelley Jr WE. The evolution of laparoscopy and the revolution in surgery in the decade of the 1990s. JSLS. 2008;12(4):351–7.
3. A prospective analysis of 1518 laparoscopic cholecystectomies. The Southern Surgeons Club. N Engl J Med. 1991;324(16):1073–8.

4. NIH Conference. Gastrointestinal surgery for severe obesity. Consensus Development Conference Panel. Ann Intern Med 1991;115(12):956–61.
5. Jacobs LK, Shayani V, Sackier JM. Determination of the learning curve of the AESOP robot. Surg Endosc. 1997;11(1):54–5.
6. Baek NH, Li G, Kim JH, Hwang JC, Kim JH, Yoo BM, et al. Short-term surgical outcomes and experience with 925 patients undergoing robotic cholecystectomy during a 4-year period at a single institution. Hepatogastroenterology. 2015;62(139):573–6.
7. Breitenstein S, Nocito A, Puhan M, Held U, Weber M, Clavien PA. Robotic-assisted versus laparoscopic cholecystectomy: outcome and cost analyses of a case-matched control study. Ann Surg. 2008;247(6):987–93.
8. Vidovszky TJ, Smith W, Ghosh J, Ali MR. Robotic cholecystectomy: learning curve, advantages, and limitations. J Surg Res. 2006;136(2):172–8.
9. Ayloo S, Roh Y, Choudhury N. Laparoscopic versus robot-assisted cholecystectomy: a retrospective cohort study. Int J Surg (London, England). 2014;12(10):1077–81.
10. Kim JH, Baek NH, Li G, Choi SH, Jeong IH, Hwang JC, et al. Robotic cholecystectomy with new port sites. World J Gastroenterol. 2013;19(20):3077–82.
11. Agresta F, Campanile FC, Vettoretto N, Silecchia G, Bergamini C, Maida P, et al. Laparoscopic cholecystectomy: consensus conference-based guidelines. Langenbecks Arch Surg. 2015;400(4):429–53.
12. Nelson EC, Gottlieb AH, Muller HG, Smith W, Ali MR, Vidovszky TJ. Robotic cholecystectomy and resident education: the UC Davis experience. Int J Medical Robot. 2014;10(2):218–22.

# Masters Program Foregut Pathway: Robotic Fundoplications

George Orthopoulos, Partha Bhurtel, and Omar Yusef Kudsi

## Introduction

Gastroesophageal reflux disease (GERD) is the most common gastrointestinal-related diagnosis in the United States [1]. Its prevalence varies from 8 to 28% in Western countries and reduces health-related quality of life and imposes a significant economic burden on the healthcare system [2]. It is defined as "a condition that develops when reflux of gastric contents causes troublesome symptoms or complications [3]." Initial management of GERD consists of life style modifications and medical therapy directed at neutralizing acid. Despite improvement in surgical techniques, there is significant debate surrounding optimal surgical management. Appropriate patient selection and knowledge of principles of surgical therapy is important to obtain a good surgical outcome [4]. Minimally invasive fundoplication is the current standard in surgical approach to GERD with 3% of all fundoplications being performed laparoscopically with robotic assistance and 79% being performed by the conventional laparoscopic approach [5].

G. Orthopoulos, M.D., Ph.D. • P. Bhurtel, M.B.B.S.
Department of General Surgery, St. Elizabeth's Medical Center, Brighton, MA 02135, USA

O.Y. Kudsi, M.D., M.B.A., F.A.C.S. (✉)
General Surgery, Tufts University School of Medicine, One Pearl St., Suite 2000, Brockton, MA 02301, USA
e-mail: omar.kudsi@tufts.edu

© Springer International Publishing AG 2018
A.D. Patel, D. Oleynikov (eds.), *The SAGES Manual of Robotic Surgery*,
The SAGES University Masters Program Series, DOI 10.1007/978-3-319-51362-1_3

## Indications and Preoperative Evaluation

### Surgical Indications

Antireflux surgical procedures should be considered for definitive treatment of patients with objective evidence of reflux who [6, 7]:

- Have persistent or troublesome symptoms despite optimal medical therapy with proton pump inhibitors (PPI)
- Are responsive to, but intolerant of medical therapy (non-compliance with medications, unwillingness to life long medications, long-term expense related to medications, etc.)
- Have complications related to GERD (benign stricture, Barrett's esophagus, bleeding, ulceration)
- Have persistent atypical reflux symptoms (asthma, hoarseness, cough, etc.)

Patients most likely to have successful surgical outcome are ones who have typical symptoms of GERD, show a response to medical therapy but are unwilling or unable to take daily medications, and demonstrate increased esophageal acid exposure on pH monitoring [8].

### Preoperative Work Up

Appropriate preoperative work up, inclusive of esophagogastroduodenoscopy (EGD), pH monitoring, manometry, and barium esophagram, is necessary to delineate the extent of the disease.

- EGD can reveal valuable information regarding the anatomy of the esophagus and the gastroesophageal junction, the presence and size of hiatus hernia, and the presence and degree of esophagitis.
- pH monitoring is the gold standard to confirm the presence of acid reflux. pH monitoring and the calculation of DeMeester score (percentage of time of esophageal acid exposure to pH < 4.0) is very helpful in making a diagnosis of GERD in patients with atypical symptoms. It is imperative to document the existence of reflux disease in patients with classic symptoms of heartburn and regurgitation. Erosive esophagitis or Barrett's metaplasia symptoms are not a reliable guide to the presence of disease [9].
- Esophageal manometry can reveal esophageal dysmotility syndromes. Based on this information, the surgeon is able to design the optimal surgical approach and decide between a complete or partial fundoplication.
- Barium esophagram is performed to outline the anatomy of the esophagus and abnormalities such as a hiatus hernia, diverticulum, stricture, or a luminal mass. It helps assess esophageal length. Presence of a large (>5 cm) hiatal hernia suggests the presence of a shortened esophagus and may change choice of operation [10].

The preferred approach is minimally invasive and the main techniques performed include complete (Nissen, 360°) or partial (Toupet-posterior, 270° and Dor-anterior, 180°) fundoplication [5].

The key steps to fundoplication include formation of a gastric wrap to enhance the lower esophageal sphincter, restoration of the angle of His, and closure of the hiatal defect, if present. Crucial points of the procedure are the placement of the patient in supine, steep reverse Trendelenburg position, hiatal dissection in a clockwise fashion starting from the right diaphragmatic crus, identification and preservation of the vagi nerves, and division of the short gastric vessels prior to the fundoplication and posterior gastropexy (in case of a partial fundoplication).

Robotic-assisted laparoscopic partial fundoplications were developed to prevent or alleviate symptoms of dysphagia or gas bloating noted after complete fundoplications (e.g. Nissen fundoplication). Indications that favor partial fundoplication include patients with achalasia following Heller myotomy, myotomy after resection of an epiphrenic diverticulum, and in patients who have had previous gastric resection or have tubular stomach, due to lack of sufficient fundus to perform a full 360° wrap [11].

Although widely taught, severe esophageal dysmotility is not an indication for choosing partial over complete fundoplication. Many studies have proven that in patients with weak, but not absent, esophageal peristalsis, there is similar postoperative outcome regardless of a complete or partial fundoplication [12].

## Patient Preparation

In preparation for surgery, the patient is being kept nothing by mouth (NPO) after midnight the night before the operation. Depending on the degree of esophageal dysmotility, especially for patients with achalasia, it might be beneficial for the patient to be placed on a clear liquid diet for 24–48 h prior to the operation, to minimize the amount of retained food in the esophageal lumen. This reduces the risk of aspiration upon endotracheal intubation and facilitates the performance of intraoperative EGD if required. Good communication with the anesthesiologist is paramount before and during the case and occasionally rapid sequence induction and intubation is performed.

## Patient Position and Room Setup

1. The patient is positioned in a supine position. The patient's arms can either be tucked or outstretched to ~80° and secured on padded arm boards.
2. The patient should be fully secured to the operating table in order to achieve reverse Trendelenburg position (head up approximately >30°), which will help in displacing the organs from the hiatus and optimize the exposure of the working area.

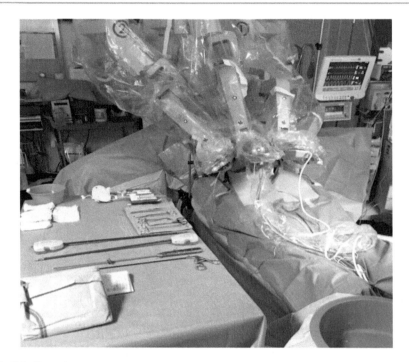

**Fig. 3.1** Operating room setup

3. The assistant usually stands on the patient's right side, but an alternative position on the left side of the patient might be elected depending on the room setup.
4. The monitor is placed either at the patient's feet on the left side or at the patient's left shoulder, depending on the position of the assistant (Fig. 3.1).
5. Antibiotics with gram-negative and gram-positive coverage are administered at induction of anesthesia as they have shown to decrease the risk of postoperative wound infection.

## Trocar Position

1. After pneumoperitoneum is established, usually by using the Veress needle in the left hypochondrium, the initial port is inserted in the abdominal cavity. Correct placement of the 8 mm camera port is of utmost importance. The typical supraumbilical port position is 12 cm caudad to the xiphoid and 2 cm to the patient's right. For larger patients, port is placed 15 cm caudal to the xiphoid and 2 cm to the right. The distance might need to be re-adjusted especially if the procedure includes a large hiatal hernia repair [13].
2. The two 8 mm trocars for the robotic arms are placed on the same horizontal line and 8 cm lateral to the camera port in the left and right upper quadrant close to the mid-clavicular line. The third 8 mm trocar for the third robotic arm is inserted

**Fig. 3.2** Potential configurations of trocar positioning. ①②③ robotic arm ports, *MCL* midclavicular line, *SUL* spinal umbilical line

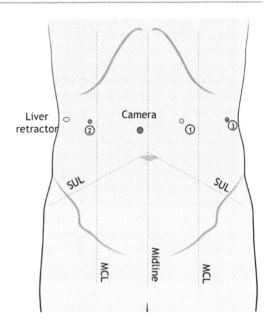

in the left anterior axillary line (Fig. 3.2). Depending on surgeon preference, a liver retractor could be utilized [5, 14].

3. Following port placement, the patient is placed in a reverse Trendelenburg position with an angle of >30° and the robotic cart is brought into the field. With the Si system, the robot must be parked at the head of the table, whereas with the Xi system, the robot can be parked at the patient's side as this platform includes an overhead boom allowing the arms to rotate as a group into any orientation. This allows for direct access to the patient by the anesthesia team. The console and vision cart are located safely away from the robot to allow for adequate movement of the arms and adequate room for the anesthesia team. The monitor is either at the foot of the table or mounted on the wall depending on the operating room setup. Appropriate adjustments of the operating table might need to be applied to prevent obstruction of the Anesthesiologist.

## Steps of Complete (Nissen) Fundoplication [5, 11, 14–17]

1. The operation begins with a hiatal dissection. First, retract the anterior epigastric fat pad and the stomach downward and towards the left lower quadrant using a Cadiere grasper. The gastrohepatic ligament is divided, using the electrocautery hook (Fig. 3.3), along the edge of the caudate lobe and the dissection plane is moved cephalad until the junction between the right crus of the hiatus and the phrenoesophageal membrane is encountered. Extra care is taken to preserve the anterior vagus nerve and especially the nerve of Latarjet and any aberrant left hepatic arteries, if present, are divided between clips (Fig. 3.4).

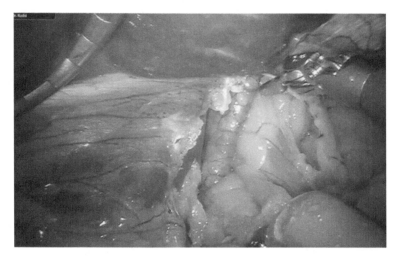

**Fig. 3.3** Dissection of gastrohepatic ligament

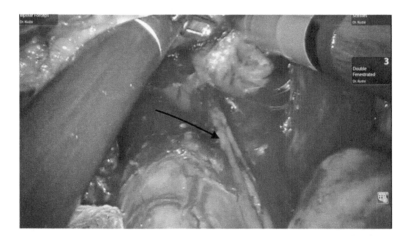

**Fig. 3.4** Identification of anterior vagus nerve

2. The right anterior phrenoesophageal ligament and the peritoneum overlying the anterior esophagus are incised superficially in order to prevent any injuries to the esophagus or anterior vagus. This incision is extended to the left crus and the esophagus is peeled off the right crus providing access to the mediastinum. The posterior vagus is identified and preserved (Fig. 3.5) and the dissection is extended circumferentially and in a clockwise fashion within the mediastinum. If a hiatal hernia is encountered, the hiatus is fully dissected and the esophago-gastric junction is reduced into the abdomen. Eventually, using sharp and blunt dissection, 4 cm of intra-abdominal esophagus are mobilized anteriorly and pos-teriorly from the right and the left crural limbs (Fig. 3.6). Complete excision of the sac should be performed. Subsequently, the robotic instruments are switched

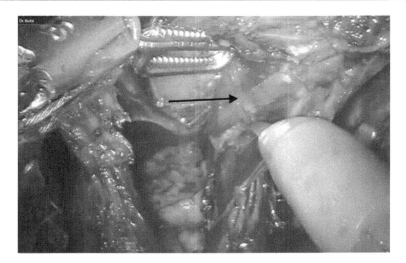

**Fig. 3.5**  Identification of posterior vagus nerve

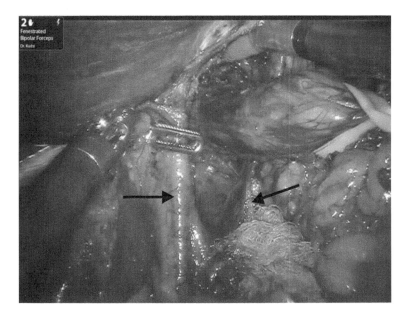

**Fig. 3.6**  Mobilization of esophagus from right and left crura

to two needle drivers and the hiatus is closed using non-absorbable sutures (2-0) (Fig. 3.7). Occasionally, a biologic mesh could be applied for reinforcement with promising results.

3. A point along the upper third of the gastric fundus (approximately 10–15 cm from the angle of His) is selected to begin ligating the short gastric vessels with an ultrasonic coagulator or bipolar vessel sealer (Fig. 3.8), in order to achieve

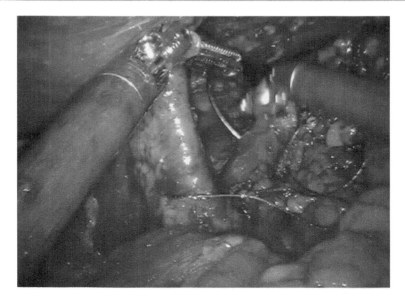

**Fig. 3.7** Primary closure of the hiatus

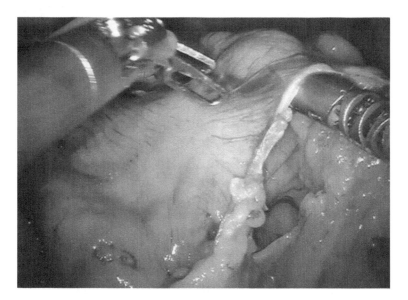

**Fig. 3.8** Division of the short gastric vessels

mobilization of the fundus for the creation of the posterior partial fundoplication. The ligation is continued up to the level of the left crus.

4. The anterior epigastric fat pad is removed from the distal esophagus and cardia to ensure appropriate visualization of the exact placement of the wrap. A retro-esophageal window is created and the posterior wall of the mobilized fundus is

grasped and passed behind the posterior vagus and posterior distal esophagus in a "shoeshine"-like maneuver.

5. Permanent 2-0 sutures are used to secure the fundoplication. The two sides of the fundus are sutured together and a small bite of the esophagus is also taken. The wrap faces the patient's right side in its final position. The first suture is most cephalad and is placed up on the esophagus at least 2–3 cm above the gastro-esophageal junction. The next suture incorporates a small bite of the esophagus and is placed 1 cm distal. The third suture only incorporates the fundus and is placed another centimeter distal (Fig. 3.9).

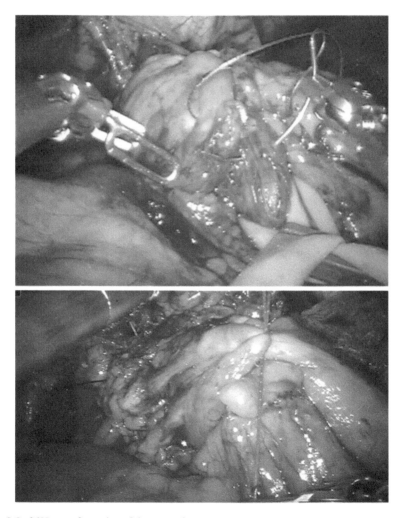

**Fig. 3.9**  360° wrap formation of the stomach

## Steps of Partial Posterior (Toupet) Fundoplication [5, 11, 14–16]

The basic steps of the partial fundoplication are identical to the steps for the posterior complete fundoplication, as described above. The differences include the creation of the fundoplication that is being performed as listed below:

1. The gastric fundus is grasped and retracted towards the midline, exposing the posterior hiatus. The superior aspect of the posterior fundus is sutured to the inferior right crus. Two coronal sutures are placed at 10 and 2 o'clock securing the fundus wrap to the hiatus (bougie might be helpful in this particular step).
2. Finally, two to three interrupted sutures are placed from the esophagus to the left and right fundus, leaving the anterior esophagus open and approximately 270° of the posterior esophagus wrapped. If an esophageal myotomy has been performed, as part of achalasia treatment, the edges of the fundus wrap are sutured to the myotomy edge.

## Steps of Anterior (Dor) Fundoplication

The basic steps of the anterior fundoplication are identical to the steps for the posterior partial fundoplication, as described above. The differences include the creation of the fundoplication that is being performed as listed below [18]:

1. Two rows of sutures are applied, one left and one right. The uppermost suture on the left side incorporates the fundus of the stomach, the esophageal wall, and the left pillar of the crus. The second and third sutures incorporate the stomach and the esophageal wall.
2. The fundus of the stomach is folded in a way so that the greater curvature is positioned next to the right pillar of the crus. Two to three sutures are placed between the fundus and the right pillar in an apical position, and finally, the right row is performed by placing two additional sutures between the superior aspect of the fundoplication and the edge of the esophageal hiatus.

## Postoperative Management

Following the completion of the procedure, the patient is transferred to the post-anesthesia recovery unit and is admitted to the surgical floor. A clear liquid diet may be initiated when post-anesthesia nausea has resolved. A soft mechanical diet is usually started on postoperative day 1 and the patient is maintained on that diet for 2–3 weeks after the operation. If no significant dysphagia is encountered, a regular diet can be instituted. Initial pain management is achieved with IV narcotics and a patient-controlled analgesia technique. Transition to oral narcotics pain medications is usually accomplished within 24 h after the procedure and most of the patients are getting discharged home on postoperative day 1 on pain control medications and anti-emetics.

## Intraoperative Complications

Fundoplications are usually categorized as low-risk procedures, but they can be associated with perioperative complications that increase significantly the morbidity and mortality of the procedure [11].

## Perforation

The most dreaded complication is perforation, which can occur during the placement of the trocars, hiatal dissection, and placement of the bougie. It can also be a result of a thermal injury by electrocautery that occurred at some point during the procedure. Intraoperative identification of an injury can be usually repaired primarily. If the injury is in the suture line, you should repair it primarily with coverage of the gastric fundus if possible. A closed suction drain may be left in place.

## Bleeding

Bleeding is usually minor and easily controlled. Most commonly, it occurs during division of the short gastric vessels that arise from the spleen. However, the incidence is <1% and the bleeding is usually easily controlled with ultrasonic coagulator or vessel sealer.

## Pneumothorax

During mediastinal dissection, there is risk of tearing the pleura. The incidence is <1% and the pneumothoraces are usually small and rarely require any further intervention. Often, surgeon could place a clip to approximate the parietal pleura. It is important to notify the anesthesiologist and, in case peek pressure is high, to decrease intra-abdominal carbon dioxide pressure to facilitate ventilation.

## Postoperative Complications

### Herniation

In approximately <1% of the patients, the gastric fundus can herniate through the hiatus. The patient usually presents with epigastric pain and tachycardia and is verified by a contrast study. Herniation noted in the immediate postoperative period is treated with immediate reoperation, reduction, and repeat closure of the crural defect. It's important to identify the technical error and rule out short esophagus and/or the need for lengthening procedure.

## Persistent Nausea and Vomiting

Severe postoperative nausea has been reported in up to 60% of patients after antireflux surgery and ~3–5% are experiencing episodes of emesis during their postoperative hospitalization. The patients who retch or vomit during the early postoperative period are at increased risk of disrupting the crural closure or herniate the newly fundoplicated wrap. If these symptoms persist for 7–10 days, the patient should undergo a barium esophagogram to evaluate the integrity of the fundoplication and if disruption is identified reoperation is indicated.

## Dysphagia

All patients are expected to have some degree of dysphagia, regurgitation, or inability to swallow appropriately in the early postoperative period. This is usually the consequence of postsurgical edema and inflammation that can delay the transit of food during swallowing. During that time, patients are advised to consume small, frequent, and soft meals with plenty of fluids. Subsequently, these symptoms usually resolve after the first few weeks in the vast majority of patients and approximately 3% of the patients will continue to report dysphagia after 6 months. In the population that has persistent symptoms for more than 6–12 weeks, a barium esophagogram should be performed. If an abnormal passage of barium is identified at the level of the gastroesophageal junction, endoscopic balloon dilations are recommended. Of note, the incidence of these symptoms is lower in patients who underwent partial posterior compared to complete fundoplication and, when endoscopic dilations are required, the result is usually curative [19]. If the dysphagia symptoms are caused by herniation of the wrap, the recommended treatment is reoperation, as discussed previously.

## Re-operative Procedures for Antireflux Surgery

Before proceeding with any surgical approach, the appropriate preoperative work up must be performed. This might include EGD, barium esophagogram, 24-h pH monitoring manometry, gastric emptying studies, and/or CT scan of the chest and abdomen, in order to identify a possible anatomical abnormality or recurrence.

Performing another surgical intervention in patients who already had antireflux surgery can be accompanied with great technical challenges. The presence of many adhesions can obscure the correct dissection plane and can limit the identification of the normal anatomic landmarks. In this situation, the use of the robot with the precision instruments and the high definition optics might provide extra benefit during the procedure, which has not yet translated to improve patients' outcomes. All patients need to undergo takedown of the original fundoplication, resection of a hernia sac, if necessary, and formation of a new fundoplication and/or assessment for the need of lengthening procedure such as Collis gastroplasty. In patients whose dysphagia is due to a tight previous Nissen wrap, creation of a partial fundoplication might be indicated.

## References

1. Shaheen NJ, Hansen RA, Morgan DR, Gangarosa LM, Ringel Y, Thiny MT, et al. The burden of gastrointestinal and liver diseases, 2006. Am J Gastroenterol. 2006;101(9):2128–38.
2. Lacy BE, Weiser K, Chertoff J, Fass R, Pandolfino JE, Richter JE, et al. The diagnosis of gastroesophageal reflux disease. Am J Med. 2010;123(7):583–92.
3. Vakil N, van Zanten SV, Kahrilas P, Dent J, Jones R. The montreal definition and classification of gastroesophageal reflux disease: a global evidence-based consensus. Am J Gastroenterol. 2006;101(8):1900–20; quiz 43.
4. Worrell SG, Greene CL, DeMeester TR. The state of surgical treatment of gastroesophageal reflux disease after five decades. J Am Coll Surg. 2014;219(4):819–30.
5. Tolboom RC, Broeders IAMJ, Draaisma WA. Robot-assisted laparoscopic hiatal hernia and antireflux surgery. J Surg Oncol. 2015;112(3):266–70.
6. Stefanidis D, Hope WW, Kohn GP, Reardon PR, Richardson WS, Fanelli RD. Guidelines for surgical treatment of gastroesophageal reflux disease. Surg Endosc. 2010;24(11):2647–69.
7. Kahrilas PJ, Shaheen NJ, Vaezi MF. American gastroenterological association medical position statement on the management of gastroesophageal reflux disease. Gastroenterology. 2008;135(4):1383–91.e5.
8. Campos GMR, Peters JH, DeMeester TR, Öberg S, Crookes PF, Tan S, et al. Multivariate analysis of factors predicting outcome after laparoscopic Nissen fundoplication. J Gastrointest Surg. 1999;3(3):292–300.
9. DeMeester TR, Johnson LF. The evaluation of objective measurements of gastroesophageal reflux and their contribution to patient management. Surg Clin North Am. 1976;56(1):39–53.
10. Peters JH. Modern imaging for the assessment of gastroesophageal reflux disease begins with the barium esophagram. J Gastrointest Surg. 2000;4(4):346–7.
11. Ujiki M, Shogan BD. Partial fundoplications: indications and technique. In: Swanstrom LL, Dunst CM, editors. Antireflux surgery. New York: Springer; 2015. p. 89–98.
12. Patti MG, Robinson T, Galvani C, Gorodner MV, Fisichella PM, Way LW. Total fundoplication is superior to partial fundoplication even when esophageal peristalsis is weak. J Am Coll Surg. 2004;198(6):863–9; discussion 9–70.
13. Dunn DH, Johnson EM, Kemp K, Ganz R, Leon S, Banerji N. Robotic assisted operations for gastroesophageal reflux. In: Kim KC, editor. Robotics in general surgery. New York: Springer; 2014. p. 33–54.
14. Melotti G, Trapani V, Frazzoni M, Varoli M, Piccoli M. Anti-reflux procedures and cardioesophagomyotomy. In: Spinoglio G, editor. Robotic surgery. Milano: Springer; 2015. p. 51–8.
15. Morelli L, Guadagni S, Mariniello MD, Pisano R, D'Isidoro C, Belluomini MA, et al. Robotic giant hiatal hernia repair: 3 year prospective evaluation and review of the literature. Int J Med Robot. 2015;11(1):1–7.
16. Wykypiel H, Wetscher GJ, Klaus A, Schmid T, Gadenstaetter M, Bodner J, et al. Robot-assisted laparoscopic partial posterior fundoplication with the DaVinci system: initial experiences and technical aspects. Langenbecks Arch Surg. 2003;387(11–12):411–6.
17. French G, Khaitan L. Laparoscopic Nissen fundoplication. Oper Tech Gen Surg. 2006;8(3):119–26.

18. Patti MG, Molena D, Fisichella PM, Whang K, Yamada H, Perretta S, et al. Laparoscopic Heller myotomy and Dor fundoplication for achalasia: analysis of successes and failures. Arch Surg. 2001;136(8):870–7.
19. Almond LM, Wadley MS. A 5-year prospective review of posterior partial fundoplication in the management of gastroesophageal reflux disease. Int J Surg (London, England). 2010;8(3):239–42.

# Masters Program Foregut Pathway: Robotic Heller

**4**

Amareshewar Chiruvella, Christopher Crawford, Crystal Krause, and Dmitry Oleynikov

## Introduction

Achalasia is a rare primary esophageal motility disorder that is characterized by the absence of peristalsis and a defective relaxation of the lower esophageal sphincter (LES), resulting in impaired bolus transport and food stasis in the esophagus. The first description of achalasia was provided in 1674 by Willis, and in 1888, Einhorn hypothesized that the defect was secondary to the absence of opening of the cardia. In 1937, Lendrum first proposed that the syndrome was caused by incomplete relaxation of the LES and coined the term after the Greek word "*khalasis*," meaning failure to relax. Over the years, the diagnosis of this rare yet debilitating primary motility disorder has evolved from the use of swallow studies alone to the application of conventional manometry using water-perfused, catheter-based systems, to the usage of solid-state, multichannel catheters/high resolution manometry (HRM). With the advent of HRM, we have been able to classify this disease process into three subtypes that vary with respect to disease prognosis and response to treatment. Detailed discussion about the different achalasia subtypes and manometric interpretation is beyond the scope of this chapter. In the following pages, we will briefly describe the different diagnostic and treatment options that are currently available for achalasia, with a more comprehensive depiction of robotic-assisted Heller myotomy.

A. Chiruvella, M.D. • C. Crawford, M.D.
Advanced Gastrointestinal/Minimally Invasive Surgery, University of Nebraska Medical Center, Omaha, NE, USA

C. Krause, Ph.D.
Surgery, University of Nebraska Medical Center, Omaha, NE, USA

D. Oleynikov, M.D., F.A.C.S. (✉)
Gastrointestinal, Minimally Invasive and Bariatric Surgery, The Center for Advanced Surgical Technology, University of Nebraska Medical Center, Omaha, NE, USA
e-mail: doleynik@unmc.edu

© Springer International Publishing AG 2018
A.D. Patel, D. Oleynikov (eds.), *The SAGES Manual of Robotic Surgery*,
The SAGES University Masters Program Series, DOI 10.1007/978-3-319-51362-1_4

## Pathophysiology

Achalasia can be classified into primary and secondary forms. While the cause for primary achalasia is yet unknown and a subject of debate, every hypothesis accounts for the loss of ganglia within the esophageal myenteric plexus. The myenteric plexus is comprised of both excitatory and inhibitory motor neurons. The esophageal myenteric plexus releases acetylcholine, which produces smooth muscle contraction, and the myenteric plexus releases nitric oxide and vasoactive intestinal polypeptide, producing smooth muscle relaxation. It is the imbalance between the density of these two groups of neurons that leads to impaired relaxation of the LES due to unopposed cholinergic stimulation of the LES [1]. Three etiologies have been proposed [1]:

1. A degenerative process of the neurons
2. Viral infections such as measles, varicella-zoster virus, and herpes
3. Autoimmune cause with antibodies against the myenteric neurons

Secondary achalasia can either be isolated to the esophagus or be part of a generalized motility disorder affecting other portions of the GI tract. It is important to rule out causes of pseudoachalasia prior to embarking on treating achalasia per se.

## Clinical Features

Achalasia is a relatively uncommon primary motility disorder with an incidence of 1 in 100,000 individuals and a prevalence of 10 in 100,000. The disease usually presents between 30 and 60 years of age and is equally distributed between males and females, without racial predilection [2].

The classic presentation of most patients is with progressive dysphagia to solids and liquids (90%) associated with regurgitation of undigested food or saliva (45%). The second most common symptom is heart burn (75%) followed by non-cardiac chest pain with intake of food (20–40%). This was corroborated in a single-center review by Tsuboi et al. over a period of 24 years (1984–2008) and found that patients with achalasia most commonly presented with dysphagia and heart burn [3–5]. Respiratory symptoms are also common due to decreased esophageal clearance resulting in aspiration of food or liquid. Chronic aspiration is seen in 20–30% of patients, and around 33% complain of sore throat or hoarseness. Around 5–10% of patients have unintentional weight loss.

This disease process also confers a 40–100 times increased risk of squamous cell cancer of the esophagus compared to the non-achalasia patient [6, 7].

## Therapeutic Modalities

While no cure currently exists for this disease process, all present-day therapeutic approaches aim to reduce the LES pressure. These can be classified into non-surgical and surgical treatments:

Non-surgical Treatment

1. Pharmacotherapy—Calcium channel blockers and Nitrates
2. Injection of botulinum toxin
3. Pneumatic dilation (PD)

Surgical Treatment

1. Peroral Endoscopic Myotomy (POEM)
2. Heller Myotomy

In this chapter, we will focus on the surgical treatment of achalasia by Heller myotomy.

## Non-surgical Treatment

### Pharmacotherapy

The most commonly used agents are calcium channel blockers (CCB) and nitrates. Nifedipine has been found to decrease LES pressure by 13–49% and improve patient symptoms by 0–75%. Its duration of effect is 30–120 min and used 30–45 min before meals in 10–30 mg doses for best response. Sublingual isosorbide dinitrate has been effective in reducing LES pressure by 30–65%, leading to symptomatic improvement ranging from 53 to 87%. It is administered in 5 mg doses, 10–15 min before meals, and has a shorter duration of action at 30–90 min [2, 8].

The clinical response to these agents is of short duration as drug tolerance develops rapidly. Symptomatic improvement is incomplete and causes undesirable side effects of headache, hypotension, and leg edema, thus limiting their use. These drugs are only considered for patients who cannot or refuse to undergo other invasive therapies and for those in whom even botulinum toxin injection has failed. Other agents that have been used are PDE five inhibitors such as sildenafil, anticholinergics, beta adrenergic agonists, and theophylline, but none of these agents have been shown to be as effective as the endoscopic or surgical therapies.

### Injection of Botulinum Toxin

Botulinum toxin is a presynaptic inhibitor of acetylcholine release from the nerve endings. The toxin cleaves the SNAP-25 protein, which is involved in the fusion of the presynaptic vesicles containing acetylcholine with the neuronal plasma membrane. This inhibition of exocytosis of acetylcholine causes a short-term paralysis of the LES.

The treatment, however, is limited in efficacy and is associated with an approximately 50% reduction in the basal LES pressure. The average duration of action is around 3–4 months [9]. The standard approach is to inject 80–100 units in four quadrants, just above the Z line. Doses higher than 100 units have not been found to be effective. While 75% of patients have an initial response, the therapeutic effect wears off to less than 60% at 1 year. About 50% of patients relapse and require repeat treatments at 6–24 months [10–12]. Repetitive injections of botox into the LES can incite a fibrotic reaction, obscuring the sub-mucosal plane thus making future myotomy difficult. Due to these limitations, botulinum toxin injections should be considered only in elderly patients who are not candidates for pneumatic dilation, laparoscopic Heller myotomy, or peroral endoscopic myotomy.

## Pneumatic Dilation

Pneumatic dilation (PD) is considered an effective non-surgical option to treat achalasia. The principle lies behind the use of air pressure for intra-luminal dilation and disruption of the circular muscle fibers of the LES. Csendes and colleagues (1989) performed a randomized trial comparing pneumatic dilatation to myotomy with anterior fundoplication. After a 5-year follow-up, 73% of patients in the dilatation group reported absent or mild dysphagia compared to 98% in the surgical group. The most serious complication with PD is esophageal perforation, with an incidence of approximately 1.9% [13, 14]. Hence, all patients who undergo a PD should be counseled about the possible need for an emergent surgical intervention in the rare event of an uncontrolled perforation. As with botulinum toxin injections, subsequent myotomy may be complicated by prior pneumatic dilations.

## Surgical Treatment

### Per Oral Endoscopic Myotomy

Per oral endoscopic myotomy (POEM) is a novel endoscopic procedure performed under general anesthesia. After suctioning the esophagus, the Z line is identified and at around 10–15 cm from the Z line, an initial submucosal injection is made to safely access the mucosa-submucosal plane to create a submucosal tunnel. During the procedure, multiple such injections of diluted contrast agent (e.g. methylene blue) are performed to a total volume of 100–150 cc. A 1.5 cm mucosal incision is then made with either a triangular tip knife or a hybrid knife and a submucosal tunnel is carefully extended to 3 cm into the gastric cardia. As the operator advances into the cardia, the vessel density and diameter of the tunnel increases and the mucosa becomes thinner, lending itself to a higher risk of perforation. Different centers across the world vary in the choice of site for the myotomy. Myotomy positions include anterior (11 or 2 o'clock), posterior (5 or 7 o'clock), and lateral (3 or 8 o'clock). The total length of a standard myotomy is around 10–12 cm, including the 2–3 cm of cardiomyotomy. After the myotomy is completed, hemostasis is achieved and the mucosotomy is closed either with endoscopic clips, OVESCO clips, endoscopic suturing devices, or fully covered self-expanding metal stents.

Inoue et al. published the first series of patient outcomes after this procedure in 2010, showing promising early results in the treatment of achalasia [15]. Following this, several studies by Swanstrom et al., von Rentien et al., and Bhayani et al. have shown comparable outcomes to surgical myotomy with significant improvements in LES pressure, Eckardt scores, and postoperative morbidity at least in the short term [16–18].

## Heller Myotomy and Its Evolution

The first reported treatment of achalasia was to pass a piece of curved whalebone with a sponge at the distal end through the esophagus by Willis in 1674. Heller described the first surgical myotomy as a treatment for achalasia in 1914. The original procedure involved myotomies over the anterior and posterior walls of the esophagus via a thoracotomy incision. In 1923, Zaaijer modified this technique and used only an anterior myotomy with excellent results in eight patients [19].

During the 1960s and 1970s, esophageal myotomy was performed through an open approach, either left trans-thoracic or trans-abdominal. The initial myotomy as proposed by Ellis et al. extended to only 5 mm onto the gastric wall. In his personal 22 year experience, Ellis reported the use of a transthoracic short myotomy without an antireflux procedure in 179 patients. The overall improvement rate was 89% with marked reflux in only 5% of patients [20]. Compared to the trans-thoracic myotomy, the trans-abdominal approach was found to result in a significantly higher incidence of postoperative reflux. The proposed mechanisms for the latter include a longer myotomy onto the gastric wall, division of the phreno-esophageal ligament, and greater mobilization of the esophagus.

Dor, in 1962, proposed the addition of a partial anterior fundoplication to a long myotomy to minimize the risk of post-operative reflux. Several studies have evaluated the outcome of open trans-abdominal myotomy and anterior fundoplication. One such study by Bonavina et al. was done on 206 patients who underwent a trans-abdominal Heller myotomy (8 cm on the esophagus and 2 cm on the stomach) along with a Dor fundoplication for the treatment of achalasia. 93.8% of patients had complete or near complete resolution of symptoms [21]. 3.6% of patients had recurrent dysphagia and abnormal acid exposure with 24 h pH monitoring was present only in 8.6% of patients. Richards et al. demonstrated through a randomized prospective study that addition of a Dor fundoplication after Heller myotomy reduces pathologic reflux, as measured by 24 h pH studies, from 47 to 9% and has no measurable impact on postoperative dysphagia [22].

With the advent of minimally invasive techniques in the early 1990s, the first minimally invasive myotomy was performed in the US in 1991 [23]. This was initially performed via a left thoracoscopic approach, replicating the technique described by Ellis, with a 7 cm myotomy extending onto the gastric wall for only 5 mm. The shortcomings of this approach, however, were as follows: (1) need for single lung ventilation, (2) inadequate exposure of the GE junction, (3) high incidence of postoperative reflux due to absence of a fundoplication, and (4) postoperative discomfort secondary to the chest tube. This led to the advent of the laparoscopic Heller myotomy (LHM) with Dor fundoplication. Several studies have compared these two approaches and the laparoscopic approach was found to be associated with better postoperative pain control, shorter length of stay, better relief of dysphagia, and lower incidence of postoperative gastroesophageal reflux [24–27]. One of these studies was done by Patti et al., reviewing outcomes in 60 patients who underwent thoracoscopic (30 patients) or LHM with anterior fundoplication (30 patients). Median hospital stay was 42 h in the laparoscopic group and 84 h in the thoracoscopic group. Resolution of dysphagia was seen in 87% of thoracoscopic and 90%

of laparoscopic group patients. Abnormal reflux was seen on 24 h pH testing in 60% of the thoracoscopic group and in only 10% of the laparoscopic group [25].

The type of fundoplication used after a myotomy has been debated as well. An anterior 180° Dor, a posterior 270° Toupet, and a floppy 360° Nissen have all been proposed. Rebecchi and colleagues performed a randomized controlled trial comparing Dor versus Nissen fundoplication in 144 patients who underwent a Heller myotomy. No significant difference was seen with respect to reflux, but dysphagia was significantly more common in the Nissen group [28].

With the advent of robotic surgery, robotic-assisted Heller myotomy (RAHM) has now taken the stage as an emerging standard of care for achalasia. Although its laparoscopic counterpart is more widespread, RAHM has shown equivalent outcomes. Horgan et al. conducted a multi-institutional retrospective review of 121 achalasia patients. Fifty-nine patients underwent a robotic myotomy and 62 underwent a conventional LHM. Although the mean operative time was longer in the robotic group, esophageal perforations occurred more commonly in the laparoscopic group (16% vs. 0%) [29]. Similar results were achieved with respect to relief of dysphagia. Another study by Huffman et al. found a lower rate of esophageal perforations in the robotic group (0% vs. 8%) and higher postoperative quality of life indices [30]. It is likely that the better visualization provided by the robot along with the enhanced degrees of freedom allows a more controlled dissection of the individual muscle fibers resulting in a better technical outcome. Contrary to this, other studies have not shown a difference in intraoperative complications or postoperative course, while projecting higher operative costs with the use of the robot.

Nevertheless, with the continued research and development in the field of robotics, it is undeniable that the robot is here to stay and familiarity with this technique is essential for future surgeons.

## Preoperative Evaluation

Patients with achalasia are typically referred for symptoms of dysphagia or regurgitation. A thorough history and physical are necessary for all patient evaluations. We use a standard questionnaire for all patients that is entered both into the patient medical record and a research database. The questionnaire goes through a detailed description of the patient's symptoms and their duration, including the extent of dysphagia, regurgitation, reflux, chest or abdominal pain, and associated symptoms such as pulmonary or pharyngeal complaints. Symptoms typical for achalasia include progressive dysphagia beginning with intolerance to bulky solid foods such as bread, raw vegetables, and chunks of meat. This progresses to difficulty with swallowing even water, and some patients can feel the sensation of food accumulating in their esophagus and passing very slowly.

The first diagnostic test is typically a contrast esophagram under fluoroscopy, to evaluate esophageal anatomy and clearance of contrast. The classic finding of

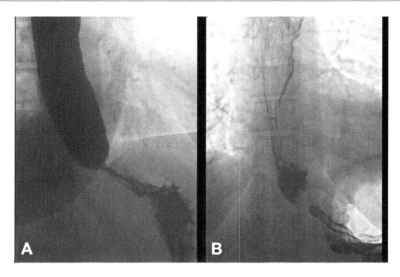

**Fig. 4.1** Preoperative and postoperative images of achalasia. (**a**) This contrast esophagram demonstrates the findings of a hypertensive lower esophageal sphincter with a proximally dilated esophagus, showing a "bird's beak" narrowing; (**b**) Postoperative esophagram at 1 year follow-up

achalasia is the bird's beak esophagus, which shows a large distal esophagus tapering to a smooth point at the gastroesophageal (GE) junction (Fig. 4.1a). The distal esophagus can become markedly dilated, which is called a sigmoid esophagus. Upper endoscopy is necessary to rule out the presence of any lesions that may cause pseudo-achalasia, such as an esophageal neoplasm, and to evaluate for any concurrent pathology.

All patients require manometry to confirm the diagnosis. Conventional manometry relied on the absence of relaxation of lower esophageal sphincter. High-resolution manometry of the esophagus allows calculation of the integrated relaxation pressure (IRP), which is a 4 s mean calculated in reference to gastric pressure. A median IRP > 15 mmHg in the presence of 100% failed peristalsis is diagnostic of achalasia. Spastic achalasia and achalasia with esophageal compression are variants that can involve hypercontractile findings on manometry, but these subtypes as well as classical achalasia can all be treated with an esophagomyotomy. Frequently, the manometry will show little more than a lower esophageal sphincter that fails to relax and no significant peristaltic activity in the body of the esophagus (Fig. 4.2).

Patients are not routinely tested with pH monitors, as our standard approach entails a partial fundoplication. A circumferential fundoplication will cause dysphagia in a patient with poor peristaltic function, such as those with achalasia. Conversely, completely defeating the lower esophageal sphincter without providing any anti-reflux mechanism is associated with high rates of esophagitis.

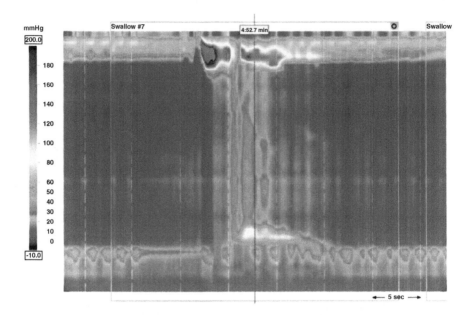

**Fig. 4.2** This high-resolution manometry shows a lower esophageal sphincter that fails to relax with aperistalsis of the body of the esophagus

## Operative Planning

Our standard approach is always trans-abdominal [31, 32]. This can be performed as a combination of laparoscopic technique with robotic assistance or a purely robot-assisted approach. In our practice, the initial approach to the dissection is laparoscopic, but the actual myotomy is performed with the da Vinci Surgical System (Intuitive Surgical, Sunnyvale, CA). The da Vinci System provides a magnified stereoscopic image to the surgeon seated at a console away from the patient, which we find to be very useful in establishing the plane of dissection beneath the muscular layer and avoiding iatrogenic mucosal perforation. The da Vinci System provides six degrees of movement with a wristed action that allows delicate sweeping movements to create this plane. It also dampens any tremors and can be scaled to allow very fine movements by the surgeon as the muscle is elevated and divided.

All patients undergo standard pre-operative evaluation for general anesthesia and laparoscopy. They are placed on a clear liquid diet for 3 days to decrease the amount of retained food in the esophagus. They are given a clear liquid protein supplement during this time. A type and screen for blood is not routinely obtained. All patients are given pre-operative intravenous antibiotics within an hour of incision. Mechanical and chemical prophylaxes are given for venous thromboembolism prevention. Patients are placed supine on the operating table with a foot board in place to allow steep reverse Trendelenburg positioning without shifting. A Foley catheter and an orogastric tube are placed. The arms are tucked at the sides, and the lower legs and shoulders are padded. A thigh strap is placed, and the lower legs and shoulders are taped to the operating table. The overhead monitor is placed over the patient's head to allow the operating surgeon and assistant to look at the same screen. Our practice is to set the room up so that the robot may be docked from the head of the bed, with the anesthesia equipment to one side and the surgical equipment to the other side, as shown in Fig. 4.3.

Access to the abdomen is gained with a Veress needle to create pneumoperitoneum, and an optical 12 mm trocar is placed. This camera port is not placed in the midline, but rather in line with the diaphragmatic hiatus, to facilitate triangulation around the hiatus. This is about 3 cm to the patient's left of the umbilicus, 15 cm inferior to the xiphoid process. Two 8 mm ports are placed along the left costal margin, as close to the rib as possible. The lateral left costal margin port is placed as far lateral as possible to prevent collision of the robot arms. A Nathanson liver retractor is placed inferior to the xiphoid process to elevate the left lobe of the liver to visualize the hiatus, and it is fixed to a post on the operating table. An 8 mm port is placed to the patient's right of the epigastrium, and the trocar is advanced through the falciform ligament, which prevents the falciform ligament from hanging in front of the instrument being advanced into the abdomen (Fig. 4.4). The patient is then placed in steep reverse Trendelenburg position, with the patient's right side tilted down. The robot is docked at this time. The operating assistant stands on the patient's left side and provides lateral retraction of the fundus of the stomach. Alternatively, this could be performed by the third working arm of the robot. The

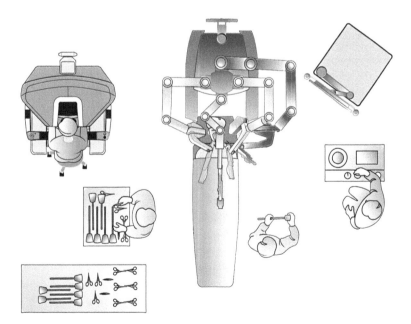

**Fig. 4.3** The robot is docked from the head of the bed, with the assistant at the patient's left

**Fig. 4.4** The camera port is off-midline in order to be in line with the hiatus, and the other ports are positioned to allow triangulation focused at the hiatus

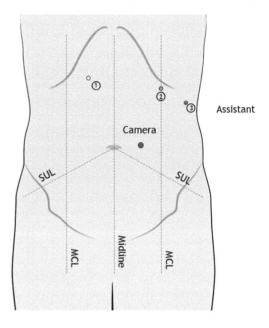

surgeon begins with an atraumatic grasping device in the left hand and a monopolar cautery hook in the right hand. This is used to divide the phrenoesophageal ligament to expose the angle of His. The left pillar of the crus must be visualized, and dissection is carried anteriorly toward the midline. The lesser sac is then entered through the lesser omentum, and the right pillar of the crus is identified. This dissection is carried anteriorly up to the level of the contralateral side. The anterior vagus nerve is adherent to the esophagus and must be identified and mobilized to allow for a complete myotomy. The anterior vagus lies on the esophagus at the 1 o'clock position and crosses toward the lesser curvature (Fig. 4.5). It has attachments on the medial and lateral side that must be divided separately to fully mobilize it. Limited use of thermal energy is important to prevent nerve damage. The phrenoesophageal ligament and esophageal fat pad are divided in the midline to expose the muscular layers at the GE junction, taking care to note the position of the vagus nerve as it passes through this fat pad.

The fundus of the stomach may require some mobilization to allow for the partial fundoplication, particularly in the obese male patient. The short gastric vessels should be divided with an energy device (the authors prefer a bipolar sealing/cutting device) along the greater curvature of the stomach. This typically requires division of the first short gastric vessels. A posterior dissection and identification of the posterior vagus nerve are not necessary and should be avoided in order to maintain the native anatomy of the hiatus. The esophagus is exposed at least 8 cm above the GE junction. The esophagus is then lightly scored with a monopolar hook cautery to demarcate the site of the myotomy, with a goal of a 7 cm esophagomyotomy and a 3 cm gastromyotomy, including the sling fibers at the GE junction.

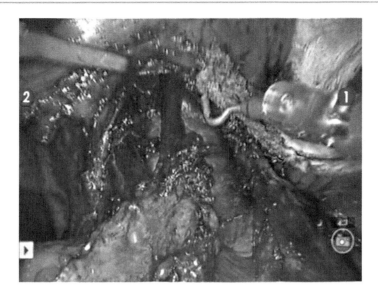

**Fig. 4.5** The left/anterior vagus nerve can be seen crossing from the anterior esophagus to the lesser curvature of the stomach

A lighted 56 French bougie is placed through the mouth and advanced into the stomach, with the purpose of illuminating the areas with an incomplete myotomy as the operation proceeds. A gentle twisting motion usually allows the bougie to pass into the stomach, taking care not to perforate the GE junction, which is often angulated in achalasia patients. The myotomy is initiated at the GE junction, as this region is easily visualized, and the myotomy can be extended in either direction from that point. Muscle fibers along the scored line at the GE junction are then elevated and gently spread, until the submucosal plane between the mucosa and muscle fibers is identified. The left hand grasps and elevates these fibers anteriorly, and the hook is used to gently push the mucosa posteriorly and then cauterize the muscle fibers, taking care not to allow stray energy to pass onto the esophageal mucosa (Fig. 4.6). This "lift and spread" method is continued cephalad, cauterizing the muscle fibers that do not split with gentle blunt dissection. Most fibers split with blunt dissection alone. Esophageal mucosa will bulge anteriorly once the muscle fibers are divided, and the light from the bougie should be visible. Persistent muscle fibers will appear as stripes across the mucosa with the light shining (Fig. 4.7). Once the proximal extent of the myotomy is complete, the dissection is continued down onto the stomach. The sling fibers at the GE junction are an important adjunct to the LES, so they must be divided to provide a complete myotomy. The completed myotomy should show light clearly shining through the mucosa (Fig. 4.8).

At the completion of the myotomy, an anterior Dor fundoplication is created. The first step is to re-create the angle of His by tacking the medial gastric fundus to the left pillar of the crus with a 2-0 silk (Fig. 4.9). The medial edge of the gastric

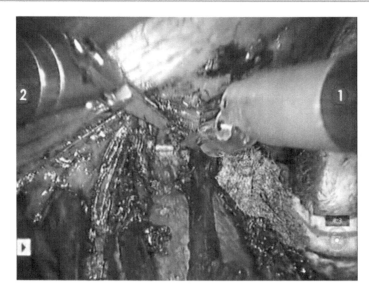

**Fig. 4.6** The longitudinal and circular muscle fibers of the esophagus are elevated anteriorly, and the mucosa is gently depressed to create a plane of dissection

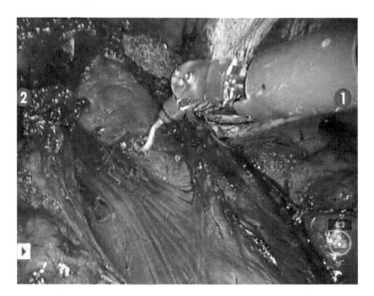

**Fig. 4.7** Residual muscle fibers are backlit by the lighted bougie, allowing improved visualization of an incomplete myotomy

fundus is then sewn to the lateral cut edge of the myotomy with two 2-0 silk sutures. The gastric fundus is then folded over the esophagus for the anterior fundoplication. The greater curvature of the gastric fundus is then sewn to the medial cut edge of the myotomy with two 2-0 silk sutures (Fig. 4.10).

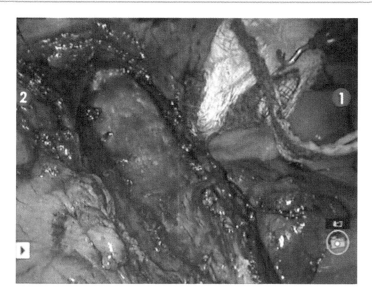

**Fig. 4.8** This depicts a completed myotomy, with bulging mucosa in between the cut edges of the muscle

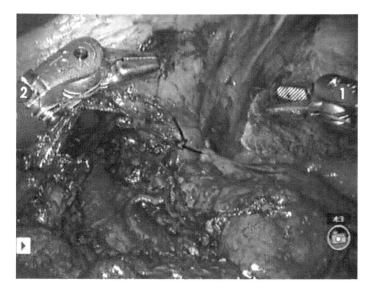

**Fig. 4.9** The medial aspect of the gastric fundus is sutured to the left pillar of the crus to re-approximate the angle of His

The bougie is then removed, and a completion endoscopy is performed. The endoscope should pass easily through GE junction without any pressure or angulation. The endoscope should be retroflexed to evaluate the fundoplication for any twisting or corkscrew effect on the esophagus. A saline leak test can also be performed. The ports are then removed, and the operation is complete.

**Fig. 4.10** A partial anterior (Dor) fundoplication is created. Reprinted from [32]

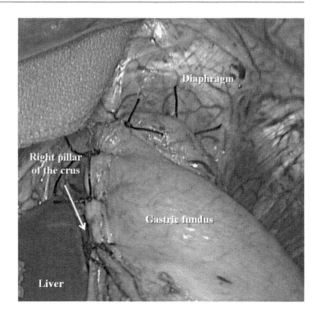

This operation may also be performed completely with the robot. Our practice is to perform the initial dissection laparoscopically, as the haptic feedback is particularly useful in the dissection while entering the mediastinum.

## Post-operative Care

Patients are admitted to our standard surgical floor and given a clear liquid diet the same day as surgery. Analgesia is provided with scheduled intravenous ketorolac and intermittent oral opioids. Antiemetics are scheduled to prevent retching, which could potentially disrupt the fundoplication. Patients are typically given ondansetron and metoclopramide intravenously. We do not routinely check any laboratory studies, and no routine postoperative imaging is obtained. The morning of postoperative day one, patients are advanced to a full liquid diet and are discharged home. They are to advance to a pureed diet at home and then move onto more solid foods, but they are counseled to continue avoiding bulky solid foods such as bread, raw vegetables, and chunks of meat.

## Outcomes

Patients typically report an immediate improvement in their dysphagia when they begin drinking clear liquids. They are seen in our clinic 2 weeks after surgery and again at 6 months to evaluate their symptoms. All patients undergo a contrast esophagram 1 year after their operation (see Fig. 4.1b). The purpose of this is to provide early notice of recurrent disease, which allows for early re-intervention. It is relatively rare for patients to require a secondary intervention, but the initial course of treatment after a failed myotomy would include endoscopic therapy such as botulinum toxin injection or pneumatic dilation. If this fails to provide symptomatic relief, then repeat myotomy should be considered.

## References

1. Hirano I. Pathophysiology of achalasia. Curr Gastroenterol Rep. 1999;1(3):198–202.
2. Vaezi MF, Pandolfino JE, Vela MF. ACG clinical guideline: diagnosis and management of achalasia. Am J Gastroenterol. 2013;108(8):1238–49. Quiz 1250
3. Pandolfino JE, Gawron AJ. Achalasia: a systematic review. JAMA. 2015;313(18):1841–52.
4. Sinan H, et al. Prevalence of respiratory symptoms in patients with achalasia. Dis Esophagus. 2011;24(4):224–8.
5. Tsuboi K, et al. Insights gained from symptom evaluation of esophageal motility disorders: a review of 4,215 patients. Digestion. 2012;85(3):236–42.
6. Leeuwenburgh I, et al. Long-term esophageal cancer risk in patients with primary achalasia: a prospective study. Am J Gastroenterol. 2010;105(10):2144–9.
7. Ravi K, Geno DM, Katzka DA. Esophageal cancer screening in achalasia: is there a consensus? Dis Esophagus. 2015;28(3):299–304.
8. Gelfond M, Rozen P, Gilat T. Isosorbide dinitrate and nifedipine treatment of achalasia: a clinical, manometric and radionuclide evaluation. Gastroenterology. 1982;83(5):963–9.
9. Ghosh B, Das SK. Botulinum toxin: a dreaded toxin for use in human being. J Indian Med Assoc. 2002;100(10):607–8, 610–2, 614.
10. Annese V, et al. A multicentre randomised study of intrasphincteric botulinum toxin in patients with oesophageal achalasia. GISMAD Achalasia Study Group. Gut. 2000;46(5):597–600.
11. Pasricha PJ, et al. Intrasphincteric botulinum toxin for the treatment of achalasia. N Engl J Med. 1995;332(12):774–8.
12. Torresan F, et al. Treatment of achalasia in the era of high-resolution manometry. Ann Gastroenterol. 2015;28(3):301–308.
13. Vaezi MF. Achalasia: diagnosis and management. Semin Gastrointest Dis. 1999;10(3):103–12.
14. Vaezi MF, et al. Botulinum toxin versus pneumatic dilatation in the treatment of achalasia: a randomised trial. Gut. 1999;44(2):231–9.
15. Inoue H, et al. Peroral endoscopic myotomy (POEM) for esophageal achalasia. Endoscopy. 2010;42(4):265–71.
16. Bhayani NH, et al. A comparative study on comprehensive, objective outcomes of laparoscopic Heller myotomy with per-oral endoscopic myotomy (POEM) for achalasia. Ann Surg. 2014;259(6):1098–103.
17. Swanstrom LL, Rieder E, Dunst CM. A stepwise approach and early clinical experience in peroral endoscopic myotomy for the treatment of achalasia and esophageal motility disorders. J Am Coll Surg. 2011;213(6):751–6.
18. von Renteln D, et al. Peroral endoscopic myotomy for the treatment of achalasia: a prospective single center study. Am J Gastroenterol. 2012;107(3):411–7.
19. Zaaijer JH. Cardiospasm in the aged. Ann Surg. 1923;77(5):615–7.
20. Ellis Jr FH. Oesophagomyotomy for achalasia: a 22-year experience. Br J Surg. 1993;80(7):882–5.
21. Bonavina L, et al. Primary treatment of esophageal achalasia. Long-term results of myotomy and Dor fundoplication. Arch Surg. 1992;127(2):222–6; discussion 227.
22. Richards WO, et al. Heller myotomy versus Heller myotomy with Dor fundoplication for achalasia: a prospective randomized double-blind clinical trial. Ann Surg. 2004;240(3):405–12; discussion 412–5.

23. Shimi S, Nathanson LK, Cuschieri A. Laparoscopic cardiomyotomy for achalasia. J R Coll Surg Edinb. 1991;36(3):152–4.
24. Graham AJ, et al. Laparoscopic esophageal myotomy and anterior partial fundoplication for the treatment of achalasia. Ann Thorac Surg. 1997;64(3):785–9.
25. Patti MG, et al. Comparison of thoracoscopic and laparoscopic Heller myotomy for achalasia. J Gastrointest Surg. 1998;2(6):561–6.
26. Patti MG, et al. Minimally invasive surgery for achalasia: an 8-year experience with 168 patients. Ann Surg. 1999;230(4):587–93; discussion 593–4.
27. Rosati R, et al. Laparoscopic approach to esophageal achalasia. Am J Surg. 1995;169(4):424–7.
28. Rebecchi F, et al. Randomized controlled trial of laparoscopic Heller myotomy plus Dor fundoplication versus Nissen fundoplication for achalasia: long-term results. Ann Surg. 2008;248(6):1023–30.
29. Horgan S, et al. Robotic-assisted Heller myotomy versus laparoscopic Heller myotomy for the treatment of esophageal achalasia: multicenter study. J Gastrointest Surg. 2005;9(8):1020–9; discussion 1029–30.
30. Huffmanm LC, et al. Robotic Heller myotomy: a safe operation with higher postoperative quality-of-life indices. Surgery. 2007;142(4):613–8; discussion 618–20.
31. Bochkarev V, Ringley CD, Oleynikov D. Robotic-assisted operative techniques in general surgery. Oper Tech Genral Surg. 2005;7:188–200.
32. Oleynikov D, Martin RF, editors. Surgical approaches to esophageal disease. Surg Clin North Am. 2015;95(3):i.

Paul A.R. Del Prado and James G. Bittner IV

## Introduction

There are two general types of hiatal hernia: sliding and paraesophageal. The sliding hiatal hernia (Type I) is defined by a cephalad displacement of the esophagogastric junction and proximal stomach through the hiatus into the posterior mediastinum. The stomach is covered anteriorly by peritoneum, whereas the posterior stomach is bare. In most patients, the esophagus is normal in length, and the hernia reduces easily in the upright position. The other major type of hiatus hernia is termed a paraesophageal hernia (PEH), of which there are three subtypes. Type 2 PEH is one in which the esophagogastric junction remains in place below the diaphragm but the stomach herniates into the chest next to the esophagus and is covered completely by peritoneum. Initially, only the gastric fundus herniates through the hiatus, until finally the entire stomach enters the chest giving the appearance of the "upside-down stomach or gastric volvulus." Type 3 PEH is one in which the esophagogastric junction is displaced above the diaphragm while a PEH with herniation of colon, spleen, or pancreas is termed Type 4 [1].

Patients with PEH may be asymptomatic or present with a myriad of symptoms including postprandial dyspnea, early satiety, dysphagia, heartburn, epigastric pain, or associated conditions such as gastroesophageal reflux disease (GERD), esophagitis and/or gastritis, gastric volvulus with incarceration or strangulation, and even gastric rupture. Diagnosis of PEH is confirmed with endoscopic and/or radiologic

P.A.R. Del Prado, M.D.
Maricopa Integrated Health System, Pheonix, AZ, USA
e-mail: l.delprado@vcuhealth.org

J.G. Bittner IV, M.D. (✉)
Virginia Commonwealth University, Medical College of Virginia, Richmond, VA, USA
e-mail: james.bittner@vcuhealth.org

© Springer International Publishing AG 2018
A.D. Patel, D. Oleynikov (eds.), *The SAGES Manual of Robotic Surgery*,
The SAGES University Masters Program Series, DOI 10.1007/978-3-319-51362-1_5

studies. The management of patients with PEH may include proton pump inhibitor therapy, endoscopic treatment, and/or surgical intervention. Controversy exists as to whether PEH should be managed by simple reduction of the hernia with excision of the sac and closure of the hiatus, or whether all patients should have an antireflux procedure in addition. The following chapter will discuss the indications and minimally invasive techniques for repair of PEH and concomitant prevention of gastroesophageal reflux.

## Indications for Operation

When considering patients for minimally invasive paraesophageal hernia repair, it is important to assess the patient thoroughly, taking care to fully elucidate patient symptoms, concomitant medical conditions, and determine the feasibility and type of repair [1]. To this end, the Society of Gastrointestinal and Endoscopic Surgeons (SAGES) published Guidelines for the Management of Hiatal Hernia to aid surgeons and patients in the decision-making process. The guidelines that specifically address the indications for repair of PEH are summarized below.

## SAGES Guidelines for Management of Hiatal Hernia

- Asymptomatic hiatal hernia (Type I) does not, in and of itself, necessitate elective repair; however, elective repair may be indicated for patients with GERD [1].
- Patients with a symptomatic PEH should undergo repair, especially for acute obstructive symptoms. However, repair of asymptomatic PEH may not always be indicated, taking into account the patient's age and comorbidities. Patients with asymptomatic PEH may be observed and managed expectantly, noting that progression from an asymptomatic to a symptomatic PEH occurs infrequently. The annual probability of developing acute symptoms requiring emergent operation is calculated to be approximately 1% [2–6].

## Operative Management

When the patient meets indication for operative repair of PEH, the surgeon must take into consideration all aspects of perioperative management. These perioperative considerations may include ensuring appropriate equipment is readily available to conduct the operation safely, discussing rapid sequence intubation or gastric decompression with an anesthesia colleague, and maintaining the technical skills necessary for quality outcomes, tracked longitudinally. Before describing the operative technique of robot-assisted laparoscopic (RAL) repair of PEH, it is necessary to detail the operating room setup, equipment, patient positioning, and trocar placement and docking strategies to ensure a safe and effective operation.

## Room Setup

At the time of this writing, one robotic platform is approved for use in the United States (da Vinci® Surgical System, Intuitive Surgical, Sunnyvale, CA), so the following descriptions will all relate to that platform and its various models (S, Si, and Xi). The orientation of the operating table within the operating theater may vary depending on the model and mobility of robotic equipment as well as room size. Assuming a square-shaped operating room, the operating table is located centrally. When using the S or Si models, there are several ways to set up the operating room. The anesthesia equipment and providers can be located at the patient's head and the robotic platform docked in parallel to the bed on either the patient's left (preferred) or right side. Another approach is to turn the operating table 90° from the anesthesia equipment and dock the robotic platform over the patient's head. When using the Xi model, the specific orientation of the operating table and room setup is less critical. With the Xi and its ability to side-dock or parallel dock, the anesthesia equipment and providers can remain at the patient's head, and the robotic platform is docked from the patient's left (preferred) or right side (Fig. 5.1).

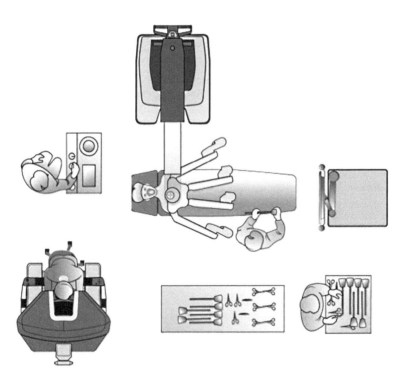

**Fig. 5.1** An operating room setup for robot-assisted laparoscopic paraesophageal hernia repair using a side docking technique. The operating room could be set up similarly when using a parallel docking technique with the robotic platform on the patient's *left side*

The robotic console can be located anywhere in the operating room, but thoughtful consideration should be given to cord management so as to not create a hazardous work environment for those moving about the operating room. One method to ensure a safe walking and working environment is to secure the console cords to the wall or temporarily the floor. The operating surgeon should adjust the robotic console and chair in advance of the procedure to optimize comfort and ergonomics.

When the robotic platform is docked on the patient's left side, the bedside assistant or co-surgeon is most commonly positioned on the patient's right side, where an accessory trocar may be placed to facilitate the operation. The equipment table and surgical scrub technician/nurse are positioned on the patient's right side, near the feet. This position allows the surgical scrub technician/nurse unrestricted access to the bedside assistant or co-surgeon as well as the robotic equipment and tower. Using this room setup, the robotic tower is positioned on the patient's right side near the feet (Fig. 5.1). If ceiling-mounted monitors are available, these should be oriented to allow the surgical scrub technician/nurse and bedside assistant or co-surgeon an unrestricted and preferably in-line view. Additional monitors can be oriented for the staff and/or trainees as needed.

## Patient Positioning

Patient positioning can be made easier when using a specific operating table that allows for bed movement during the operation (TruSystem® 7000dV OR Table Package, TRUMPF Medizin Systeme GmbH & Co, Saalfed, Germany); however, a robot-specific operating table is not required. First, the patient is placed supine on the operating table with the right arm on an armboard and the left arm padded and tucked. This position is used if the robotic platform will be docked on the patient's left side. If the patient is obese or other reasons prohibit tucking the left arm, then the arm can be secured to an armboard with the shoulder abducted. It is important to communicate patient positioning with the anesthesia team, specifically if arms will be tucked, as the anesthesia provider may elect to place additional intravenous access or reposition the blood pressure cuff.

After placement of sequential compression devices, a padded footboard is secured to the bed to prevent the patient from slipping when in reverse Trendelenburg position. Additionally, a strap or tape across the pelvis or upper thigh is used to secure the patient to the bed. Usually, a lower body-warming blanket is used to maintain the patient's temperature during the operation. An orogastric tube to decompress the stomach and a urinary catheter to decompress the bladder may be placed at the discretion of the surgeon. Caution is encouraged knowing that there may be significant difficulty in cases of gastric volvulus. Once the patient is secured to the bed, it is advisable to place the patient in steep reverse Trendelenburg to assure there is no undue pressure on extremities or shifting of patient position before the bed is again leveled and the abdomen prepped. As a routine, flexible upper gastrointestinal endoscopy is performed at the completion of the operation to inspect the fundoplasty. The location of the endoscopy tower must be considered when orienting the equipment in the room as well.

## Trocar Positioning

After the abdomen is prepped from the nipples to the pubis and laterally to the operating table, sterile drapes are secured to the skin. The first 8 mm robotic trocar is located 12–15 cm inferior to the xyphoid and approximately 1–2 cm left of midline, as this location allows for adequate camera distance from the robotic arms but also permits easy visualization high in the mediastinum. A robotic trocar without the obturator is pressed against the skin at this location to mark the site and size of incision. Injection of local anesthetic precedes an 8 mm transverse incision, insertion of a Veress needle, saline drop test, and establishment of pneumoperitoneum to 15 mmHg. When the patient is deemed low risk an 8 mm robotic trocar can be inserted directly; however, in higher risk patients it is advisable to perform trocar placement under laparoscopic visualization. This may necessitate the setup of a 5 mm laparoscope and/or tower.

While robotic trocar positioning is dictated by surgeon and patient factors, there are several generalizable strategies for robotic trocar placement that differ from laparoscopic trocar placement for the repair of PEH (Fig. 5.2). First, robotic trocars should be placed at least 8 cm apart from one another whenever possible to minimize robotic arm collisions. Second, the robotic arms and instruments are often longer than most laparoscopic instruments; so robotic trocars can be placed further from the target anatomy. In fact, if the robotic trocars are placed too close to the target anatomy, it my limit degrees of freedom and impede usability of the robotic instruments. Third, the robotic trocars can be positioned in a more crescent-shaped orientation rather than a staggered "W" orientation, which some surgeons adopt for laparoscopic repair of PEH.

The robotic trocar position most conducive to repair of small and large PEH, fundoplasty, and/or gastropexy is illustrated in Fig. 5.2, which shows a relatively universal location for robotic and accessary trocars for repair of PEH. In addition to the camera trocar, additional 8 mm robotic trocars are placed under direct visualization at the following locations: right upper quadrant (anterior axillary line, 3–4 cm inferior to the costal margin), left upper quadrant (anterior axillary line, 3–4 cm inferior to the costal margin), left flank (mid axillary line, 3–4 cm inferior to the costal margin). All these trocars should be at least 8 cm from one another whenever possible. If needed, an accessory trocar is placed in the right abdomen, between the right upper quadrant trocar and the camera trocar. Most often, this trocar is a 10–12 mm disposable trocar. When available, constant pneumoperitoneum, smoke/steam evacuation, and valve-free access to the peritoneal cavity is possible through a specialized trocar (AirSeal® System, SurgiQuest Inc., Milford, CT) and may minimize loss of pneumoperitoneum that can occur when passing needles or other devices. Lastly, a disposable 5 mm trocar is placed in the hypogastrium to dilate a track for passage of the medium-sized Nathanson liver retractor blade. Once the trocars are liver retractor are placed and secured, respectively, the patient is positioned in steep reverse Trendelenburg.

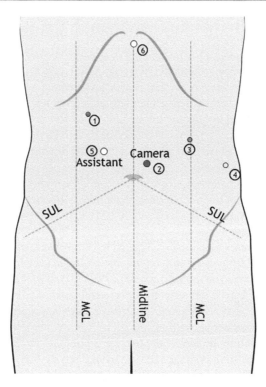

**Fig. 5.2** The typical location of robotic (1, 2, 3, and 4) and accessory trocars for robot-assisted laparoscopic paraesophageal hernia repair. Trocar 1 is used for an atraumatic Cadiere grasper, trocar 2 is meant for the camera, trocar 3 allows passage of the harmonic scalpel, bipolar electro-surgery device, needle driver, or other robotic instruments, and trocar 4 is used for an atraumatic grasper. Trocar 5 serves as an accessory trocar to allow easy passage of suture and hiatal graft/mesh, retraction of tissues, and/or removal of specimens. Trocar 6 is used to dilate a track through the abdominal wall so as to facilitate passage of the Nathanson liver retractor

## Robotic Platform Docking and Instrumentation

The specifics of docking vary depending on the platform (S, Si, or Xi). A complete description of docking for the S/Si and Xi platforms is beyond the scope of this chapter; however, a brief detail of docking the Xi system follows. In advance, the robotic platform is draped (all four arms) and oriented according to the docking location (patient's left, right, etc.) and the operative field (upper abdomen, pelvis, etc.). Once oriented (patient left side, upper abdomen field), the robotic platform is positioned and the arms centered over the camera trocar. At this time (Xi only), the camera trocar is docked (arm 2) and the 30° camera inserted to facilitate automatic reorientation of the remaining robotic arms. Then, all remaining robotic trocars are docked to the platform and instruments inserted, taking care to avoid injury to sur-rounding structures. Various strategies exist to improve mobility of robotic arms in relation to one another depending on the platform; however, it is important to assure before beginning the operation that the robotic arms do not apply pressure to or injury the patient outside of the sterile field.

The instruments preferred for the operation will vary by surgeon preference but with experience the following instruments seem to facilitate the operation by minimizing instrument exchanges. The operation begins with Cadiere grasper placed through the right upper quadrant trocar (arm 1), a Cadiere or fenestrated bowel grasper passed through the left flank trocar (arm 4), and ultrasonic shears placed through the left upper quadrant trocar (arm 3). Alternatively, a bipolar electrosurgery device can be used in place of ultrasonic shears depending on surgeon preference. For suture repair of the PEH with or without fundoplasty, the energy device is exchanged for a robotic needle driver (arm 3). If an accessory trocar is used, sutures can be cut using disposable endoshears, which may be less expensive than the robotic scissors; however, if an accessory trocar is not placed then the robotic scissors can be used to cut sutures.

## Operative Technique

Using the robotic Cadiere graspers (or alternative atraumatic graspers), the stomach and other contents of the PEH are manually reduced, taking care to notice the tension on these structures (Fig. 5.3). In the opinion of the authors, it is critical that surgeons performing RAL PEH repair can safely and effectively evaluate tension on tissues without the use of haptic feedback, a critical part of the learning curve. While dissection may begin on the right or left crus of the diaphragm, herein is detailed the procedure beginning with dissection of the right crus of the diaphragm.

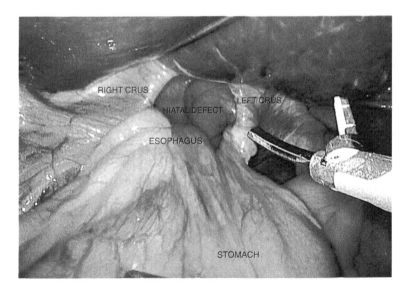

**Fig. 5.3** An initial paraesophageal hernia prior to manual reduction

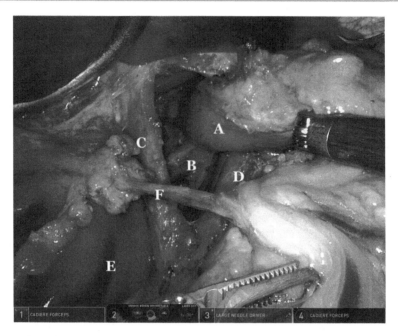

**Fig. 5.4** Retraction of the gastrohepatic ligament with atraumatic Cadiere graspers (arm 1) and division using harmonic shears (arm 3). Both the caudate lobe of the liver and inferior vena cava (IVC) appear posterior to the divided gastrohepatic ligament. A dissected hiatus with normal anatomical variant left intact: (**a**) esophagus; (**b**) posterior mediastinum; (**c**) right crus of diaphragm; (**d**) left crus of diaphragm; (**e**) caudate lobe of liver; (**f**) accessory left hepatic artery

Using an atraumatic grasper (arm 4), the stomach is retracted caudad and to the patient's left, exposing the gastrohepatic ligament. Using ultrasonic shears (arm 3), the gastrohepatic ligament is divided, taking care to avoid injury to the vagus nerve coursing along the lesser curve of the stomach and any variant anatomy (replaced left hepatic vessels). Both the right crus of the diaphragm and the inferior vena cava posterior to the caudate lobe of the liver are identified.

The right crus is gently retracted laterally utilizing a Cadiere grasper (arm 1) allowing for incision of the peritoneal sac by ultrasonic shears (arm 3). When incising the peritoneal sac along the right crus of the diaphragm, it is best to leave the crus covered by its investing peritoneum whenever possible. Dissection moves from posterior to anterior long the right crus, across the phrenoesophageal ligament, until reaching the anterior aspect of the left crus of the diaphragm. Care should be taken to identify and protect anatomical variants whenever possible (Fig. 5.4). The PEH sac is dissected from surrounding tissues using a combination of blunt dissection and ultrasonic shears. Care is taken to identify and protect the posterior vagus nerve during dissection of the right crus of the diaphragm. One way to identify the right/posterior vagus nerve is to find the point near the gastroesophageal junction, where the vagal nerve fibers begin to decussate. Once identified, maintaining a plane of dissection lateral to the right/posterior vagus nerve, specifically keeping the nerve against the esophagus, is a method to avoid injury to this important structure.

Once the right crus of the diaphragm is dissected, the left crus of the diaphragm is dissected taking care to minimize the risk of injury to the spleen or bleeding from the short gastric vessels. To expose the posterior portion of the left crus of the diaphragm, the short gastric vessels are transected using ultrasonic shears. The connective tissue posterior to the fundus often requires transection to allow full exposure of the left crus. Importantly, the posterior aspect of the PEH sac should be incised from the crus and completed reduced from the mediastinum as well as the anterior PEH sac. Identification and protection of the left/anterior vagus nerve is critical during this dissection. Excessive rotation of the esophagus during left sided crural dissection must be avoided to prevent unrecognized injury to the posterior vagus. Ultimately, the decussation of crural fibers posteriorly serve as a landmark to ensure the entire hiatus is dissected, as to allow for adequate closure of the defect with or without reinforcement.

Dissection in the mediastinum posterior to the esophagus is best initiated above the diaphragm if possible so as to avoid esophageal injury; however, initial creation of a retroesophageal window inferior to the diaphragm is performed. Anterior and inferior retraction of the esophagus facilitates dissection of the posterior attachments within the mediastinum. Specific to RAL PEH repair, care must be taken to retract the esophagus by grasping the esophageal fat pad and/or hernia sac, placing an instrument through a retroesophageal window with gentle anterior displacement, and/or utilizing a Penrose drain around the distal esophagus. A robotic instrument (arm 4) passed posterior to the esophagus with gentle anterior retraction of the esophagus facilitates the dissection of the posterior mediastinum without using a Penrose drain.

During esophageal mobilization within the hiatus, feeding vessels from aorta are divided using ultrasonic shears to achieve hemostasis. Areolar tissue may be divided up to the level of the inferior pulmonary vein. Once the hernia sac is completely reduced from the mediastinum and the esophagus mobilized to ensure at least 2–3 cm of intra-abdominal length, with care taken to avoid injury to the parietal pleura and subsequent capnothorax, the hernia sac is divided or excised in part or whole. Care must be exercised to avoid injury to the vagus nerves when removing the esophageal fat pad and hernia sac.

Next, attention is turned to re-approximating the crura (Fig. 5.5). Beginning posteriorly, the left and right crus of the diaphragm are approximated using permanent suture. While there are various methods of crural closure, the method here uses a series of horizontal mattress stitches with nonabsorbable braided polyester suture (0-Ethibond Excel® Suture, Ethicon, Inc., New Brunswick, NJ). Key portions of crural closure include beginning the closure at the most posterior aspect of the hiatus, taking significant bites of muscle (including peritoneum) and approximating tissue without undue tension. When suturing the crura, care should be taken to avoid injury to the caudate lobe of the liver, inferior vena cava, and esophagus.

During closure of the crural defect, the esophagus remains retracted using a robotic instrument (arm 4) and sutures are passed through an accessory trocar (when no accessory trocar is used a robotic instrument must be removed to pass sutures). An experienced bedside assistant or co-surgeon exchanges used for new sutures through an accessory trocar, cuts sutures with disposable endoshears, and facilitates retraction using laparoscopic atraumatic graspers as needed.

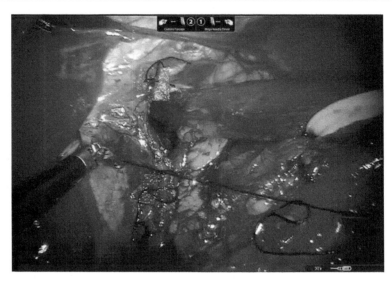

**Fig. 5.5** Posterior reapproximation of the crura of the diaphragm by horizontal mattress stitches using nonabsorbable braided polyester suture. Note the anterior and inferior retraction of the esophagus using an atraumatic grasper (arm 4) placed carefully through the retroesophageal window

In the majority of RAL PEH repairs, a posterior closure of the hiatus is sufficient. At times, a large gap between the crura anterior to the esophagus may be present despite closure of the posterior hiatus. In such situations, closure of the hiatus anterior to the esophagus may be warranted, but care should be taken to avoid injury to the anterior vagus nerve and esophagus. When this is deemed necessary, the defect is approximated using a simple interrupted stitch with nonabsorbable braided polyester suture.

## Adjunct Procedures

Additional maneuvers may be used to decrease tension on the crural closure including relaxing incisions of the diaphragm (partial or complete, right or left) and left capnothorax. These procedures can be performed using the same robotic instruments used for dissection of the hiatus and mediastinum. Moreover, procedures for esophageal lengthening such as wedge fundectomy or Collis gastroplasty can be performed with assistance of the robotic platform. Either a laparoscopic stapler-cutter inserted through an accessory trocar or a robotic stapler-cutter (Si and Xi) inserted through a robotic 12 mm trocar and controlled from the robotic console can be used for wedge fundectomy or Collis gastroplasty. However, with extensive mobilization of the esophagus from surrounding mediastinal tissues, it is the experience of the authors that the need for a formal esophageal lengthening procedure is

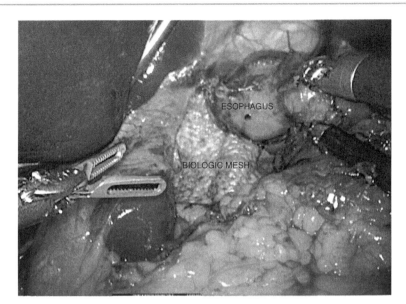

**Fig. 5.6** A U-shaped biologic graft placed for reinforcement of the hiatus after robot-assisted laparoscopic paraesophageal hernia repair and Nissen fundoplasty. The biologic graft can be secured to the hiatus in various ways; in this case, the graft was secured using fibrin sealant

infrequent even for repair of initial giant PEH. In addition, esophageal lengthening procedures may increase the risk of postoperative complications such as dysphagia and staple line leak. When indicated, the robotic platform and robotic stapler facilitates performance of wedge fundectomy over a Bougie as the esophageal lengthening procedure of choice.

Reinforcement of the hiatus with a biologic graft or bioabsorbable synthetic mesh can be performed using the robotic platform (Fig. 5.6). In the opinion of the authors, safe options for fixation of the graft or mesh include suture alone, fibrin sealant/glue alone, or a combination thereof. Robot-assisted retraction of the stomach leaves two hands for operating, so reinforcement of the hiatus can be performed before or after fundoplasty, although the latter is preferred when fibrin sealant/glue is used for fixation. Newer robotic platforms provide for console surgeon-controlled injection of fibrin sealant/glue. It is the practice of the authors to reinforce the crural closure when the defect is large or closure appears to be under some tension, when a relaxing incision of the diaphragm is performed, as well as when patients have giant and/or recurrent PEH. After suture closure of the hiatus, reinforcement is performed using a U-shaped graft of porcine small intestine submucosa (Biodesign® Hiatal Hernia Graft, Cook Medical, Inc., Bloomington, IN) passed through the accessory trocar by a bedside assistant or co-surgeon then secured using 10 mL of fibrin sealant (TISSEEL®, Baxter Healthcare Corp., Deerfield, IL) by directing the malleable dual-cannula applicator (DUPLOTIP Applicator 320, Baxter Healthcare Corp., Deerfield, IL) with robotic Cadiere graspers.

## Nissen Fundoplasty

A partial or complete fundoplasty is employed following the great majority of RAL PEH repairs. This is based on the premise that patients with PEH are at increased risk of gastroesophageal reflux due to an incompetent lower esophageal sphincter (LES). The practice of the authors is to tailor the type of fundoplasty to the patient. In the elective setting, patient history and symptoms, radiologic studies, and most importantly high-resolution esophageal manometry are used to select patients for partial or complete fundoplasty. Of note, current evidence fails to support tailoring the fundoplasty based on high-resolution esophageal manometry. In the emergent setting, a partial fundoplasty (Toupet) is more often employed considering the age and comorbidities of the patient.

The creation of a fundoplasty requires an understanding of the anatomical relationship of the stomach (particularly posterior fundus) to intra-abdominal esophagus. A 360°, floppy Nissen fundoplasty is created around a large esophageal dilator (54–60 French). A fundoplasty is performed after complete closure of the hiatal defect, and when indicated, adjunct procedures and/or reinforcement of the hiatus. There are several published descriptions of how to reproducibly create a floppy Nissen fundoplasty, but the key element of each is to ensure adequate intra-abdominal esophageal length, avoid twisting of the gastric fundus as it passes through the retroesophageal window, and suture the correct parts of the stomach to one another.

The use of a robot-assisted approach does not change any of the critical elements of a reproducible, floppy Nissen fundoplasty. First, the operating surgeon passes a tapered-tip (Maloney) esophageal dilator (54–60 French) down the esophagus. Communication with the bedside assistant or co-surgeon and visualization of the hiatus is important to prevent injury to the esophagus during passage of the esophageal dilator. Next, a Cadiere grasper (arm 4) or a laparoscopic atraumatic bowel grasper passed through the accessory trocar may be used to retract the stomach (or esophageal fat pad if still intact) posteriorly and inferiorly along the axis of the esophagus. Another Cadiere grasper (arm 1) enters from the right upper quadrant and passes posterior to the esophagus through the retroesophageal window. This instrument is used to grasp the posterior aspect of the fundus at a location approximately 6 cm lateral and 6 cm inferior to the angle of His. The posterior aspect of the fundus is pulled from patient left to right through the retroesophageal window and a "shoe-shine" maneuver is performed to ensure the stomach is oriented properly and not twisted. The "shoe-shine" maneuver also permits assessment of any tension on the greater curve of the stomach from the short gastric vessels or omental attachments. The stomach to be used for the fundoplasty is pushed cephalad as needed to ensure that the stomach will be wrapped around the distal esophagus and not below the gastroesophageal junction.

The robotic platform, when using all four arms, permits a stabilization of the fundus near the esophageal hiatus so that the console surgeon has two arms (arms 1 and 3) with which to create the fundoplasty in a tension-free manner. It is important that the console surgeon recognize that undue tension on the stomach may result in injury. Finally, the stomach is sutured to itself as well as the esophagus using three simple interrupted stitches of nonabsorbable braided polyester sutures. This, in turn, creates a short (2.5 cm) floppy Nissen fundoplasty with the suture line at the 10 or

11 o'clock position relative to the esophagus. Additional suturing devices are not required, as the robotic needle driver allows for articulated movement and facilitates intracorporeal suturing and knot tying. Once the fundoplasty is complete, the esophageal dilator is removed carefully to inspect adequacy of the hiatal closure and correct orientation and floppiness of the fundoplasty. Although not the practice of the authors, some surgeons advocate the use of posterior gastropexy in which a nonabsorbable suture is used to secure the posterior aspect of the fundoplasty to the crus of the diaphragm.

## Toupet Fundoplasty

In situations where a partial 270° (Toupet) posterior fundoplasty is preferred, the initial steps are similar to a Nissen fundoplasty. First, the posterior fundus of the stomach is passed through the retroesophageal window as would be done for a Nissen fundoplasty. An esophageal dilator may not be necessary when performing a partial posterior fundoplasty. Second, the superior aspect of the wrapped fundus is secured to the anterior portion of each crus of the diaphragm and the proximal intra-abdominal esophagus. The inferior aspect of the wrapped fundus is sutured to the distal intra-abdominal esophagus only taking care to avoid injury to the vagus nerves. Like the Nissen fundoplasty, the 270° posterior partial fundoplasty is fashioned using simple interrupted stitches with nonabsorbable braided polyester  sutures. In total, approximately four to six stitches are required to create a Toupet fundoplasty of approximately 2.5 cm in length (Fig. 5.7).

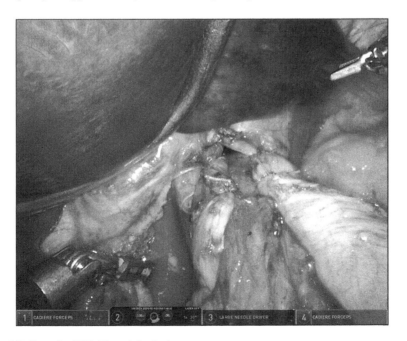

**Fig. 5.7**  Posterior 270° (Toupet) fundoplasty

## Gastropexy/Gastrostomy

Both suture gastropexy and gastrostomy placement are means to anchor the stomach to the anterior abdominal wall. While safe, RAL PEH repair plus suture gastropexy in lieu of an antireflux procedure should be considered in emergent settings where patient condition or clinical situation may preclude fundoplasty. A gastrostomy tube can be placed using a percutaneous endoscopic or robot-assisted approach but should be considered selectively in patients for whom it is necessary to provide both fixation and allow access to the stomach (gastroparesis, head and neck cancer, etc.). It is the opinion of the authors that suture gastropexy and/or gastrostomy are needed infrequently.

## Postoperative Management

Most patients are admitted to a surgical ward (with or without cardiac monitoring), started on a liquid diet, and encouraged to ambulate. Pain is usually minimal and controlled with oral narcotics augmented by intravenous non-narcotic as well as narcotic pain medications as needed. In an effort to minimize nausea and gas bloating in the immediate postoperative period, it is the practice of the authors to schedule non-drowsy antiemetic medication and liquid simethicone during the hospital stay and discharge patients with both medications for home use. By the end of the first postoperative day, most patients are advanced to a full liquid diet and discharged to home with instructions to begin a puree/soft diet for 2 weeks. Patients without evidence of esophagitis on intraoperative upper endoscopy are discharged without proton pump inhibitors, while those with ongoing esophagitis or Barrett's esophagus are discharged with a proton pump inhibitor and instructed to take the medication for 1 month.

## Summary

Experienced surgeons who have overcome their learning curve on the robotic platform can perform robot-assisted laparoscopic paraesophageal hernia repair with fundoplasty safely. The robotic-platform may make transition from open to minimally invasive PEH repair technically less demanding. For surgeons who perform laparoscopic PEH repair, the robotic platform may allow for more stable or better visualization as well as facilitate intracorporeal suturing and knot tying. Depending on the surgeon, the different ergonomics of the robotic console may serve as an advantage. The potential benefits of RAL PEH repair compared to conventional laparoscopic PEH repair is yet unproven [7–9].

# References

1. Kohn GP, Price RR, DeMeester SR, et al. Guidelines for the management of hiatal hernia. Surg Endosc. 2013;27:4409–28.
2. Stylopoulos N, Gazelle GS, Rattner DW. Paraesophageal hernias: operation or observation? Ann Surg. 2002;236:492–500.
3. Allen MS, Trastek VF, Deschamps C, Pairolero PC. Intrathoracic stomach: presentation and results of operation. J Thorac Cardiovasc Surg. 1993;105:253–8.
4. Hallissey MT, Ratliff DA, Temple JG. Paraoesophageal hiatus hernia: surgery for all ages. Ann R Coll Surg Engl. 1992;74:23–5.
5. Pitcher DE, Curet MJ, Martin DT, Vogt DM, Mason J, Zucker KA. Successful laparoscopic repair of paraesophageal hernia. Arch Surg. 1995;130:590–6.
6. Gantert WA, Patti MG, Arcerito M, et al. Laparoscopic repair of paraesophageal hiatal hernias. J Am Coll Surg. 1998;186:428–32.
7. Seetharamaiah R, Romero RJ, Kosanovic R, et al. Robotic repair of giant paraesophageal hernias. JSLS. 2013;17:570–7.
8. Morelli L, Guadagni S, Mariniello MD, et al. Robotic giant hiatal hernia repair: 3 year prospective evaluation and review of the literature. Int J Med Robot. 2015;11:1–7.
9. Falkenback D, Lehane CW, Lord RV. Robot-assisted oesophageal and gastric surgery for benign disease: antireflux operations and Heller's myotomy. ANZ J Surg. 2015;85:113–20.

# Masters Program Hernia Pathway: Robotic Ventral Hernia Repair

Conrad Ballecer, Jarvis Walters, and Brian E. Prebil

## Introduction

Robotic hernia repair is an emerging laparoscopic technique born from well-established principles set by open and conventional laparoscopic technique. Its growing popularity in the United States is often attributed to enhanced 3D visualization, precision, and enhanced surgeon ergonomics. Inherent limitations of conventional "straight-stick" laparoscopy make operating high on the anterior abdominal wall difficult. Overcoming such difficulties may further the adoption of MIS technique.

There is a growing body of literature which promotes keeping mesh out of the intraperitoneal cavity secondary to serosal adhesions and intestinal erosions with intraperitoneal mesh (IPOM) which may complicate subsequent abdominal operations [1, 2]. The robotic platform enables exploitation of the individual layers of the abdominal wall. Virtually, any well-established surgical plane of the abdominal wall can be exploited and dissected for the subsequent placement of mesh in a preperitoneal, retromuscular, and even onlay position, effectively protected from the visceral cavity by the body's own autologous tissue. While this approach has been demonstrated with conventional laparoscopy, it remains technically challenging [3].

C. Ballecer, M.D., F.A.C.S.
Center for Minimally Invasive and Robotic Surgery, Maricopa Integrated Health System, 2601 E Roosevelt St, Phoenix, AZ 85008, USA

J. Walters, D.O.
Department of Surgery, Maricopa Integrated Health System, 2601 E. Roosevelt Street, Phoenix, AZ 85008, USA

B.E. Prebil, D.O. (✉)
Surgery, Arrowhead Hospital, 14155 N. 83rd Ave., Suite 105, Peoria, AZ 85381, USA
e-mail: bprebil@cmirs.com

© Springer International Publishing AG 2018
A.D. Patel, D. Oleynikov (eds.), *The SAGES Manual of Robotic Surgery*,
The SAGES University Masters Program Series, DOI 10.1007/978-3-319-51362-1_6

In this chapter, we introduce the robotic trans-abdominal preperitoneal (rTAPP) approach for hernias of the anterior abdominal wall.

## Surgical Anatomy

A clear understanding of the layers of the abdominal wall is imperative to properly execute this technique. The basic principles of the r-TAPP ventral hernia repair are based on conventional laparoscopic TAPP for inguinal hernias in which (1) the peritoneum is incised and dissected off the transversalis fascia, (2) the hernia sac is reduced, (3) and a mesh is placed within this retroinguinal space. For hernias of the anterior abdominal wall, the peritoneum is dissected from the posterior sheath, the hernia sac is reduced and a large space is opened to accommodate well-overlapping mesh. The size of the preperitoneal mesh is based on the original size of the defect adhering to well-established principles of maintaining at minimum 4–5 cm overlap in all directions.

This approach is best suited for smaller or medium size hernias (<6 cm) that do not require component separation in order to reconstitute the linea alba. It can also be readily adapted to repair hernias in atypical locations such as flank, suprapubic, retrosternal, and subxiphoid defects.

The authors contend three major advantages to placing mesh in a preperitoneal position:

1. Eliminates the requirement for placing costlier coated intraperitoneal mesh (IPOM)
2. The mesh incorporates on both sides, eliminating need for full-thickness transfascial suture fixation which is associated with both acute and chronic postoperative pain [4, 5]
3. Minimizes bowel-associated complications with leaving mesh in an intraperitoneal position, i.e., adhesions and bowel fistula

## Preoperative Considerations

A thorough history and physical is mandatory to formulate and execute an effective preoperative plan. Specifically, certain comorbidities, such as diabetes, obesity, smoking, prior abdominal surgeries including hernia repairs, and prior history of abdominal wall infection may critically affect the operative approach as well as the risk/benefit ratio for surgical intervention versus watchful waiting.

Many primary umbilical hernias detected on physical exam warrant no preoperative further workup. CT scan of the abdomen and pelvis may be ordered for atypical hernias or small to moderate incisional hernias in order to correctly diagnose and delineate the size, position, and content of the hernia defect.

## r-TAPP Hernia Repair for Umbilical or Small Mid-Abdominal Incisional Hernia Repair

### Patient Prep and Positioning

Standard operative protocols are utilized including SQIP antibiotic dosing, body hair clipping, and placement of sequential compression devices. The patient is positioned supine with arms tucked at the sides. In patients with small torsos, it is helpful to position the patient under the kidney rest at the level of the umbilicus (Fig. 6.1). The patient is strapped securely to the bed to allow for Trendelenburg tilting and lateral rotation of the table. After obtaining safe intraperitoneal access, the kidney rest is raised which increases the distance between the costal margin and the anterior superior iliac spine. This allows for port placement with adequate separation. Patient positioning should be finalized prior to docking of the robot. Foley catheterization is not generally required unless the surgeon expects a prolonged case or the hernia defect extends to the lower abdomen.

### Port Positioning, Docking, and Instrumentation

The ports are positioned with the established principles of triangulation similar to conventional laparoscopy (Fig. 6.2). It is important to place the trocars as far from the defect as possible without sacrificing range of motion based on potential collisions with the upper and lower extremities.

As in any minimally invasive surgery, the first step is to gain safe intra-abdominal access which may be difficult in the re-operative abdomen. Sites of previous

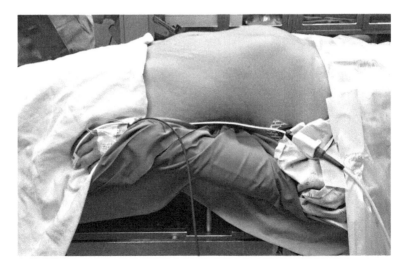

**Fig. 6.1**  Kidney rest positioning

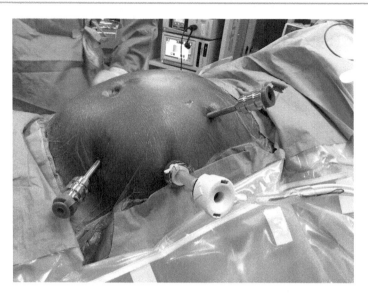

**Fig. 6.2** rTAPP port position

operative intervention will certainly influence the strategy. Optical entry with a 5 mm trocar at Palmer's point with or without initial Veress needle insufflation in the left upper quadrant is generally safe.

A 12 or 8 mm trocar for the camera is placed as far lateral to the ipsilateral edge of the defect. As a general rule, we place the camera trocar a minimum of 15 cm away from the ipsilateral edge of the hernia defect. This allows for visualization, dissection, and instrumentation on the side closest to the ports. An 8 mm robotic trocar is placed in the lower lateral abdomen and the initial 5 mm optical trocar is then replaced with an 8 mm trocar. Final configuration of the trocars for an SI robot is typically in a V configuration (Fig. 6.2). Additional trocars on the contralateral abdomen or an assist trocar is typically unnecessary, but this may vary depending on surgeon comfort.

Following port placement and satisfactory patient positioning, the robot is docked directly over the lateral abdomen and in line with the trocar sites (Fig. 6.3). Instrumentation includes a grasper, monopolar scissors, and a needle driver. A 30° up scope is used to begin the case and may need to be switched to a 0 or 30° down when progressing to the contralateral abdomen.

## Adhesiolysis and Developing a Preperitoneal Plane

As with conventional laparoscopy, the anterior abdominal wall is meticulously cleared of all adhesions to delineate the full extent of the defect as well as uncover any other sites of herniation. Care must be taken to avoid not only injury to intraperitoneal viscera, but also to avoid injury to the peritoneum which may complicate preperitoneal dissection. If bowel manipulation is required, a lower grip strength grasper is utilized to avoid iatrogenic serosal injury.

**Fig. 6.3** rTAPP docking
for midline abdominal wall
hernias

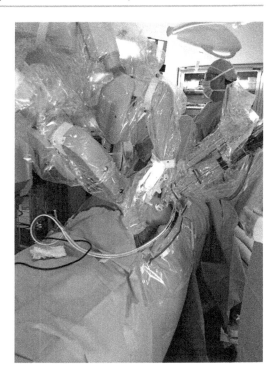

Starting a minimum of 5 cm from the edge of the defect the peritoneum is incised using scissors (Fig. 6.4). This will allow for the placement of mesh with a minimum of 5 cm overlap on the side ipsilateral to the working ports. Ideally, the incision is often made within the visible preperitoneal fat that underlies the rectus muscle. The plane of dissection is more readily entered in this manner without causing disruption of the overlying posterior sheath. The preperitoneal plane is developed widely in a cephalad to caudad direction with a combination of meticulous blunt and sharp dissection. Sweeping with the blunt edge of the scissors is an effective technique to separate the peritoneum from the posterior sheath. Cautery is sparingly applied to avoid thermal injury which may result in peritoneal defects. The hernia sac is reduced and further dissection continues laterally (Fig. 6.5). Wide preperitoneal dissection is performed to allow for the placement of a large mesh based on the original size of the defect (Fig. 6.6). If the preperitoneal space is deemed inaccessible, the procedure may be converted to placement of an intraperitoneal coated mesh subsequent to primary closure of the defect.

## Primary Closure of Defect

After the preperitoneal space is widely dissected, the hernia defect is primarily closed with absorbable suture (Fig. 6.7). In order to minimize operative time, the author prefers to use knotless barbed suture in a running fashion. The subcutaneous tissue situated at the dome of the defect is incorporated within the primary closure.

**Fig. 6.4** Peritoneal incision

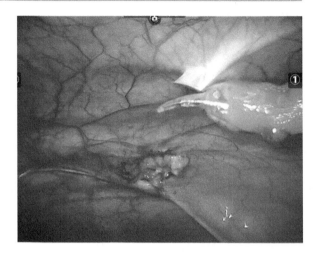

**Fig. 6.5** Reducing the hernia sac

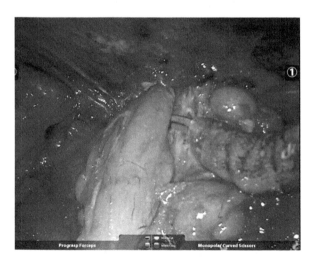

This effectively obliterates the anterior dead space minimizing the risk of seroma formation. Desufflation of the abdominal cavity to a pressure of 6–8 mmHg may facilitate primary closure.

## Mesh Placement, Fixation, and Reperitonealization

An appropriately sized uncoated mesh is introduced into the abdominal cavity via the 8 mm trocar. The mesh is placed flat against the abdominal wall and fixated with either tacks or sutures placed at cardinal points (Fig. 6.8). A minimum of fixation points are used to accomplish flush approximation of mesh against the abdominal wall.

**Fig. 6.6** (a, b)
Preperitoneal dissection

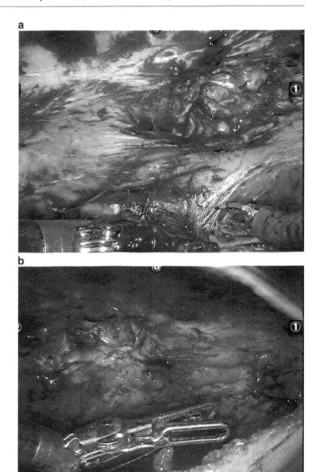

Following adequate fixation, the peritoneum is re-approximated to completely cover the mesh with either running suture or tacks (Fig. 6.9). Peritoneal rents should be repaired to prevent bare mesh exposure to the visceral content. The fascia for all 10 mm or greater trocar sites are closed with absorbable suture under direct vision.

## rTAPP Repair of Atypical Hernias

### Introduction

Atypical hernias such as suprapubic and retrosternal hernias are classically more difficult to repair due to anatomical constraints in dissection as well as limited points of fixation due to bony prominences. Wide preperitoneal dissection is required to gain adequate overlap of reinforcing mesh following defect closure.

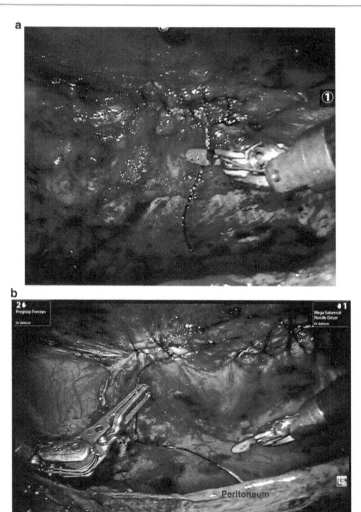

**Fig. 6.7** (**a, b**) Primary defect closure

Suprapubic hernias require wide dissection of the retropubic space, bladder mobilization, and entry into the space of Retzius.

## rTAPP Repair of Suprapubic Hernias

### Patient Positioning, Trocar Placement, and Docking

The repair of suprapubic hernias require a wide dissection of the retropubic and space of Retzius to accommodate an adequately sized mesh which extends well beyond the area of the parietal defect. This may require exposure of the myopectineal orifice bilaterally in order to achieve the minimum 5 cm overlap in all directions.

**Fig. 6.8** (**a, b**) Mesh
placement and fixation

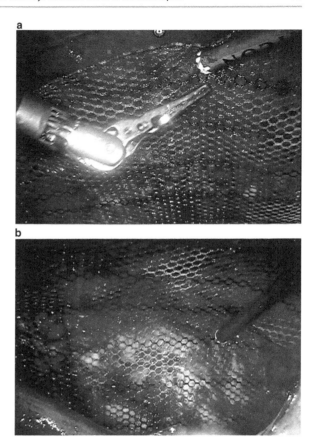

Therefore, a thorough comprehension of the anatomy of these spaces is required to both minimize the risk of iatrogenic injury and to affect a durable repair which minimizes the potential of recurrence.

A three-way Foley is placed to distend the bladder for proper identification. The patient is placed in a supine lithotomy position. The camera port is placed at least 15 cm above the most cephalad aspect of the suprapubic defect. Two instrument ports are placed in line with the camera trocar (Fig. 6.10). The patient is placed in Trendelenburg, and the robot is docked between the legs which enables complete evaluation and dissection of the bilateral retropubic spaces (Fig. 6.11).

**Operative Steps**
A preperitoneal plane is incised a minimum of 5 cm cephalad to the superior aspect of the hernia defect. Dissection is carried laterally to encompass lateral umbilical ligaments in order to accommodate a large sheet of overlapping mesh.

The hernia sac is identified and reduced. The superior dome of the bladder may occupy the hernia sac. Therefore, careful dissection is performed to avoid bladder injury. Instillation of 200–300 mL of saline into the Foley may help facility proper

**Fig. 6.9** (a) Tack
reperitonealization of
mesh. (b) Suture
reperitonealization of mesh

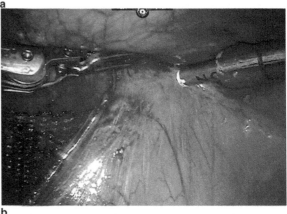

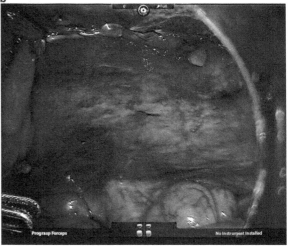

identification of the bladder (Fig. 6.12). The retroinguinal space (space of Bogros) is developed bilaterally to expose Cooper's ligament. Posterior mobilization of the bladder reveals the space of Retzius (Fig. 6.13). This space can be dissected inferiorly to insure adequate overlap of mesh inferior to the caudal aspect of the hernia defect. For larger suprapubic hernias, the bilateral retropubic spaces are exposed (Fig. 6.14).

The hernia defect is primarily closed with a running barbed suture (Fig. 6.15). Partial desufflation of the abdominal cavity may be required to facilitate defect closure. An adequately sized mesh is introduced into the preperitoneal space. Absorbable tacks or sutures are placed to secure the mesh to the abdominal wall. A series of interrupted sutures are used to secure the mesh to Cooper's ligament bilaterally, as well as the symphysis pubis (Fig. 6.16). Upon completion of mesh fixation, the mesh is reperitonealized with running suture or tacks.

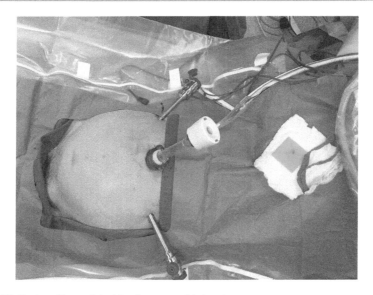

**Fig. 6.10**  Port position and docking for suprapubic hernias

## rTAPP Repair of Morgagni Hernias

### Clinical Anatomy

As the rTAPP approach can be employed for hernias of the lower abdomen, upper abdominal hernias are amenable to the robotic preperitoneal technique. To illustrate this versatility, we describe the rTAPP repair of anterior diaphragmatic hernias such as the hernia of Morgagni.

Morgagni or retrosternal hernias are considered rare forms of congenital diaphragmatic defects located immediately adjacent to the xiphoid process of the sternum. Its hernia content can include omentum, liver, or any portion of the GI tract, all of which must be reduced safely prior to preperitoneal dissection. Patient positioning and operative steps are similar to rTAPP repair of high epigastric and subxiphoid hernias.

### Patient Positioning, Trocar Placement, and Docking

Patient is placed supine with the arms tucked and padded. The camera port can generally be placed at the paraumbilical position assuming the umbilicus is situated at least 15 cm away from the xiphoid process (Fig. 6.17). Two 8 mm instrument trocars are then placed 10 mm apart from the camera port. The patient is placed in a reverse Trendelenburg position, and the robot is docked over the left or the right shoulder which allows for unimpeded access to both the left and right upper quadrants (Fig. 6.18). A 30° up camera is utilized to effectively view the anterior abdominal wall.

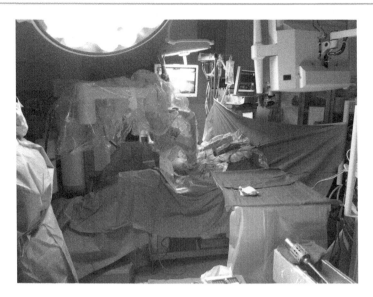

**Fig. 6.11** Docking for suprapubic hernias

**Fig. 6.12** Bladder
distension

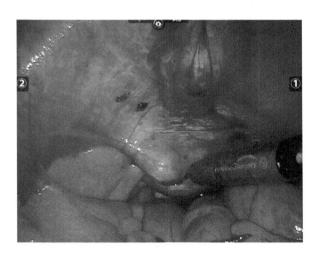

## Operative Steps

As described above, meticulous adhesiolysis is performed to clear the anterior
abdominal wall while avoiding injury to the peritoneum. The hernia content of the
diaphragmatic defect is carefully reduced.

Incision of the peritoneum is performed at least 5 cm caudal to the xiphoid process (Fig. 6.19). Part of the preperitoneal dissection includes mobilizing the falciform ligament off the abdominal wall providing a source for peritoneal tissue for the
eventual reperitonealization of mesh. Once the hernia sac is encountered, it is
reduced completely. Preperitoneal dissection is continued cephalad to the defect
including the central tendon to allow for adequate superior overlap.

**Fig. 6.13**  Space of
Retzius

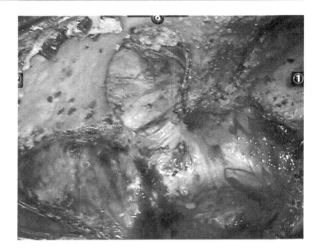

**Fig. 6.14**  (**a**, **b**) Wide
bilateral myopectineal
dissection

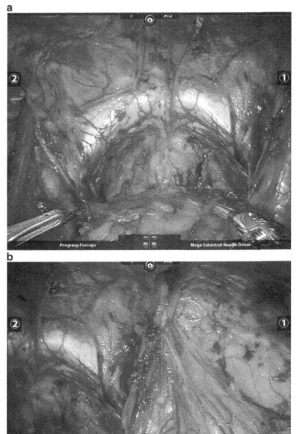

**Fig. 6.15** Primary defect
closure

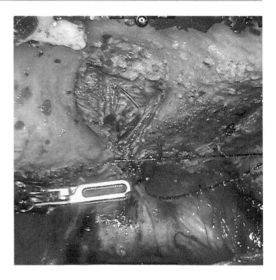

**Fig. 6.16** Mesh placement
and fixation

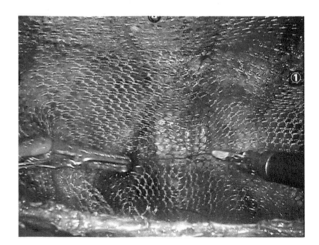

Primary closure of the defect is performed with either running barbed suture or interrupted sutures (Fig. 6.20). Suitable mesh is chosen based upon the size of the original defect. Mesh is placed within the preperitoneal pocket. Either tacks or sutures are employed to secure the mesh to the abdominal wall. Sutures are placed above the level of the costal margin. Subdiaphragmatic sutures are carefully placed at cardinal points for superior fixation of mesh (Fig. 6.21). The mesh is then reperitonealized by reapproximating the peritoneal flap with either suture or tacks.

**Fig. 6.17** Morgagni
hernia port placement

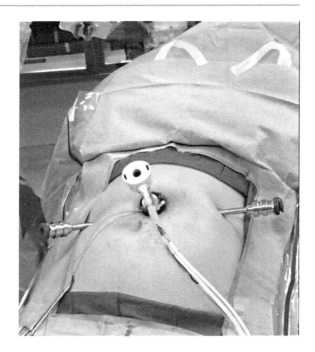

**Fig. 6.18** Morgagni
hernia docking position

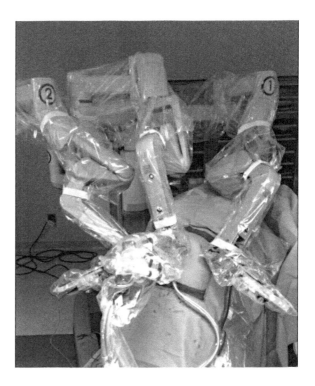

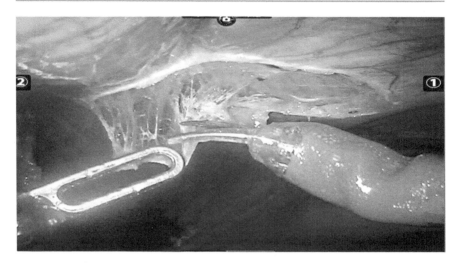

**Fig. 6.19**  Peritoneal incision for Morgagni hernia

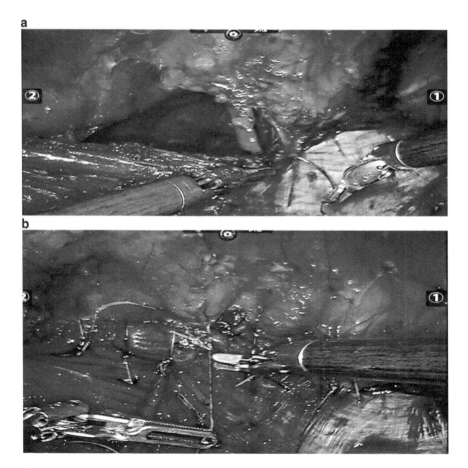

**Fig. 6.20**  (**a**, **b**) Diaphragmatic defect closure

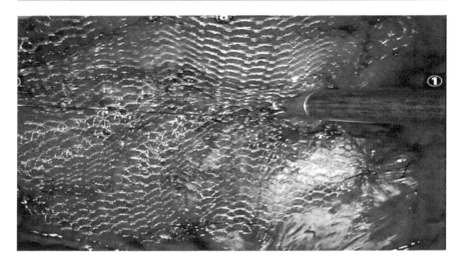

**Fig. 6.21**   Subdiaphragmatic suture fixation

## Conclusion

The rTAPP approach in the repair of abdominal wall and diaphragmatic hernias is reproducible for smaller defects not requiring component separation. Not only is this approach readily reproducible, but it is also versatile. This is evidenced by its effectiveness in the repair of virtually any hernia in any location not requiring myofascial advancement releases.

Potential advantages of the technique include minimizing the risk of mesh exposure to the intraperitoneal content, the ability to use a less expensive uncoated mesh, and potentially decreasing postoperative pain by utilizing less abdominal wall fixation as compared to that of traditional IPOM.

The rTAPP approach should be considered as another viable and reproducible option in the repair of abdominal wall hernias. It is important to note that the dissection of a preperitoneal plane may be inaccessible due to numerous reasons including prior surgical interventions and the requirement of mesh explantation. As in all surgical endeavors, it is important to be well versed in other options and techniques of repair.

## References

1. Halm JA, De Wall LL, Steyerberg EW, Jeekel J, Lange JF. Intraperitoneal polypropylene mesh hernia repair complicates subsequent abdominal surgery. World J Surg. 2007;31:423–9.
2. Gray SH, Vick CC, Graham LA, Finan KR, Neumayer LA, Hawn MT. Risk of complications from enterotomy or unplanned bowel resection during elective hernia repair. Arch Surg. 2008;143:582–6.
3. Prasad P, Tantia O, Patle NM, Khanna S, Sen B. Laparoscopic transabdominal preperitoneal repair of ventral hernia: a step towards physiological repair. Indian J Surg. 2011;73:403–8.

4. Colavita PD, Tsirline VB, Belyansky I, Walters AL, Lincourt AE, Sing RF, Heniford BT. Prospective, long-term comparison of quality of life in laparoscopic versus open ventral hernia repair. Ann Surg. 2012;256:714–22.
5. Liang MK, Clapp M, Li LT, Berger RL, Hicks SC. Patient satisfaction, chronic pain, and functional status following laparoscopic ventral hernia repair. World J Surg. 2013;37:530–7.

# Masters Program Hernia Pathway: Robotic Inguinal Hernia Repair

Sam E. Kirkendall and Sachin S. Kukreja

## Introduction

While guidelines for details regarding laparoscopic transabdominal preperitoneal (TAPP) and totally extraperitoneal (TEP) inguinal hernia repairs are available [1], there is a paucity of research regarding utilization of the robotic platform for repair. Both TAPP and TEP are acceptable treatment options for inguinal hernia repair without appreciable differences in both short- and long-term outcomes. For the robotic platform, the TAPP approach is the preferred method given the space limitations and arm position issues encountered. Many of the recommendations listed below are from the International Endohernia Society (IEHS) guidelines regarding TAPP and personal experience with the robotic approach.

## Preoperative Evaluation

### Selection

If the clinician is unsure whether a hernia exists or an additional contralateral hernia is present, an ultrasound examination with valsalva or a non-contrast CT of the pelvis can be informed. Likewise, a TAPP approach allows for a rapid assessment of the contralateral side. The patient should be counseled preoperatively on the possibility of bilateral hernia repair.

S.E. Kirkendall, M.D.
Department of Surgery, University of Texas Southwestern Medical Center, Dallas, TX, USA

S.S. Kukreja, M.D. (✉)
Department of Surgery, University of Texas Southwestern Medical Center, Dallas, TX, USA

North Texas Veterans Affairs, Dallas, TX, USA
e-mail: kukreja.sachin@gmail.com

© Springer International Publishing AG 2018
A.D. Patel, D. Oleynikov (eds.), *The SAGES Manual of Robotic Surgery*,
The SAGES University Masters Program Series, DOI 10.1007/978-3-319-51362-1_7

For a patient who has had a previous open hernia repair and presents with recurrence, the TAPP approach provides several advantages over a repeat open approach. These include a recurrence rate similar to a primary repair, lower complication rate with less sick leave, and less acute and chronic pain compared with the Lichtenstein repair [2], while allowing an operation through fresh tissue planes. In the event that a plug was previously placed in either the indirect or direct spaces, this may be excised as it can also be a cause of chronic pain in some individuals. In addition, the incidence of wound and mesh infections in the recurrent hernia are lower. For these reasons, a laparoscopic approach for a recurrent hernia is preferable to an open repair [2].

In a patient who has had a previous posterior repair (TAP or TEPP) and presents with a recurrence, approaching the recurrence via TAPP is still an option; however, it should be reserved for surgeons who are very comfortable with the fundamentals of the TAPP repair. Longer operative times and morbidity are associated with this situation; however, in the hands of qualified laparoscopic surgeons, the recurrence rates are comparable to Lichtenstein repair [2]. Though this situation has not been specifically studied utilizing the robotic platform, the improved fine motor skills and wristed instruments may provide an additional advantage over traditional laparoscopic surgery.

In a patient with a previous transabdominal radical prostatectomy, TAPP is an option, though there is a longer operative time with increased morbidity [2]. In these patients, this probably remains the best option in most patients if they have not had a previous anterior approach to an inguinal hernia.

## Contraindications

- Inability to tolerate pneumoperitoneum
- Ascites
- Gross contamination
- Previous lower abdominal surgery (relative)

## Counseling

The patient should be counseled on the risks of the procedure. These are discussed in detail in the complications section later in the chapter.

The patient with a clinically unilateral hernia should be counseled about the possibility of finding a contralateral hernia at time of laparoscopy. An unexpected bilateral hernia is found in 10–25% of patients and 28.6% of these patients will progress to symptoms with a year [2, 3]. If a patient is found to have unexpected bilateral inguinal hernias, both hernias should be fixed.

## Optimization

A patient must be able to undergo general anesthesia and tolerate pneumoperitoneum to have a robotic inguinal hernia repair. If unable to do so due to medical comorbidities, then an anterior, open approach under local anesthetic would be the preferred technique.

## Robotic TAPP

### Positioning

Place the patient supine on the operating table. Tuck both arms.

Prior to docking the robotic arms, place in the patient in 15-degree Trendelenburg. If it is a unilateral hernia, you can tilt the bed 15-degrees away from side of the hernia.

### Perioperative Management

Have the patient void immediately prior to entering the operating room to avoid need for a Foley catheter. Foley can be used alternatively, particularly with patients who may have sliding hernias or advanced age with incomplete voiding. If difficult dissection is anticipated or hernia has a scrotal component, a Foley catheter can be placed. It is important to have a decompressed bladder during the case to avoid the risk of bladder injury. Restricting the peri- and postoperative quantity of intravenous fluids can reduce need for Foley catheter and reduce postoperative urinary retention. Ideally, this would be kept to <500 cc IVF total.

There is no evidence for a difference in surgical site infections (SSIs) between hair removal or no removal. However, there is a higher incidence of SSIs with shaving compared to clipping [2]. Therefore, use clippers if you choose to remove hair at the surgical site.

### Antibiotic Prophylaxis

There is no definitive evidence to recommend routine use of antibiotic prophylaxis [2]. It can be considered when risk factors for mesh infection exist (age > 75, steroid usage, immunosuppressive conditions and therapy, obesity, diabetes, malignancy, long operation time, and urinary catheter).

### Trocar Placement and Docking

Initial entry is made via the umbilicus or periumbilical region. In our practice, the camera port can be placed transumbilical by making a vertical incision within the umbilicus, taking care not to extend the incision below the inferior umbilicus. Then use a blunt clamp to identify the umbilical opening, gain entry into the peritoneum, and enlarge the defect to accommodate the camera trocar. The type of trocar utilized for the camera will vary depending on the robotic platform utilized. We usually use a 12 mm Hassan trocar at the umbilicus to facilitate mesh insertion and dock either the camera through this (Si) or an 8 mm trocar piggyback (Xi). It is possible to simply use an 8 mm in this position on the Xi and insert the mesh through this; however, we find that we often have to enlarge the incision to close the fascia at the end and that the mesh can become quite distorted when inserted through an 8 mm cannula.

Intra-abdominal inspection is first performed after placement of the umbilical camera trocar and insertion of the camera. Two additional trocars will be placed symmetrically on either side of the umbilicus. Position the working trocars 2 cm cephalad to the umbilicus and >10 cm laterally. Avoid placing too far laterally as this will impede suturing at the level of the ASIS as well as flap creation in this area. In patients with a short umbilicus to pubis distance, it may be necessary to place all trocars higher to enable adequate peritoneal flap creation. One pitfall to avoid in creation of the trocar sites is cutting the skin wider than the diameter of the trocar for lateral 8 mm cannulas. Laterally, the incision can be "mapped" by pressing the trocar (without obturator) against the skin and then keeping the incision within this diameter. This cannot be done within the folds of the umbilicus so one must be mindful of making a small incision in this area (Fig. 7.1).

**Fig. 7.1** Port placement

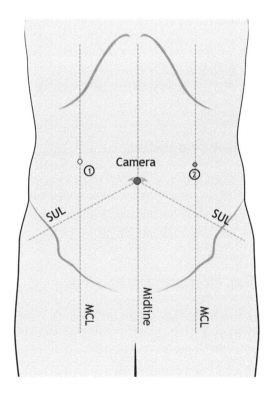

If mesh size and laterality is known at this point, mesh is inserted into the abdomen and placed immediately beneath the camera. For bilateral hernias, it can be helpful to mark the mesh so as to not confuse the two pieces of mesh.

Prior to docking the robot place the patient in 15-degree Trendelenburg position. If using the Si platform, the robot can be brought from the patient's feet and positioned parallel to the bed, particularly if a unilateral hernia is present. Alternatively, the patient can be positioned in a split-leg position and the robot is brought between the legs. Though ideally the robotic platform would be at a right angle to the target pathology, it is acceptable for the robot to be off to the side with arms angled over the patient in this instance (Fig. 7.2).

If using the Xi platform, dock the robot as convenient with room setup.

Place each instrument under direct visualization. We begin the case with a Cadiere grasper in the left port and a scissor with monopolar cautery on the right.

## Opening of Peritoneum

The peritoneal incision is started 4–5 cm above the internal ring. We include the transversalis fascia in the flap thereby exposing the rectus muscle in the midline. This is carried laterally to the ASIS (anterior superior iliac spine) (Fig. 7.3). Take care to avoid injury to the inferior epigastric vessels and dissect bluntly to keep them elevated anteriorly along the rectus muscle.

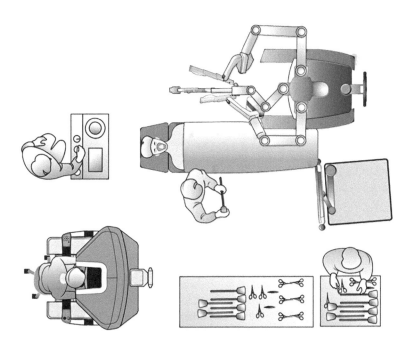

**Fig. 7.2** Si docking in supine position

**Fig. 7.3** Opening of
peritoneum

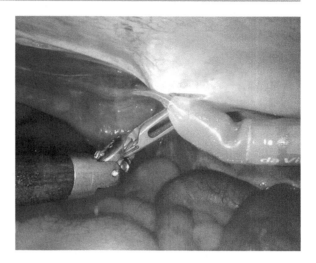

If performing a bilateral hernia repair, we recommend extending the peritoneal incision across the midline to the contralateral ASIS and dissecting out the entire preperitoneal space to provide superior visualization and room. Some surgeons advocate separate peritoneal incisions and dissections as it is felt this makes closure simpler, although, by starting the closure in the midline and moving laterally is not problematic and is at the surgeons' discretion, provided dissection is sufficient to allow for midline mesh overlap. Bringing down the entire preperitoneal flaps facilitates mesh placement in the setting of bilateral inguinal hernias.

## Dissection

It is important to not only get through the peritoneum but through the transversalis fascia as well to dissect in the areolar plane between the transversalis fascia and the transversus abdominus muscle. In up to 20% of patient, the muscle will be fused to the fascia laterally and will have to be separated from the transversalis fascia to maintain the proper plane. For a unilateral hernia, the extent of dissection will be medially 1–2 cm past symphysis pubis to the contralateral side, laterally to the ASIS, and caudally 5 cm below the ileopubic tract. At the medial portion of the dissection, identify the pubis symphysis/pubic tubercle then follow this laterally to Cooper's ligament, which is then followed several centimeters inferolaterally to clear off the overlying tissue.

Be aware of the "corona mortis" in this area, a crossing vein between the iliac vein obturator veins. Leave undisturbed or carefully divide with electrocautery. Unintentional disruption can lead to troublesome bleeding (Fig. 7.4).

Medially, look for direct defects. If present, reduce with traction and electrocautery. Lipomas in this area should be excised. If a large direct hernia defect is present, the transversalis fascia can be imbricated to reduce the incidence of postoperative seroma [2], though this is controversial and may result in nerve entrapment (Fig. 7.5).

**Fig. 7.4** Corona mortis. (Courtesy of James G. Bittner IV, MD)

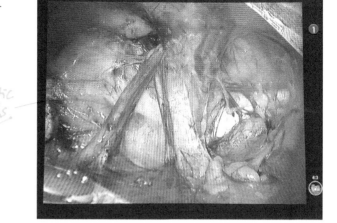

spermatic vessels.

**Fig. 7.5** Reduction of direct defect

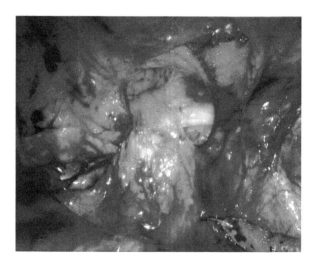

Identify the indirect hernia sac and initiate the dissection laterally. The spermatic vessels and cord structures can be identified in this area and reduced inferiorly. Continue to reduce the indirect hernia sac at the level of the ring with usage of electrocautery as necessary once clear planes have been established to reduce risk of injury to cord structures (Fig. 7.6).

One should be able to get completely around the sac; this should be done to further isolate off the cord structures (Fig. 7.7).

Avoid creating peritoneal defects onto the sac; however, these can be repaired at the conclusion of the dissection with a 3-0 vicryl suture.

In situations where reduction of the hernia sac is difficult, an additional 5 mm port may be placed in the upper abdomen on the patient's right or left depending on the comfort of the bedside assistant. The assistant can apply constant traction to the

**Fig. 7.6** Lateral dissection
with indirect sac dissection

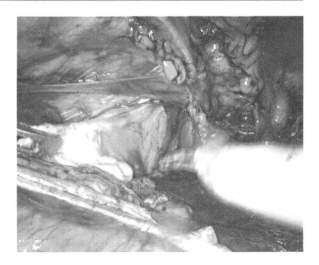

**Fig. 7.7** Indirect sac
reduced

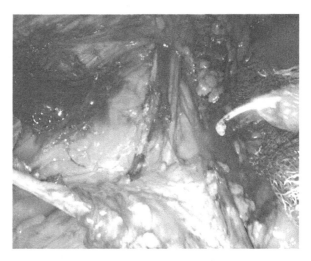

hernia sac while the surgeon works to reduce it off the cord. Complete reduction of the hernia sac is possible in most cases and recommended whenever it is feasible. This does not appear to substantially increase the risk of hematomas or testicular ischemia [2].

In situations where the hernia sac is quite large and redundant, the resulting defect is often quite small. To perform high ligation, it is preferable to establish a window anterior to the cord structures prior to division to ensure their safety. After fully encircling the sac and ensuring that the cord structures are isolated, the sac can be divided at the level of the internal inguinal ring. The distal portion is left open while the proximal portion is ligated. There is a higher risk of a postoperative hydrocele when leaving the distal portion of the sac so complete reduction is recommended when possible but high ligation is a good alternative when necessary.

Other tips include the following: 1. The peritoneal sac should be retracted completely off of the cord structures back to the level of the peritoneum, approximately mid psoas laterally and to the iliacs medially (Fig. 7.7).

2. Cord lipomas should be fully reduced and excised if they are encountered as this can mimic a hernia recurrence postoperatively.

3. Round ligament in females is typically left intact but can be taken if needed. There is some thought that transection increases pelvic floor dysfunction.

Overall, you should define the "critical view" in the setting of laparoscopic inguinal hernia: the peritoneal flap is completely reduced, cooper's ligament is exposed, the direct space has been explored, and the cord or round ligament can be seen entering the internal ring. All lipomas have been reduced as well.

## Mesh

Mesh is typically placed prior to docking into the abdomen to aid in efficiency. It is placed through the midline trocar (usually 12 mm); however, it is possible to slowly advance it through an 8 mm, though this may result in tearing or disfigurement of the mesh. The mesh chosen should be a monofilament, have a pore-size of at least 1.0–1.5 mm, and have a tensile strength of >16 N/cm [2].

Polypropylene mesh (Bard © 3Dmax) is our preference. The shape is helpful with orientation, placement, and to reduce the need for anchoring. Large (10.8 × 16 cm) is generally utilized. X-Large (12.4 × 17 × 3 cm) may be preferable with a large hernia defect or in large patients. Some practices have transitioned to self-gripping polyester mesh for which we have limited experience but feel that it can be safe and may have the benefit of not requiring fixation.

There was previously a tendency by surgeons performing a laparoscopic repair to cut a slit in the mesh to allow cord structures to pass. This may however lead to recurrence and also scarring and pain associated with the cord structures, potentially with testicular ischemia. There does not appear to be any increased adverse occurrences associated with leaving the mesh intact and that is our recommended practice for the robotic platform.

There is ample evidence to support equal recurrence rates comparing fixation vs. non-fixation of mesh with lower incidence of chronic pain after non-fixation. However, non-fixation was frequently performed in hernias <3 cm; therefore, it is recommended to fixate mesh with hernia defects>3 cm [2]. This may be particularly true in the case of direct defects. An advantage to the robotic platform is the ability to place sutures (rather than utilizing a tacking device). We generally place two 3-0 vicryl simple interrupted sutures medially in the rectus muscle and 1 laterally, superior to the ASIS, into the transversus musculature. No sutures or tacks are placed into the midline bony or ligamentous structures. As with the laparoscopic approach, it is imperative to avoid fixation inferior to the iliopubic tract to avoid risks associated with triangle of pain and triangle of doom. Fibrin glue is an acceptable alternative for mesh fixation, which may result in lower chronic pain rates [2].

For unilateral hernias, the mesh should overlap the pubic symphysis on the affected side. For bilateral hernias, the meshes should overlap at midline (Fig. 7.8).

## Peritoneal Closure

Complete closure of the peritoneum is very important. Leaving gaps or defects carries an increased risk of bowel contact with prosthetic mesh material and/or bowel obstruction (Fig. 7.9).

An advantage of the robotic over laparoscopy is the ease of closing with a running suture. Commonly, a laparoscopic closure is performed with tacks which is not only more expensive but could lead to higher levels of postoperative pain if placed in an inappropriate area.

Closure is performed with an absorbable, barbed suture. The suturing is generally easier if performed backhand as this maximizes range of motion. Take the first bite along the inferior lip of peritoneum then the superior portion. Next, run the needle through the looped end of the barbed suture. Then continue suturing backhand in an inferior to superior direction. Every 2–4 throws tighten the suture to eliminate spacing between the peritoneum. Tightening every throw is unnecessary and inefficient.

When a bilateral inguinal hernia repair results in a large peritoneal flap to close, start medially making sure to approximate a similarly oriented medial portion of the inferior and superior peritoneal flaps. A pitfall at this point is approximating the closure too medially or laterally leaving too much or not enough peritoneum at the end of the closure.

**Fig. 7.8** Mesh overlap

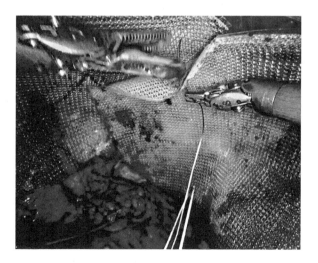

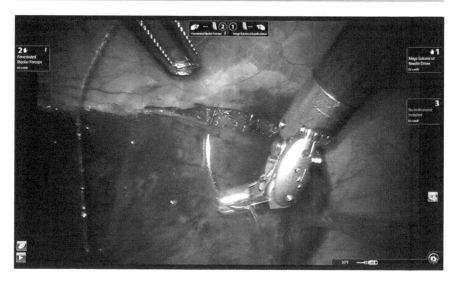

**Fig. 7.9** Closure of peritoneum. (Courtesy of Steven G. Leeds, MD)

If having difficulties with the peritoneal closure, reduce the pneumoperitoneum to 8 mmHg to facilitate closure. Additionally, the superior peritoneal flap can be mobilized further to facilitate closure. It is important to note that the inferior edge of the mesh should not fold up during peritoneal closure. If this happens, either the inferior dissection was inadequate, or the mesh size or position is inappropriate.

## Trocar Closure

It is recommended to close the umbilical incision and any lateral incisions ≥10 mm. The lateral working arms on the robotic platform are 8 mm and do not need to be closed. The skin incisions are closed with a single 4-0 vicryl subcuticular suture and covered with dermabond. For the umbilical wound, a 2 × 2 cm gauze is placed within the umbilical depression and covered with a tegaderm. This is left in place for 1 week. Long-acting local anesthetic can be infiltrated at the trocar sites though definitive evidence regarding its efficacy is lacking and it appears similar to placebo [2].

## Special Cases

### Incarcerated or Strangulated Hernia

Though approaching the incarcerated or strangulated inguinal hernia via a robotic approach is not an absolute contraindication, the surgeon must be experienced and comfortable with the robotic repair of non-incarcerated inguinal hernias prior to undertaking these cases.

In irreducible hernias, prior reduction is NOT mandatory. The preperitoneal dissection can be performed in a similar fashion. This can allow identification of the ring and a relaxing incision to be made as necessary. The hernia ring can be enlarged through a ventromedial incision for direct defects and a ventrolateral incision for indirect defects. Additionally, the bedside assistant can aid in reduction through manual pressure from the outside of the patient through the internal ring or direct space. There are only case series regarding the usage of TAPP for incarcerated femoral hernias though it does appear feasible. Division of the lacunar ligament may be required for reduction of hernia contents.

Compromised bowel noted during a TAPP can be resected at the end of the repair to give the bowel time to declare its viability. This waiting period can lead to a lower incidence of bowel resection. Bowel resection at the time of placing polyester mesh (even if in the preperitoneal space) is controversial and we do not advocate for it at this time. Should a bowel resection be necessary, the hernias can be closed primarily posteriorly, an anterior tissue repair can be undertaken, or a biologic posterior repair can be entertained.

Robotic (or laparoscopic) hernia repairs are more difficult to perform in the setting of peritonitis or frank bowel necrosis. An open approach with tissue repair and laparotomy as necessary for control of intestinal necrosis is prudent.

## Direct Hernias and Large Hernias

There are higher recurrence rates associated with larger defects, particularly direct ones. Therefore, it is recommended that with larger hernia openings (>3–4 cm) a XL (12.4 × 17.3 cm) mesh be used rather than the standard Large (10.8 × 16 cm). If a large direct defect is present, consideration should be given to fixing the mesh medially to pubic symphysis, Cooper's ligament, and rectus muscle. Also, some will close the direct space but this does risk nerve entrapment. In large indirect defects (>4–5 cm), we recommended increasing overlap by 1–3 cm at the ASIS. Fibrin fixation to the psoas can be considered (Fig. 7.10).

Avoid lightweight mesh as it may be pushed into the defect. Ensure careful usage of electrocautery to avoid scrotal hematomas.

## Recurrent Hernia

If the previous hernia repair was via an anterior approach, then the mesh should not interfere with posterior placement, unless a plug was placed during the previous operation. Plug location can be highly variable and even adherent to the iliac vessels and may be best left in place in many situations if it doesn't interfere with placement of your new mesh.

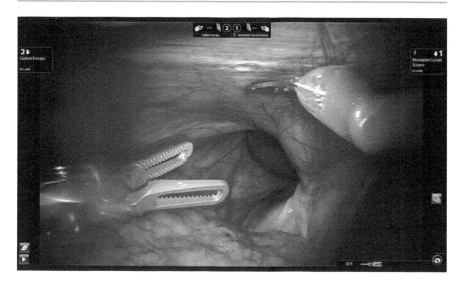

**Fig. 7.10**   Large indirect defect. (Courtesy of Steven G. Leeds, MD)

If the previous hernia repair included a plug that interferes with the posterior mesh lying flat, some authors advocate using electrocautery to cut away the protruding portion down to the level of the internal inguinal ring.

It is possible to perform repeat posterior approaches in a patient who has a recurrence after a minimally invasive repair; however, this should only be attempted by a surgeon with considerable experience (Figs. 7.11 and 7.12).

If the previous hernia repair included a posteriorly placed mesh, it is recommended to leave that mesh in place to avoid injuries to the surrounding structures and rather conform the new mesh to overlay the existing mesh and cover the remaining defect [2].

## Inguinal Hernia Repair with Concurrent Robotic-Assisted Radical Prostatectomy

A significant proportion of patients needing a robotic-assisted radical prostatectomy (RALP) are noted to have an inguinal hernia. There has been concern about situations where a patient is undergoing an RALP and an inguinal hernia is discovered intraoperative, or a patient needing an RALP is noted to have an inguinal hernia during the preoperative evaluation. Concomitant inguinal hernia repair utilizing the robotic platform during RALP is safe and effective and has not been shown to have increased risk of wound infection, fluid collection, or chronic pain [4].

If noted preoperatively or prior to the urologists initiating their dissection, it is helpful to adjust the flap typically created for prostatectomy. Rather than bringing the flap down only to the level of the median umbilical ligaments, the flap needs to be extended laterally past the indirect spaces (4 cm superior) to the ASIS. Typically, port placement for the prostatectomy is also suited for inguinal hernia repair. It is

**Fig. 7.11** Indirect recurrence with posterior mesh in place

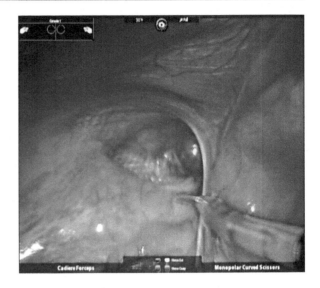

**Fig. 7.12** Exposed posterior mesh in recurrent hernia

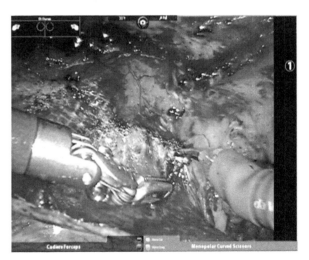

important to obtain consent for hernia repair preoperatively if possible and prudent to ensure a clean urinalysis prior to mesh placement.

The ability to perform a totally extraperitoneal (TEP) robotic inguinal hernia repair at the time of robot-assisted endoscopic extraperitoneal radical prostatectomy (R-EERPE) has been shown to be feasible. These authors performed it through a five trocar setup with a camera at the umbilicus, an assistant arm near the right ASIS, and three robotic arms (one on the right and two left) along an imaginary line drawn between umbilicus and ASIS. They showed similar outcomes to laparoscopic TEP at time of R-EERPE [5]. This method is not extensively described and requires significant expertise and further investigation.

## Postoperative Care

- Foley, if placed, is removed immediately before the patient wakes up.
- All patients are expected to void >250 mL spontaneously prior to discharge.
- They are to expect bruising of the groin and penis (if applicable).
- A folded gauze is placed within the umbilicus depressing the incision and covered with a tegaderm. This is removed by the patient at 1 week.

## Cost Considerations

There are several advantages that the robotic platform allows over pure laparoscopic that can decrease cost below even laparoscopic approaches in some situations.

- Specific instrument selection—minimize the instruments that are opened. For a standard hernia repair, there shouldn't be a need for anything other than a Cadiere or fenestrated bipolar, scissors, and needle driver.
- Do not use a tacker device. If choosing to secure the mesh use 3-0 vicryl (or equivalent) and for peritoneal closure use absorbable barbed suture (V-loc at our institution). In some circumstances, securing the mesh may not be necessary.
- Not using the balloon dissector as commonly used for TEP leads to lower overall costs.
- Robotic TAPP allows for reusable trocars whereas many practices use disposable ones for the laparoscopic approach. A Hassan may still be used at the umbilicus.

## Complications

### Bleeding

At various points during the repair, there are pitfalls that can lead to significant bleeding, made more dramatic by the magnification properties of laparoscopy. It is imperative to recognize these complications and act quickly.

If the disrupted vessel is believed to be a main trunk of the iliac vasculature, an immediate conversion to an open procedure with vascular control and repair is recommended.

If the bleeding is coming from a smaller side-branch vessel, several adjunctive measures can be utilized. First, attempt to get control of the vessel. Reaching a grasper into a bloody pool is rarely successful and often can worsen the situation. Do not hesitate to place on additional trocar for the assistant to utilize a suction irrigator. This additional port should be placed cephalad and between the camera port and the working arm on the side of the bleed.

A gauze sponge can be brought into the abdomen and used to apply pressure to the bleeding area while the trocar is being placed. Use the sponge to mop up old blood once the bleeding is controlled.

Once adequate suction is available, the vessel should be grasped to control the bleeding. If the vessel appears small, electrocautery can be attempted. If the vessel appears larger and can be identified, a robotic clip applier can be utilized to ligate the vessel.

If there is any question or difficulty in controlling, the bleeding do not hesitate to convert to an open procedure.

## Pain

Chronic pain is of particular concern after inguinal hernia repair. Generally, an endoscopic approach will have a lower incidence of acute and chronic pain compared to an open procedure [2]. History of other pain syndromes and preoperative pain are both risk factors for chronic pain syndrome. Other risk factors for chronic pain include recurrence, younger age, and female gender [2]. The risk of chronic, substantial postoperative pain at 1 year can be estimated using the Carolinas Equation for Quality of Life (CeQOL) app available on iPad/iPhone and Android platforms. This predicts postoperative chronic pain risk based on data from the International Hernia Mesh Registry.

## Recurrence

In surgeons with sufficient experience, the risk of recurrence of laparoscopic repair does not exceed that of open repair. The limited data regarding robotic repair suggests similar results. If an early recurrence occurs, an immediate return to the operating room is suggested. Otherwise, an anterior approach should be performed at a later date.

## Bladder Injury

There is a risk of bladder injury, especially in patients who have not been adequately decompressed (which includes voiding immediately preoperatively) or in preoperative fields. If sufficient experience exists, the surgeon can repair this robotically with postoperative bladder drainage. Additionally, methylene blue can be injected for confirmation if bladder injury is suspected but not certain.

## Scrotal Hematomas

These are more common in patients with bleeding disorders. They can generally be prevented by assuring complete hemostasis. Most scrotal hematomas can be treated conservatively with ice, scrotal support, pain management, and observation though some large scrotal hematomas will require evacuation.

## Hydrocele

Postoperative hydroceles are uncommon but can occur. It is important to differentiate a hydrocele from a postoperative seroma which will generally improve with conservative management.

## Orchitis and Testicular Ischemia

The incidence is reported to be low, 0.1%, and this is in a population where the sac is routinely removed despite size. If a very large inguino-scrotal hernia is encountered and excessive dissection is required, then it is recommended to divide the sac at the internal ring, leaving the distal end open.

## Sexual Dysfunction

Inguino-scrotal pain during intercourse and ejaculatory pain occurs in a small percentage of men. The incidence does not appear to be different for laparoscopic vs. open approaches.

## Infertility

In males of reproductive age, bilateral vas deferens injury will lead to infertility. This is prevented with meticulous dissection and careful preservation of cord structures. Unilateral vas deferens injury can lead to secondary infertility from exposure of spermatozoa causing formation of antisperm antibodies [2].

## Other

There are reports of mesh erosion into both the bladder and vas deferens; however, the incidence if low enough that it is relegated to sporadic case reports and possibly due to an unrecognized injury at the time of surgery.

Urinary tract infection is highest in patients who have had a urinary catheter placed. Antibiotic prophylaxis should be considered in patients at higher risk as discussed previously.

## Controversies

Occult contralateral hernias should be fixed if discovered at the time of surgery. If no opening is visible in patients with a strong clinical suspicion of hernia a pre-peritoneal exploration should be performed to rule out other pathologies, especially a cord lipoma [2].

## Conclusion

The utilization of robotic technology for the posterior, minimally invasive approach to inguinal hernias appears safe and effective compared to laparoscopy. The improved ergonomics and articulation associated with the robotic platform may allow surgeons to offer a minimally invasive repair for inguinal hernias instead of the traditional open repair. The platform may also allow surgeons already proficient with minimally invasive techniques to tackle more difficult cases.

## References

1. Bittner R et al. International Endohernia Society. Updates of guidelines of laparoscopic (TAPP) and endoscopic (TEP) treatment of inguinal hernia. Surg Endosc. 2014;29:289–321.
2. Bittner R et al. Guidelines for laparoscopic (TAPP) and endoscopic (TEP) treatment of inguinal hernia. [International Endohernia Society (IEHS)]. Surg Endosc. 2011;25:2773–843.
3. Thumbe VK, Evans DS. To repair or not to repair incidental defects found on laparoscopic repair of groin hernia. Surg Endosc. 2001;15:47–9.
4. Kyle CC, Costello AJ. Outcomes after concurrent inguinal hernia repair and robotic-assisted radical prostatectomy. J Robot Surg. 2010;4:217–20.
5. Qazi HAR, Stolzenburg JU. Robot-assisted laparoscopic total extraperitoneal hernia repair during prostatectomy: technique and initial experience. Cent Eur J Urol. 2015;68:240–4.

Puraj P. Patel and Alfredo M. Carbonell II

## Introduction

The development of robotic transversus abdominis release in hernia surgery is the direct result of a number of contributing efforts, beginning with the well-established open Rives retromuscular hernia repair [1]. This technique established the concept of broad coverage of the hernia defect a layer deep to the anterior fascia. The development of laparoscopic techniques in other areas of general surgery led to the laparoscopic incisional and ventral hernia repair with intraperitoneal mesh placement. It was originally theorized as an evolution of the initial concept of wide coverage, described by Rives [2]. Naturally, with the advent of robotic surgery [3], various new techniques in hernia repair have been successfully demonstrated [4, 5]. Recently, a robotic technique to reproduce every open step of the Rives retromuscular repair has been developed.

The open technique was adapted to the robot and first performed utilizing the da Vinci® system, by Abdalla [6] in 2012. We have developed a modified approach to the original robotic technique described. We are able to perform a retrorectus dissection, with or without the addition of a transversus abdominis release, or posterior component separation. We then suture the posterior rectus sheaths closed in the midline, followed by polypropylene mesh placement in the retrorectus space, and closure of the abdominal wall defect. Compared to open retromuscular incisional hernia repair, the robotic approach is associated with a shorter length of hospital stay and a lower incidence of wound infection [7]. This chapter will detail our approach to patient selection, operative technique of our method of repair, and pearls and common pitfalls with the use of the da Vinci® Si system

P.P. Patel, D.O. • A.M. Carbonell II, D.O., F.A.C.S., F.A.C.O.S. (✉)
Division of Minimal Access and Bariatric Surgery, Greenville Health System,
University of South Carolina School of Medicine-Greenville, 701 Grove Rd,
Greenville, SC 29605, USA
e-mail: acarbonell@ghs.org

© Springer International Publishing AG 2018                          103
A.D. Patel, D. Oleynikov (eds.), *The SAGES Manual of Robotic Surgery*,
The SAGES University Masters Program Series, DOI 10.1007/978-3-319-51362-1_8

(Intuitive Surgical; Sunnyvale, CA, USA). It is crucial that surgeons have a clear understanding and experience performing the open Rives retrorectus repair and TAR before it is attempted robotically.

## Patient Selection

Patients with prohibitive wound risk factors such as smokers, diabetics, and obese patients are well suited for the robotic approach since it mimics an open repair with the wound morbidity of a laparoscopic approach. Although in our experience, defects as wide as 16 cm have been repaired with the robotic approach, generally, defects between 6 and 10 cm are best suited for this approach. Midline defects are best, but lateral defects in the flank and lumbar regions are also amenable and will not require docking the robot twice. Patients with thin abdominal wall musculature are ideal due to their increased abdominal wall elasticity and compliance. These features help with visualization under pneumoperitoneum and allow for simple defect closure.

## Patient Positioning

The patient is positioned supine with the arms out at 90°. The patient's arms are not tucked since this would interfere with the ability to place the ports lateral and also impair movement of the robotic arms. The bed is flexed so the angle between the patient's costal margin and iliac crest is widened (Fig. 8.1). This step allows for a wider area in the lateral abdomen for horizontal port placement.

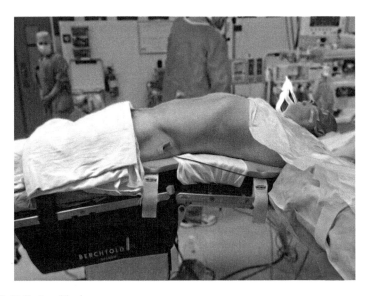

**Fig. 8.1** Patient positioning

## Gaining Access

Intraperitoneal access is gained with a 5 mm optical viewing trocar at the tip of the 11th rib along the right costal margin. Once pneumoperitoneum is established, a 12 × 150 mm balloon tip trocar and 8 mm bariatric length robotic trocar are placed along the lateral right side along the midaxillary line. The initial 5 mm entry trocar is switched to a similar 8 mm bariatric length robotic trocar (Fig. 8.2).

## Lysis of Adhesions

A diagnostic laparoscopy is performed, and a lysis of adhesions is carried out similar to the laparoscopic technique, prior to docking the robot. If an area of around 2–3 cm is clear in front of the robotic trocars, the lysis of adhesions can be carried out with robotic assistance.

## Docking the Robot

The robot is docked with the sidecart perpendicular to the patient bed. The center column is aligned with the patient's anterior superior iliac spine (Figs. 8.3 and 8.4). This allows working room for the assistant at the bedside between the sidecart and the patient's right arm. Adhesiolysis can be completed at this time.

## Left Retrorectus Dissection

The hernia defect is identified (Fig. 8.5) and measured intracorporeally using a ruler.

**Fig. 8.2**  Port placement

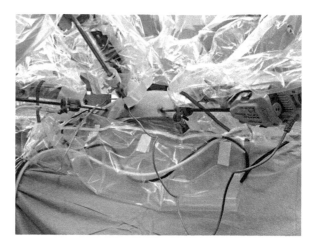

**Fig. 8.3** Initial docking
position

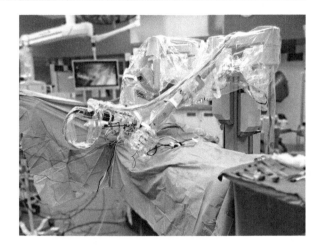

**Fig. 8.4** Docking diagram

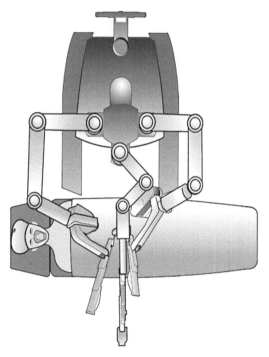

The Rives retromuscular repair commences by incising the posterior rectus sheath vertically, close to the edge of the hernia. The dissection is extended at least 5–7 cm above and below the hernia to allow for sufficient mesh overlap. The retrorectus dissection commences by peeling the posterior rectus sheath away from the posterior aspect of the rectus muscle (Fig. 8.6).

Care is taken to preserve the segmental innervation to the rectus muscle, which enters the retromuscular plane at its most lateral aspect. Identification of these nerves signifies the extent of the lateral dissection.

**Fig. 8.5** Hernia defect

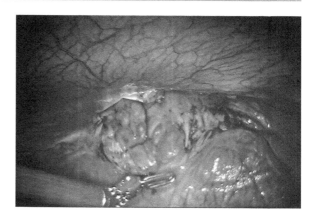

**Fig. 8.6** Left retrorectus dissection. (*A* cut edge of posterior sheath, *B* left rectus muscle, *C* hernia defect)

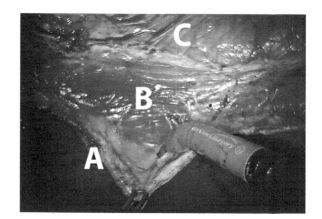

## Left TAR

Once the lateral edge of the rectus sheath is reached, the transversus abdominis muscle is identified below the posterior sheath. The TAR is most easily begun in the upper abdomen, near the costal margin where the transversus abdominis muscle is more robust; however, the TAR can also be initiated in the lower abdomen (Fig. 8.7).

The division of the muscle is the extended inferiorly, where it becomes less muscular and more aponeurotic. This will divide the transversus abdominis muscle along its entire length. It is critical that the line of transection remain medial to the neurovascular bundles. Once the muscle is divided, the pre-transversalis fascia or preperitoneal plane will be exposed. Both the peritoneum and transversalis fascia are visible below the muscle. Lateral dissection can continue in either of these planes. The preperitoneal plane usually separates more easily, but the peritoneum can be extremely thin. The pre-transversalis plane is more difficult to develop but may be necessary if the peritoneum is too thin. A blunt dissection is performed from medial to lateral, peeling the peritoneum or transversalis fascia away from the cut transversus abdominis muscle (Fig. 8.8).

**Fig. 8.7** Beginning the TAR (*A* posterior sheath deflected, *B* left TAR, *C* left rectus muscle anterior)

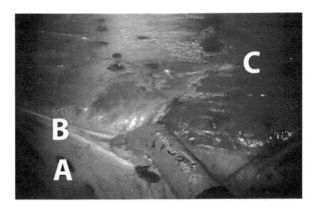

**Fig. 8.8** Developing the TAR (*A* peritoneum, *B* cut edge of left transversus abdominis muscle, *C* left rectus muscle)

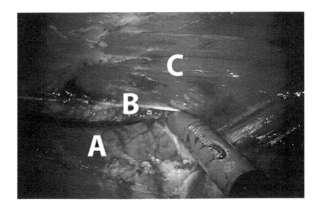

This space is dissected, lateral, until the peritoneal flap with the attached posterior sheath rests easily upon the visceral contents below, with no tension. This will create an extensive medialization of the posterior rectus sheath with peritoneum attached, laterally, for visceral sac closure later in the procedure. Small tears in the peritoneum during this dissection may be unavoidable and can be suture repaired.

## Sizing and Introducing Mesh

Using a similar configuration to the right side, identical trocars are placed into the retrorectus or preperitoneal space on the contralateral or left side of the abdomen (Fig. 8.9).

The dissected plane is measured vertically along the anterior abdominal wall with a ruler, ensuring at least a 5–7 cm overlap above and below the hernia defect. This will be the proposed vertical dimension of the mesh. With the ruler flat against the peritoneal flap, the horizontal measurement extends from the junction of the peritoneum and the muscle (lateral most extent of dissection) to the left medial edge of the hernia defect marked with a spinal needle. Since only one side of the

**Fig. 8.9** Contralateral port placement (*A* cut edge of posterior sheath, *B* preperitoneal space, *C* left rectus muscle)

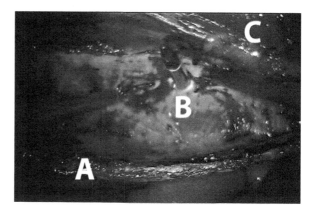

**Fig. 8.10** Mesh positioning

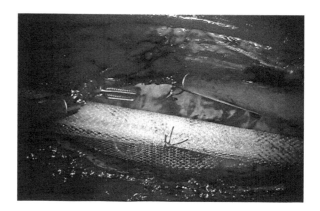

retromuscular and preperitoneal dissection has been performed at this juncture, this horizontal measurement will need to be doubled to actually reflect the horizontal dimension of the mesh.

A wide-pore mid-weight polypropylene mesh is chosen and cut to the measured size. The mesh is rolled along its vertical axis, leaving a 2 cm portion of mesh unrolled. An absorbable suture is placed into the mesh roll to prevent unrolling of the mesh during positioning. The mesh roll is now introduced into the dissected space through the contralateral 12 mm cannula on the left (Fig. 8.10). The mesh is positioned so that the unrolled edge lies under the contralateral cannulae. The edge is secured to the lateral abdominal wall with absorbable suture.

## Redocking and Right Dissection

The robot is undocked from the right side, the patient bed is pivoted to the opposite side, 45°, and the robot is redocked on the left side (Fig. 8.11).

**Fig. 8.11** Redocking
diagram

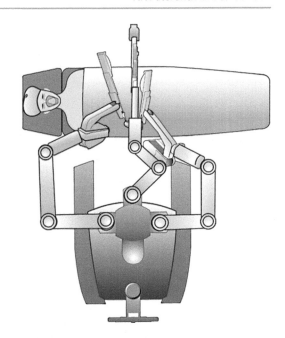

**Fig. 8.12** Right TAR (*A*
posterior sheath deflected,
*B* Right TAR, *C*
neurovascular bundle)

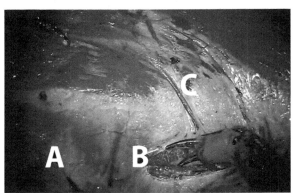

The retrorectus and TAR dissection is repeated on the right side (Fig. 8.12). As
the peritoneal flap is mobilized laterally, the initial (right side) cannulae are repositioned into the preperitoneal space and the flap is further developed until it lies in
contact with the viscera, similar to the left side. The peritoneal defects from the
cannulae are closed with absorbable suture.

## Closing Posterior Sheath and Deployment of Mesh

The posterior rectus sheaths are now suture-approximated in the midline, utilizing a
23 cm, 2-0, absorbable, self-fixating, barbed suture on a GS-22 needle (V-Loc™
180, Covidien, Minneapolis, Minnesota, USA) (Fig. 8.13). At this juncture, the visceral sac is completely closed.

**Fig. 8.13** Closing posterior sheath

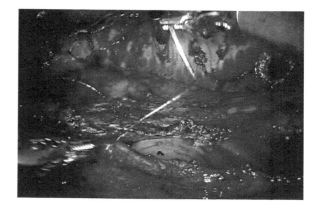

**Fig. 8.14** Deployment of mesh

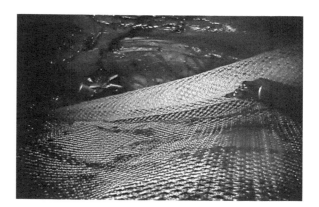

The suture holding the mesh roll is cut and the mesh is unrolled towards the patient's right side (Fig. 8.14). The mesh should lie flat against the closed posterior sheath and occupy the entire retromuscular dissected space. Similar to the left side, the right edge of the mesh is secured to the lateral abdominal wall with absorbable suture. Additional superior and infection fixation of the mesh can be performed, if desired.

## Closing the Anterior Fascial Defect

The anterior rectus sheath and hernia defect are now suture-approximated with a 45 cm, #1, absorbable, self-fixating, barbed suture on a CT-1 needle (Stratafix™ Symmetric PDS™ Plus; Ethicon™, Somerville, New Jersey, United States) (Figs. 8.15 and 8.16).

Decreasing the intra-abdominal pressure to 8–10 mmHg will help to facilitate closure. Should there be excessive tension, the bedside assistant may place two to three figure-of-eight sutures with a suture passer device to bring the defect together, facilitating the running suture closure.

**Fig. 8.15** Closing the
hernia defect

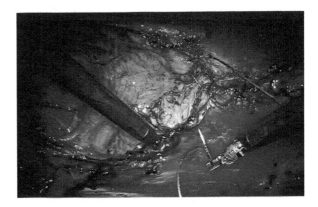

**Fig. 8.16** Final mesh
position

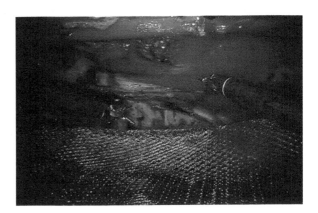

The robot is now undocked, and the laparoscope is inserted to inspect and ensure the mesh is lying flat. The trocars are then removed and the procedure ended. The trocar sites do not require fascial closure since the mesh extends beyond the fascial incisions in the retromuscular plane.

## Conclusion

Currently, the most popular form of robotic ventral hernia repair is a suture closure of the hernia defect with intraperitoneal onlay placement of mesh. We feel that the robotic platform is more effectively used for performing a retromuscular incisional hernia repair as originally described by Rives and Stoppa. Additionally, a posterior component separation technique, or transversus abdominis release (TAR) can be performed if additional release is necessary.

# References

1. Rives J, Pire JC, Flament JB, Convers G. [Treatment of large eventrations (apropos of 133 cases)]. Minerva Chir. 1977;32:749–56.
2. LeBlanc KA, Booth WV. Laparoscopic repair of incisional abdominal hernias using expanded polytetrafluoroethylene: preliminary findings. Surg Laparosc Endosc. 1993;3:39–41.
3. Wilson EB. The evolution of robotic general surgery. Scand J Surg. 2009;98:125–9.
4. Allison N, Tieu K, Snyder B, Pigazzi A, Wilson E. Technical feasibility of robot-assisted ventral hernia repair. World J Surg. 2012;36(2):447–52.
5. Gonzalez AM, Romero RJ, Seetharamaiah R, Gallas M, Lamoureux J, Rabaza JR. Laparoscopic ventral hernia repair with primary closure versus no primary closure of the defect: potential benefits of the robotic technology. Int J Med Robot. 2015;11(2):120–5.
6. Abdalla RZ, Garcia RB, Costa RIDD, de Luca CRP, Abdalla BMZ. [Modified robot assisted Rives/Stoppa videosurgery for midline ventral hernia repair]. Arq Bras Cir Dig. 2012;25(2): 129–32.
7. Warren JA, Cobb WS, Ewing J, Carbonell AM. Prospective, observational, cohort study of robotic Rives-Stoppa retrorectus incisional hernia repair. Hernia. 2015;19(S1):S181.

# Masters Program Bariatric Pathway: Robotic Sleeve Gastrectomy

Dina S. Itum and Sachin S. Kukreja

## Introduction

Sleeve gastrectomy is a partial gastrectomy that was initially performed as the first component of a two-staged bariatric surgery known as biliopancreatic diversion with duodenal switch. It was performed in high-risk bariatric patients and also in super-super-obese (Body Mass Index (BMI) $\geq$ 60) as a risk-reductive measure. However, it was observed that many patients did so well after the first stage (sleeve gastrectomy) that the second stage was unnecessary. Recent data have suggested that stand-alone sleeve gastrectomy has equivalent or in some cases superior outcomes relative to Roux-en-Y Gastric Bypass in the outcomes of weight loss, diabetes remission rates, and improvement in overall obesity-related comorbidities, such as hypertension, obstructive-sleep apnea, and hyperlipidemia [1–4]. A significant improvement in quality of life has also been evident following sleeve gastrectomy [5–8]. In light of these data, sleeve gastrectomy has been performed at increasing frequency in obese patients desiring a weight-reduction surgery and is now the most commonly performed bariatric surgery procedure in the United States.

The American Society for Metabolic and Bariatric Surgery estimates that 99,781 patients underwent a sleeve gastrectomy in 2014. This equates to 51.7% of bariatric operations performed that year. Though laparoscopic sleeve gastrectomy is less

D.S. Itum, M.D.
GI/Endocrine Division, Department of Surgery, UT Southwestern Medical Center, Dallas, TX, USA

Department of Surgery, Dallas VA Medical Center, Dallas, TX, USA
e-mail: DINA.ITUM@phhs.org

S.S. Kukreja, M.D. (✉)
Department of Surgery, University of Texas Southwestern Medical Center, Dallas, TX, USA

North Texas Veterans Affairs, Dallas, TX, USA
e-mail: kukreja.sachin@gmail.com

© Springer International Publishing AG 2018
A.D. Patel, D. Oleynikov (eds.), *The SAGES Manual of Robotic Surgery*,
The SAGES University Masters Program Series, DOI 10.1007/978-3-319-51362-1_9

technically challenging than a Roux-en-Y Gastric Bypass, technical issues often arise as the BMI approaches 50 kg/m² and beyond. These patients have thick abdominal walls (particularly female patients) which may require excessive torque to be placed on the trocars and laparoscopic instruments, thus resulting in tissue trauma, less precise movements, and surgeon fatigue. Additionally, the hepatomegaly, excessive omental fat, and increased difficulty in gaining pneumoperitoneum in super-obese patients decreases intra-abdominal working space and may make fine dissection difficult, particularly in division of the gastrosplenic ligament and obtaining control of the ultra-short gastrics while attempting visualization of the left crus.

However, the unique characteristics of the da Vinci robot may allow surgeons to overcome some of the technical challenges inherent to operating on super-obese patients. The magnified three-dimensional view, adjustable motion scaling, and wristed instruments allow for careful and precise dissection. Furthermore, the robotic arms have enough mechanical power to overcome the torque required to maneuver surgical instruments in patients with large abdominal walls, thus mitigating surgeon fatigue and allowing for fine instrument manipulation within what is often a limited working space.

Several studies have compared the laparoscopic and robotic approaches to sleeve gastrectomy. Bhatia et al. conducted a retrospective study that included 35 patients who underwent robot-assisted sleeve gastrectomy. When comparing patients who were morbidly obese (BMI> 35) and super-morbidly obese (BMI ≥ 50), there was no significant difference in operative time, blood loss, and length of hospital stay between the two groups [9, 10]. Diamantis et al. investigated the difference in operative time and operative time to BMI ratio between the two modalities and found no difference in either measurement. Furthermore, if docking time was excluded from total operative time, the robotic cases were significantly shorter (79.5 min vs. 99.5 min) [10]. In contrast, laparoscopic operative times are significantly longer in super-obese patients compared to the morbidly obese [11, 12]. These findings all suggest that robotic surgery may mitigate the technical challenges encountered in more obese patients during traditional laparoscopic surgery. Additionally, evidence suggests that the robotic sleeve gastrectomy has a less-steep learning curve, as several authors have found that docking time and net operative time decrease significantly if the operating team has completed 10–20 cases [9, 13]. In contrast, the learning curve for laparoscopic sleeve gastrectomy is approximately 30 cases [14].

## Operative Technique

The surgical team typically consists of two surgeons, the console surgeon and the table surgeon or assistant. At teaching institutions, a resident may sit at a second console and control the third robotic arm (R3) or may direct the operation depending on experience. Additionally, the need for a bedside assistant may be minimized by utilization of the robotic stapler. In smaller operating rooms, it may be necessary to re-orient the axis of the bed in order to accommodate all of the equipment, particularly using the Si platform. Once anesthesia is induced, the patient is placed in supine

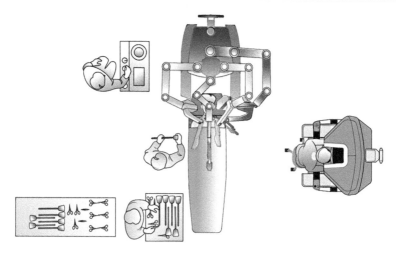

**Fig. 9.1** Schematical operating room arrangements during bariatric operations with the use of the Da Vinci Surgical System

position with his/her legs extended. The patient's right arm is typically extended and offered to the anesthesia team while the left arm is tucked along the patient's side. The robot cart is positioned over the patient's left shoulder (Si platform), as close to the operating room table as possible. With the Xi platform, the robot can alternatively be docked from either side of the patient. Care needs to be taken to provide sufficient clearance for the liver retractor of choice. In our practice, we use a simple toothed grasper from the subxiphoid position to the right crus to retract the left lobe of the liver. In patients with a larger liver, we use a Nathanson retractor with a bedside attachment to secure it to the bed rail. Alternatively, a paddle or snake retractor can be used depending on surgeon preference. The assistant stands on the patient's right side. The scrub nurse stands beside the patient's right leg. The robot monitor is situated across the assistant on the patient's left side (Fig. 9.1).

A nasogastric tube is inserted to decompress the stomach. The patient and the robot are draped in a sterile fashion. Importantly, the patient should be draped without the anesthesia drape barrier so that the robot can be docked from the patient's left shoulder.

Once positioning is complete, an optical entry is obtained into the abdomen at Palmer's Point and the abdomen is insufflated to 15 mm Hg. Alternatively, Veress entry can be utilized as appropriate depending on body habitus and surgeon comfort. All ports are placed after obtaining pneumoperitoneum, as port site placement prior to insufflation may be inaccurate. The camera port is placed 15–20 cm below the xiphoid process and slightly to the left of midline. This port is inserted into the abdominal cavity under direct visualization using a 0-degree, 10-mm laparoscope, after which four subsequent ports are placed, all under direct visualization. We prefer to use the laparoscopic stapler via a 12-mm assistant port instead of the robotic stapler for two reasons. First, the laparoscopic staple cartridges are longer (60 mm vs. 45 mm) and thus fewer staple cartridges are required to complete the operation and the risk of staple line cross-over is reduced. Secondly, we routinely buttress our staple line which is not a feature of the robotic stapler at this time.

A 12-mm working port (R1) is placed along the left-mid-clavicular line, just above the level of the camera port. The port is "double docked" with a robotic port inside in the event that we need to use this port for the laparoscopic stapler to achieve the desired angle on the sleeve, typically as we approach the Angle of His. A second 12-mm working port (R2) is placed along the right mid-clavicular line, several centimeters above the level of R1. Care must be taken to place this port below the liver margin but it is appropriate to move it more lateral toward the anterior axillary line should spacing between trocars be a concern. The angle between the camera port, R1 and R2 should be approximately 120 degrees. A third 12-mm port (R3) is placed along the left anterior axillary line at the level of the camera port (this too can be lateralized to aid in spacing; however, care must be taken to stay about the level of viscera to prevent bowel injury, particularly as this trocar can be obscured from the abdominal view in the reverse Trendelenburg position). A 12-mm assistant port is then placed halfway between the camera port and R2. A 5-mm subxiphoid incision is made to accommodate the liver retractor. Of note, in obese patients with insufflated abdomens, intra-abdominal distance is less than one would expect based on the location of the skin incisions. Thus it is critical that all ports are placed at least 10 cm apart (8 cm on the Xi) in order to prevent the robotic arms from colliding with one another (Fig. 9.2).

When docking, the robot must be positioned such that the angle between the robot column (which is at the patient's left shoulder) and the camera port is at 10°. The target anatomy, the stomach, should fall on the axis between the camera port and the robot column. The patient is placed in reverse Trendelenburg of a minimum of 20°. It is our practice to tilt the patient as much as tolerated such that we can clearly see the hiatus. The camera arm is docked first and a 30° scope is inserted into the abdomen in the 30° down position. Robotic arms 1–3 are aligned parallel to their respective ports, the target anatomy (the stomach) is identified, and the arms are docked. The essential equipment is inserted into the abdomen under direct visualization, which includes either a vessel sealer or ultrasonic shears (to R1), a fenestrated bipolar forcep (to R2) and a Cadiere grasper (to R3). The assistant typically uses an atraumatic grasper to aid in retraction or insertion of sponges or needles as necessary. All instruments are inserted into the abdomen under direct visualization. The surgery begins by first identifying the pylorus. Using the fenestrated bipolar forcep, the console surgeon grasps the greater curvature approximately 5 cm proximal to the pylorus and gently elevates it while applying medial traction. The Crow's foot can be seen penetrating the lesser curvature at this level and serves as a landmark for beginning the dissection. The atraumatic grasper (R3) is used to retract the gastrocolic ligament laterally in order to provide counter traction. We use the ultrasonic shears to divide the gastrocolic ligament at the level of the Crow's foot until the plane of the lesser sac is entered. Entering the correct plane before proceeding ensures that the posterior stomach is not inadvertently injured as the dissection is carried superiorly toward the Angle of His (Fig. 9.3). Care is taken to divide the ligament close to the greater curvature in order to avoid injury to the colon as well

**Fig. 9.2** Port placement. *C* camera port, *1/2/3* ports for robotic arms, *A* assistant port, *N* Nathanson liver retractor, *MCL* = mid-clavicular line, *SUL* spino-umbilical line

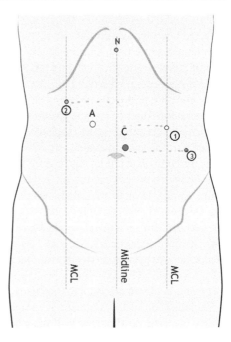

**Fig. 9.3** The lesser sac is entered by elevating the greater curvature and incising the gastrosplenic ligament in close proximity to the stomach. After entering the correct plane, gauze can be packed into the lesser sac to aid with dissection

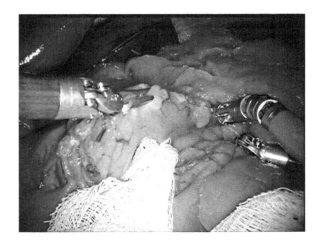

as excessive bleeding from the short gastric vessels. Once the lesser sac is entered, the surgeon can tuck the left grasper into the lesser sac and elevate the stomach in order to improve exposure. Posterior gastric adhesions must be completely divided to prevent inadvertent injury to the pancreas. Cephalad, the greater omentum and redundant gastrocolic ligament, may obstruct the console surgeon's view of the greater curvature. To reduce the impact of these structures, the surgeon can insert a sponge into the abdomen and using R3, pack the sponge into the lesser sac while applying lateral force so that the greater omentum and the gastrocolic ligament are retracted laterally toward the spleen. As the console surgeon continues to mobilize the stomach superiorly, the sponge should similarly be advanced to maintain exposure. If there is excessive omental fat, the assistant can aid with retraction.

As the dissection is carried cephalad, the fundus is mobilized away from the spleen by dividing the gastrosplenic ligament. The dissection should be taken to identify the left crus at the Angle of His and posterior attachments of the fundus need to be cleared. If necessary, dissection of the esophageal fat pad may aid with this mobilization of the fundus. Complete mobilization of the fundus is important for several reasons. First, it helps the surgeon avoid leaving a large sleeve fundus (neo-fundus), which decreases gastric restriction and could result in inadequate post-operative weight loss as well as reflux. Complete mobilization also provides adequate exposure of the gastroesophageal junction so that a staple load is not inadvertently fired across a portion of the esophagus. Lastly, it allows identification of a hiatal hernia should one be present. If a hiatal hernia is identified, it is repaired prior to proceeding with the sleeve gastrectomy in order to prevent trauma to the fresh sleeve staple line during hernia repair. We typically repair these hernias with a posterior horizontal mattress suture of 0-polyester. The hiatus is closed around a 52F bougie.

Mobilization of the stomach is complete once the lesser curvature vessels are visible from the posterior view. If the gastrocolic ligament needs to be divided further in the caudad direction, the Cadiere forcep in R3 is used to retract the greater curvature superiorly while R2 is used to retract the gastrocolic ligament laterally. The ultrasonic shears are used to complete the dissection along the greater curvature of the stomach.

Once mobilization is complete, the anesthetist advances a 40F bougie (Hurst dilator with a blunt tip) into the deflated stomach in order to assist with sleeve calibration. Once the bougie is visualized within the stomach, the surgeon assists with advancement of the bougie toward the pylorus under direct visualization, while ensuring that the bougie rests along the lesser curvature of the stomach. At this time, the assistant introduces a laparoscopic linear cutting stapler in order to fashion the gastric sleeve.

The staple height is determined based on a variety of patient factors, including BMI, gender, and the stomach thickness. The first staple load, typically a buttressed black load, is deployed across the gastric antrum, approximately 5 cm proximal to the pylorus, at a slight horizontal angle. It is our practice to make the sleeve approximately 4 cm wide opposite the incisura to minimize the possibility of distal obstruction, which may predispose the patient to leak or food intolerance. For the majority of patients, our second staple load is also a black cartridge, followed by green loads for the remainder of the stomach. In smaller patients, we may progress to reinforced gold loads as we march up the stomach. As the staples are being fired, the console surgeon should use the Cadiere grasper (R3) to retract the greater curvature laterally in order to prevent the stomach from spiraling. This helps ensure equal resection of the anterior and posterior stomach (Fig. 9.4). To prevent unintentional incorporation of the bougie into the staple line, the assistant should tighten the staple anvils around the target gastric tissue without deploying the stapler. With the staple anvils

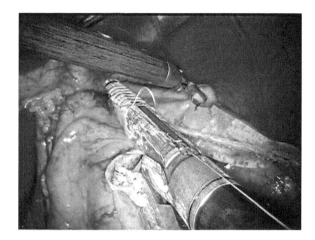

**Fig. 9.4** Lateral retraction of greater curvature helps prevent the stomach from spiraling during the stapling process

tightened, the anesthetist is asked to advance and withdraw the bougie. It is important to not "hug" the bougie in order to prevent over-pulling of the tissue which could yield stapler failure. If the bougie is freely mobile, the assistant surgeon deploys the stapler after a minimum of 15 s of tissue compression. The compression time is added in order to reduce tissue edema and allow the gastric tissue to lay flat within the tissue anvils. The assistant continues transecting the stomach along the lateral edge of the bougie, aiming toward the Angle of His. Some surgeons may opt to use the robot to oversew the staple line. The robot is well suited for this task, although the literature does not clearly delineate a benefit and there is even some literature to suggest a detrimental result. As such, it is our practice to use buttressed staples instead in order to minimize operative time.

At case completion, the gastric reservoir should measure 60–100 mL (or 20% of the initial stomach). The anesthetist fills the sleeve with diluted methylene blue and then with air to order to detect leakage from the staple line and an endoscope can be used to examine the intraluminal staple line in order to identify any bleeding or obstruction. The assistant port is serially dilated using Hagar dilators in sequence from 19 to 26F for stomach extraction. We do not remove the specimen using a bag or wound protection device. We do not routinely place a drain. The fascia is closed with 0-Vicryl suture at the assistant site before closing all skin incisions with a 4-0 Monocryl running subcuticular suture and Dermabond.

## Complications

Though complication rate statistics are not widely available for robotic sleeve gastrectomy, we believe it is safe to extrapolate laparoscopic data for cases completed robotically, as various studies have not found a difference in peri-operative or post-operative morbidity and mortality when comparing the two modalities [9, 10, 15].

For laparoscopic sleeve gastrectomy, there is a 5.2% morbidity rate and a 0.36% mortality rate, with the highest complication rates in super-obese patients, males and in patients older than 55 years [16]. The sleeve gastrectomy is the longest surgical staple line of all bariatric operations and has a reported 0–6% post-operative leak rate following laparoscopic surgery [17–22]. Proximal leaks are more common and catastrophic than distal leaks, presumably because of decreased perfusion at the cardia as well as increased pressure through a narrow low volume gastric conduit. Expert opinion states that the use of smaller bougies (<40 French) is associated with higher leak rates secondary to increased intraluminal pressure within smaller gastric sleeves [23–26]. Similarly, distal strictures are also thought to increase proximal leak rates [24]. Lastly, damage to the gastroesophageal junction during the last staple fire increases the risk of leak because esophageal tissue does not accommodate staples as well as the stomach and thus makes the staples tissue more prone to leakage. While three randomized studies revealed no difference in leak rates between reinforced and non-reinforced staple lines, other studies have shown decreased staple line leak rates when the staple line is reinforced [19, 27–30].

Another significant complication after sleeve gastrectomy is staple line bleeding, which has a reported incidence of 2–4% [30, 31]. Various authors have found that staple line reinforcement reduces the rate of bleeding and subsequent intra-abdominal collections [28, 30, 32–34]. For this reason, consensus panels recommend doing staple-line reinforcement routinely despite its controversial benefit on leak rate [24].

## Conclusion

The operative steps followed to complete a robotic sleeve gastrectomy are very similar to the laparoscopic approach. However, the robot can reduce operative time and technical challenges associated with sleeve gastrectomy, particularly in super-obese patients. The learning curve is shorter than that for laparoscopic sleeve gastrectomy and it allows novice robotic surgeons to improve their technical skills in preparation for more complex bariatric surgeries, such as the Roux-en-Y Gastric Bypass [9, 13, 14]. Though there remains much work to be done in terms of evaluating the efficacy and complications of robotic sleeve gastrectomy, it is a promising technological addition that has the potential to improve the efficacy of weight loss surgery, particularly in certain challenging subpopulations.

## References

1. Leyba JL, Aulestia SN, Llopis SN. Laparoscopic Roux-en-Y gastric bypass versus laparoscopic sleeve gastrectomy for the treatment of morbid obesity: a prospective study of 117 patients. Obes Surg. 2011;21:212–6.
2. Kehagias I, Karamanakos SN, Argentou M, Kalfarentzos F. Randomized clinical trial of laparoscopic Roux-en-Y gastric bypass versus laparoscopic sleeve gastrectomy for the management of patients with BMI < 50 kg/m². Obes Surg. 2011;21:1650–6.
3. Benedix F, Westphal S, Patschke R, et al. Weight loss and changes in salivary ghrelin and adiponectin: comparison between sleeve gastrectomy and Roux-en-Y gastric bypass and gastric banding. Obes Surg. 2011;21:616–24.

4. Karamanakos SN, Vagenas K, Kalfarentzos F, Alexandrides TK. Weight loss, appetite suppression, and changes in fasting and post-prandial ghrelin and peptide-YY levels after Roux-en-Y gastric bypass and sleeve gastrectomy: a prospective, double blind study. Ann Surg. 2008;247:401–7.

5. Alley JB, Fenton SJ, Harnisch MC, Tapper DN, Pfluke JM, Peterson RM. Quality of life after sleeve gastrectomy and adjustable gastric banding. Surg Obes Relat Dis. 2012;8:31–40.

6. D'Hondt M, Vanneste S, Pottel H, Devriendt D, Van Rooy F, Vansteenkiste F. Laparoscopic sleeve gastrectomy as a single-stage procedure for the treatment of morbid obesity and the resulting quality of life, resolution of comorbidities, food tolerance, and 6-year weight loss. Surg Endosc. 2011;25:2498–504.

7. Kafri N, Valfer R, Nativ O, Shiloni E, Hazzan D. Health behavior, food tolerance, and satisfaction after laparoscopic sleeve gastrectomy. Surg Obes Relat Dis. 2011;7:82–8.

8. Schweiger C, Weiss R, Keidar A. Effect of different bariatric operations on food tolerance and quality of eating. Obes Surg. 2010;20:1393–9.

9. Diamantis T, Alexandrou A, Nikiteas N, Giannopoulos A, Papalambros E. Initial experience with robotic sleeve gastrectomy for morbid obesity. Obes Surg. 2011;21(8):1172–9.

10. Bhatia P, Bindal V, Singh R, Gonzalez-Heredia R, Kalhan S, Khetan M, John S. Robot-assisted sleeve gastrectomy in morbidly obese versus super obese patients. JSLS. 2014;18(3)

11. Kakarla VR, Nandipati K, Lalla M, Castro A, Merola S. Are laparoscopic bariatric procedures safe in superobese (BMI $\geq$ 50 kg/m$^2$) patients? an NSQIP data analysis. Surg Obes Relat Dis. 2011;7(4):452–8.

12. Suter M, Calmes JM, Paroz A, Romy S, Giusti V. Results of Roux-en-Y gastriv bypass in morbidly obese vs superobese patients: similar body weight loss, correction of comorbidities, and improvement of quality of life. Arch Surg. 2009;144(4):312–8. discussion 318

13. Vilallonga R, Fort JM, Gonzalez O, Caubet E, Boleko A, Neff KJ, Armengol M. The initial learning curve for robot-assisted sleeve gastrectomy: a surgeon's experience while introducing the Robotic Technology in a Bariatric Surgery Department. Minim Invasive Surg. 2012;2012:347131.

14. Clinical Issues Committee of American Society for Metabolic and Bariatric Surgery. Sleeve gastrectomy as a bariatric procedure. Surg Obes Relat Dis. 2007;3:573–6.

15. Ayloo S, Buchs NC, Addeo P, Bianco FM, Giulianotti PC. Robot-assisted sleeve gastrectomy for super-morbidly obese patients. J Laparoendosc Adv Surg Tech A. 2011;21(4):295–9.

16. Sánchez-Santos R, Masdevall C, Baltasar A, et al. Short- and midterm outcomes of sleeve gastrectomy for morbid obesity: the experience of the Spanish national registry. Obes Surg. 2009;19:1203–10.

17. Ferrer-Marquez M, Belda-Lozano R, Ferrer-Ayza M. Technical controversies in laparoscopic sleeve gastrectomy. Obes Surg. 2012;22:182–7.

18. Burgos AM, Braghetto I, Csendes A, et al. Gastric leak after laparoscopic-sleeve gastrectomy for obesity. Obes Surg. 2009;19:1672–7.

19. Gagner M, Buchwald JN. Comparison of laparoscopic sleeve gastrectomy leak rates in four staple-line reinforcement options: a systematic review. Surg Obes Relat Dis. 2014;10(4):713–23.

20. Chang SH, Stoll CR, Song J, et al. The effectiveness and risks of bariatric surgery: an updated systematic review and meta-analysis, 2003–2012. JAMA Surg. 2014;149:275–87.

21. Banka G, Woodard G, Hernandez-Boussard T, et al. Laparoscopic vs open gastric bypass surgery: differences in patient demographics, safety, and outcomes. Arch Surg. 2012;147:550–6.

22. Aggarwal S, Kini SU, Herron DM. Laparoscopic sleeve gastrectomy for morbid obesity: a review. Surg Obes Relat Dis. 2007;3:189–94.

23. Rosenthal RJ, International Sleeve Gastrectomy Expert Panel, Diaz AA, Arvidsson D, Baker RS, Basso N, Bellanger D, Boza C, El Mourad H, France M, Gagner M, Galvao-Neto M, Higa KD, Himpens J, Hutchinson CM, Jacobs M, Jorgensen JO, Jossart G, Lakdawala M, Nguyen NT, Nocca D, Prager G, Pomp A, Ramos AC, Rosenthal RJ, Shah S, Vix M, Wittgrove A, Zundel N. International Sleeve Gastrectomy Expert Panel Consensus Statement: best practice guidelines based on experience of >12,000 cases. Surg Obes Relat Dis. 2012;8(1):8–19.

24. Gagner M, Deitel M, Erickson AL, Crosby RD. Survey on laparoscopic sleeve gastrectomy (LSG) at the Fourth International Consensus Summit on Sleeve Gastrectomy. Obes Surg. 2013;23(12):2013–7.

25. Aurora AR, Khaitan L, Saber AA. Sleeve gastrectomy and the risk of leak: a systematic analysis of 4,888 patients. Surg Endosc. 2012;26(6):1509–15.
26. Parikh M, Issa R, McCrillis A, Saunders JK, Ude-Welcome A, Gagner M. Surgical strategies that may decrease leak after laparoscopic sleeve gastrectomy: a systematic review and meta-analysis of 9991 cases. Ann Surg. 2013;257(2):231–7.
27. Choi YY, Bae J, Hur KY, Choi D, Kim YJ. Reinforcing the staple line during laparoscopic sleeve gastrectomy: does it have advantages? a meta-analysis. Obes Surg. 2012;22:1206–13.
28. Stamou KM, Menenakos E, Dardamanis D, Arabatzi C, Alevizos L, Albanopoulos K, Leandros E, Zografos G. Prospective comparative study of the efficacy of staple-line reinforcement in laparoscopic sleeve gastrectomy. Surg Endosc. 2011;25:3526–30.
29. Ser KH, Lee WJ, Lee YC, Chen JC, Su YH, Chen SC. Experience in laparoscopic sleeve gastrectomy for morbidly obese Taiwanese: staple-line reinforcement is important for preventing leakage. Surg Endosc. 2010;24:2253–9.
30. Shikora SA, Mahoney CB. Clinical benefit of gastric staple line reinforcement (SLR) in gastrointestinal surgery: a meta-analysis. Obes Surg. 2015;25(7):1133–41.
31. Deitel M, Gagner M, Erickson AL, Crosby RD. Third International Summit: current status of sleeve gastrectomy. Surg Obes Relat Dis. 2011;7(6):749–59.
32. Angrisani L, Lorenzo M, Borrelli V, et al. The use of bovine pericardial strips on linear stapler to reduce extraluminal bleeding during laparoscopic gastric bypass: prospective randomized clinical trial. Obes Surg. 2004;14:1198–202.
33. Consten ECJ, Gagner M, Pomp A, et al. Decreased bleeding after laparoscopic sleeve gastrectomy with or without duodenal switch for morbid obesity using a stapled buttressed absorbable polymer membrane. Obes Surg. 2004;14:1360–6.
34. Nguyen NT, Longoria M, Welbourne S, Sabio A, Wilson SE. Glycolide copolymer staple-line reinforcement reduces staple site bleeding during laparoscopic gastric bypass: a prospective randomized trial. Arch Surg. 2005;140(8):773–8.

Angela A. Guzzetta and Sachin S. Kukreja

## History

Bariatric surgery has its origins in the 1960s when jejunoileal bypass was the operation of choice. High morbidity and mortality rates caused this operation to be abandoned until the more reliable and safe roux-en-y gastric bypass (RYGB) was developed in the 1970s. With the addition of laparoscopy, the RYGB has achieved widespread acceptance as the gold standard for weight loss operations. It offers sustainable and predictable weight loss over 2 years with significant improvement in comorbidities. It has the best long-term data regarding weight loss and resolution of comorbidities making it the standard of care against which all other bariatric surgery procedures are measured.

All that being said, laparoscopic RYGB is extremely challenging to perform well. Of all the minimally invasive general surgery cases being performed today, RYGB is arguably the most difficult, requiring a great deal of skill, training, and dexterity [1]. The learning curve for a RYGB is approximately 75–100 cases [2, 3]. The learning curve refers to the number of major complications, as well as the operative time to perform the case. Expected morbidity and mortality rates are 10% and 0.1% respectively. Since all bariatric cases are closely tracked by insurance companies as well as by surgical societies, overcoming the learning curve prior to graduation from training is essential. With the boom in sleeve gastrectomy, RGYB is occupying a smaller percentage of the bariatric cases being performed nationwide. As a result, trainees

A.A. Guzzetta, M.D.
Minimally Invasive and Bariatric Surgery, Department of Surgery,
University of Texas Southwestern Medical Center, Dallas, TX, USA
e-mail: Angela.Guzzetta@UTSouthwestern.edu; drguzzetta@gmail.com

S.S. Kukreja, M.D. (✉)
Department of Surgery, University of Texas Southwestern Medical Center, Dallas, TX, USA

North Texas Veterans Affairs, Dallas, TX, USA
e-mail: kukreja.sachin@gmail.com

© Springer International Publishing AG 2018
A.D. Patel, D. Oleynikov (eds.), *The SAGES Manual of Robotic Surgery*,
The SAGES University Masters Program Series, DOI 10.1007/978-3-319-51362-1_10

are being exposed to fewer RYGB procedures in training. The number of cases required for certification in bariatric surgery has been dropped by the American Society for Metabolic and Bariatric Surgery from 100 to 50. However, this lowered requirement means that trainees may not be ready to perform this procedure in their own practice without additional training. Robotic surgery offers multiple benefits for RYGB. It decreases the anastomotic leak rate, decreases operative time, decreases overall cost of patient care, and reduces the learning curve by 90%.

## Robotic Roux-en-Y Gastric Bypass

In 2000, the United States Food and Drug Administration approved the da Vinci robotic surgical system (Intuitive Surgical, Inc., Sunnyvale, California). One year later the first robotically assisted RYGB was described [4]. The use of the robot was limited since neither staplers nor advanced thermal devices were available for the robot at that time. In 2005, the first description of totally robotically performed RYGB was published [5]. Since then, diverse experience with the robotic RYGB (RRYGB) has been described. Published results demonstrate faster operations, at a lower cost, with improved outcomes.

## Literature Supporting RRYGB

### Hand-Sewn Gastrojejunostomy

The primary benefit of the robot is in creating a hand-sewn gastrojejunostomy and the result is a decreased leak rate of that anastomosis. All RRYGB reported in the literature do a hand-sewn gastrojejunal anastomosis [5–13]. Most do a two-layer anastomosis but one group does report doing a one-layer anastomosis [1]. One group reported using braided polyester suture as the second layer but stopped the practice when they developed an increased stricture rate [14]. Since then, they have reported excellent outcomes with reduction of their stricture rate to that of reported literature.

The primary advantage of a RRYGB hand-sewn gastrojejunostomy appears to be a decreased leak rate (Table 10.1). Overall, the leak rate is 0.33% as compared to the accepted national rate of 2% during tradition RYGB. This difference may be due to several factors. The increased dexterity that accompanies use of the robot may facilitate in the creation of a more precise anastomosis. Furthermore, the improved visualization may allow for more accurate spacing of stitches.

### Additional Complications

Additional post-operative complications occur at rates similar to that of laparoscopic RYGB. These include major complications such as bleeding, anastomotic stricture, bowel obstruction, marginal ulcers, and pulmonary embolism. Minor

**Table 10.1.** Literature reports of post-operative complications and leak rates

| Study | # Patients | # Complications | # Leaks |
|---|---|---|---|
| Ayloo [9] | 80 | 2.5% | 0 |
| Deng [15] | 100 | NR | 1% |
| Hagan [16] | 143 | 16.1% | 0 |
| Hubens [1] | 45 | 11.1% | 0 |
| Mohr [5] | 75 | 22.6% | 0% |
| Moser [11] | 110 | NR | 0 |
| Myers [7] | 100 | 12% | 1% |
| Parini [12] | 17 | 0 | 0 |
| Park [14] | 105 | 9.5% | 1.9% |
| Sanchez [17] | 25 | 0 | 0 |
| Scozzari [6] | 110 | 9.1% | 1.8% |
| Tieu [8] | 1100 | 4.1% | 0.09% |
| Yu [13] | 100 | 6% | 0 |
| Total | 2110 | 6.2% | 0.33% |

*NR* not reported

post-operative complications include dehydration, edema, dysphagia, kidney insufficiency, nausea, vomiting, infection, rhabdomyolysis, and deep vein thrombosis.

## Operative Times

Increased operating room time has long been an argument against robotic surgery. The time to set up the room, dock the robot, and increased operative time have all been repeatedly used as arguments against robotic surgery. However, in the literature, the findings regarding operative times for RRYGB were mixed. Average robot setup time ranged from 7 to 30 min [1, 6]. Reported times for the RRYGB ranged from 105 to 252 min but overall time was about 177 min [5–7, 18]. In reports that compared robotic and laparoscopic cases, two reports stated that robotic RRYGB took longer, four reported robotic RRYGB were faster, and two reported no statistical difference in mean operative times [1, 5, 10, 14, 17].

Several additional points should be made regarding operative times. First, the cases reported in the literature were largely from immature robotic programs. The operating room staff, the surgeons, and the first assistants were all novices in robotic surgery in the year 2000. At that time, it was not just the surgeon undergoing a learning curve; it was the entire operative team.

Most of the cases documented in the literature from 2000 to 2010 were performed on the original da Vinci S model. This model was notoriously difficult to dock, suffered from a bulky camera, and was burdened by frequent collisions of the operating arms. All of these were improved in the 2009 release of the Si model. One study reported that their operative time decreased by 65 min after purchasing the Si model [8]. It should be noted that all of the aforementioned issues are nearly completely resolved with the 2015 release of the Xi model. The ports neatly click into place, the camera is a lean 8 mm scope, and the new linear design allows working ports to be placed closer together with nearly unlimited mobility of the arms in relation to each other.

## Costs

Robotic surgery may offer two particular cost advantages in RYGB. Because the anastomotic leak rate in RRYGB is far below that of the laparoscopic RYGB, there is a cost-saving by performing the procedure robotically. Anastomotic leaks incur significant medical costs. If the robotic leak rate remains below 2% and the laparoscopic leak rate is at or above 2%, it is cost-effective to use the robot [16]. Furthermore, the advantage of hand-sewn anastomoses furthers the cost-savings. Surgical suture is far less costly than staples. If three staple fires are used in creating the gastric pouch, and all anastomoses are hand-sewn, it is more cost-effective to perform the procedure robotically even when considering the cost of the disposables.

## Learning Curve

The robotic learning curve is another benefit of robotic surgery in bariatrics. RYGB is notorious for its learning curve of 75–100 cases. Because it mimics human hand motions, use of the robot drastically shortens the learning curve. This has been borne out in multiple studies about RRYGB [5]. The learning curve for the RRYGB was approximately ten cases [5, 17]. Indications that the learning curve has been overcome include mortality <1%, conversion to open 1–3%, major morbidity rates <5%, leak rate <2%, operative times <2 h, and robotic operative time being equal to laparoscopic operative time [3, 16, 19–22]. At teaching institutions, the learning curve appears to be the function of the attending surgeon [23]. Once the attending surgeons had overcome their own learning curves, the curves of subsequent trainees were significantly shorter than that of their prior colleague.

## Principals of Robotic Roux-en-Y Gastric Bypass

Below are some principals of the RRYGB. The literature regarding RRYGB is very supportive of the procedure. But there were several cautionary themes repeated among the reports that are mentioned below.

## There Is No Tactile Feedback

The robot is strong and there is no tactile feedback to the surgeon at the console. It will follow the commands of the operating surgeon without regard to strength of grip or tension put on tissues. This is reflected in the literature in several ways. One study attributed their stricture rate to over-tightening of the sutures at the gastroje-junostomy [14]. Another study reported a 10% conversion rate to laparoscopic or open procedures because of jejunal tears [1]. The small bowel has very little toler-ance for excessive force. As a result, we have adopted the habit of running the bowel hand-to-hand instead of hand-over-hand. Bowel is never pulled away. Instead, bowel is maintained in the left hand. The right hand grasps about 10 cm away and brings the distal loop to the left hand. The left hand drops the bowel it is holding and grasps the loop presented by the right hand. The right then goes to grasp another piece of bowel 10 cm away. Bowel is never run hand-over-hand. The time lost in this method is amply made up by not having to repair serosal or full thickness tears.

## The Robotic View Is Magnified

The robotic scope provides magnification that exceeds that of the laparoscope. This presents several challenges. First, the small bowel portion of the case is often fraught with limitations of working space. The addition of magnification can exac-erbate this issue. As a result, there is limited field of view and portions of small bowel can easily be misidentified if they move out of view and have to be retrieved. Marking the Roux limb to prevent Roux-en-O is essential when performing the case robotically [1].

The magnified view can also inhibit accurate measurement of lengths of bowel. We have found that we tend to make our biliopancreatic limb or roux limb too short when running the bowel robotically. We use a marked umbilical tape to accurately measure the distance of both limbs. The magnification must also be considered when performing hand-sewn anastomosis. One study reported an increased stricture rate with RRYGB. They attributed this to their placement of stitches too close together causing ischemia and stricture [14].

## It Is Difficult to Access Angle of His Robotically

The Angle of His poses a particular difficulty in the RRYGB. There are no bariatric length instruments for the da Vinci System. The jejunojejunostomy requires that ports be placed in the midabdomen. The low location of these ports can inhibit reach to the Angle of His. Since this dissection is essential to creating a small pouch and visibility is often limited in this area, the operating surgeon needs to be aware of this difficulty. This has been approached in three different ways. First, additional ports can be placed in the upper abdomen and the robotic arm is redocked during the case. Another approach is to perform the Angle of His dissection laparoscopically prior to docking the robot. Lastly and most commonly in our practice, the cannulas are advanced beyond their established pivot point in the abdomen wall to obtain reach. However this is dealt with, it is a consideration that should be planned for. On the Xi platform, this is rarely an issue.

## A Dedicated Robotic Operating Room Staff Is Essential

The need for operating room staff dedicated to the robot cannot be overemphasized [23]. Room turnaround for the robot has been shown to be longer than that for laparoscopic cases. This time is only lengthened with staff of limited robotic experience. Every instrument for the robot is unique to robotic surgery. In the darkened room, it can be very difficult to distinguish instruments with small tips. Frequently, the scrub nurse is the only assistant at bedside. Having one who has reasonable laparoscopic skills, good robotic knowledge, and excellent scrub skills is essential. As the surgeon is not scrubbed, they cannot directly assist with error messages of the robot. A knowledgeable scrub nurse can troubleshoot the robot without the surgeon having to leave the consul.

## Patient Selection

Patient selection for RYGB is critical to optimal outcomes. The most important factor in choosing a RYGB over other bariatric surgical procedures is patient choice. In most institutions, patients will attend a bariatric surgery seminar where all the surgical options are offered. Patients are encouraged to research these options prior to their initial consultation. When patients come in for their initial consultation, they generally know which operation they prefer. As we tell our patients, this operation is completely elective. They have no surgical issues and can live out their lives without ever having this operation. As such, it is important that they satisfied with their operation of choice. Furthermore, they should be well prepared for their course after surgery.

## Pre-operative Workup

Adequate pre-operative workup is essential to a safe and successful operative and post-operative course. This starts with the first visit. The patient should have a full history and physical examination performed. Patients who are actively smoking are not eligible for a RYGB. Targeted questions should be asked about the patient's cardiac history and health, taking note of their metabolic equivalent of daily tasks. They should be asked about their history of venous thromboembolism and the lower extremities should be examined for venous stasis changes. If they previously have had a venous thromboembolism, pre-operative retrievable inferior vena cava filter can be considered, although this is controversial. Their pulmonary function should be interrogated and the obstructive sleep apnea screening questions should be asked. Any patient with four or more positive answers needs a sleep study to evaluate for sleep apnea. Sleep apnea is a significant risk for sudden post-operative death in the bariatric population. The patient's ability to understand and cope with life changes after bariatric surgery should be evaluated. A patient who claims that their whole life will be better after bariatric surgery should be counseled about limiting expectations.

Pre-operative endoscopic evaluation has been advocated by many. The advantages include delineating gastroesophageal anatomy and obtaining gastric biopsies to determine H. pylori status which may decrease leak rate. The disadvantage is the time and cost to the patient. Others have advocated endoscopy only for patient with gastroesophageal reflux or patients over age 50, or for those who wish to have a sleeve gastrectomy.

## Immediate Pre-operative Care

Pre-operative care begins with a 2-week very low calorie diet. Patients are instructed to take one low carbohydrate, high protein drink for breakfast, one for lunch and a small, protein-rich dinner. This type of diet assists in shrinking the liver, assisting the surgeon, but has also been demonstrated to improve post-operative outcomes [24]. Patients are made NPO to solids and full liquids the night before surgery but are encouraged to drink clear liquids up until 2 h before surgery. This regimen is approved by the American Society of Anesthesiologists and has been shown to reduce patient anxiety and post-operative nausea without increasing complication rates [25].

While in holding, patients receive anticoagulation with either heparin or enoxaparin. An IV is started. For patients with a history of post-operative nausea/vomiting, or motion sickness, scopolamine patch is applied or aprepitant is administered. The patient is given 300 mg of gabapentin. Pre-operative antibiotics of cefazolin or clindamycin are administered as the patient is on the way to the operating room.

## Room Arrangement

The arrangement of the equipment in the operating room is essential when working with the robot. The robotic cart will need to come over the patient's head or left shoulder for the S and Si models (Fig. 10.1) or is side docked by the left shoulder for the Xi model (Fig. 10.2). The patient is supine with the left arm tucked, and the right arm extended. The anesthesia cart is placed to the patient's right. The robotic tower is positioned at the foot of the bed. The bedside surgeon is on the patient's left side. The scrub nurse and the sterile table is on the patient's right side.

## Operative Instruments

Standard and bariatric length laparoscopic instruments should be available. We typically use a fenestrated bipolar grasper and non-traumatic Cadiere grasper, as well as a hook cautery for the majority of the operation. Rarely is a vessel sealer or harmonic scalpel required. A large cutting needle driver is used for all suturing.

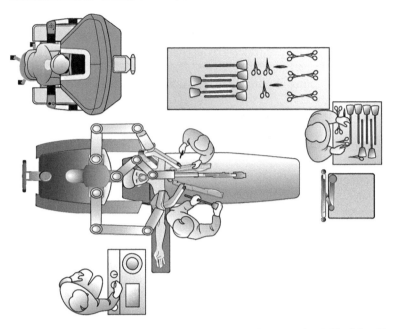

**Fig. 10.1** Operating room layout for robotic roux-en-y gastric bypass with a da Vinci S or Si robot

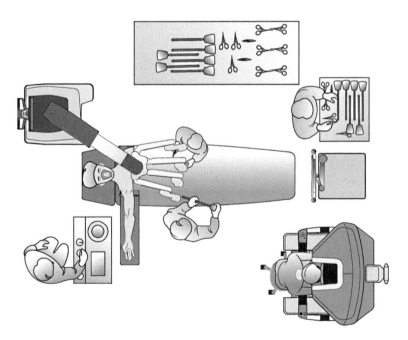

**Fig. 10.2** Operating room layout for a robotic roux-en-y gastric bypass with a da Vinci Xi robot

## Patient Positioning

The patient is positioned supine on a non-slip pad or bean bag. The left arm is tucked. Patient habitus often requires this be performed with a sled or arm board folded down to the side of the bed. The right arm is extended and securely wrapped. A footboard is placed. The legs are strapped in two separate locations to prevent bending at the knee. If desired, an additional strap can be loosely placed across the chest. A forced-air warmer is placed across the chest and arms.

## RYGB

We begin our case with an anesthesiology-performed transversus abdominus plane block. We have found that the majority of the post-operative pain in our patients is secondary to torque on the abdominal wall. Furthermore, all patients receive total intravenous anesthesia. This has significantly reduced our post-operative nausea and vomiting as well as reduced our average post-operative length of stay.

Access is gained using a Veress needle or a direct optical entry. The abdomen is insufflated to 15 mm Hg. If the patient tolerates this, raising the insufflation to 18 mmHg may provide improved visualization. Additional ports are placed. There are two schools of thought regarding this. The first limits the number of ports and favors performing an angle of His dissection laparoscopically immediately after port placement (Fig. 10.3). The second will place an additional port in the left upper quadrant to facilitate this dissection (Fig. 10.4). Figure 10.5 demonstrates port placement for a Xi robot.

After port placement, the bed is placed in reverse Trendelenburg, at a 15–25° angle. The robot is docked. The operation commences with retracting the omentum over the top of the liver until the colon is identified. The epiploicae of the colon are grasped and retracted anteriorly until the mesocolon can be grasped by the assistant and retracted anteriorly. The bowel is run proximally until the Ligament of Treitz is identified. A 50 cm long umbilical tape is used to run the bowel distal to the Ligament of Treitz. The bowel and mesentery are then divided with a linear stapler (robotic or laparoscopic). The distal portion of the divided bowel, the future Roux limb, is marked with a 2–0 silk suture. This prevents Roux-en-O and provides a way to put tension on the small bowel without causing serosal tears. A 75 cm umbilical tape is used to run the bowel for 150 cm.

A full-length 2–0 silk suture is used to approximate the biliopancreatic limb with the future common channel. Two-centimeter enterotomies are made in both limbs and a linear cutter is used to create a common channel. A hand-sewn single-layer jejunojejunostomy is created with an absorbable suture. The mesenteric defect is closed using a nonabsorbable suture. The omentum is divided allowing for a path of an anti-colic Roux limb. The future Roux limb is placed in this divide with the silk suture trailing into the upper abdomen for easy identification.

The operation now shifts to the upper abdomen and a retrogastric tunnel is created. A stapler time out is performed. This is to ensure that the only tube in the

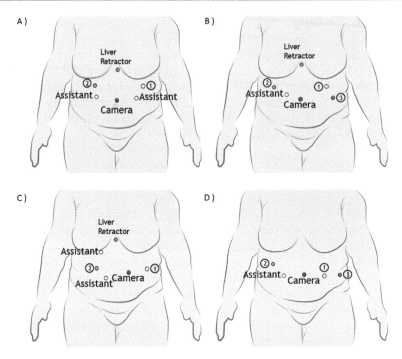

**Fig. 10.3** Port placement for a robotic roux-en-y gastric bypass with a laparoscopic dissection of the Angle of His. (**a**) Moser [4], (**b**) Yu [13], (**c**) Ayaloo [9]—Arm 2 is docked at the left-sided #2 arm for the JJ and moved to the right-sided #2 arm for the GJ, (**d**) Tieu [8]

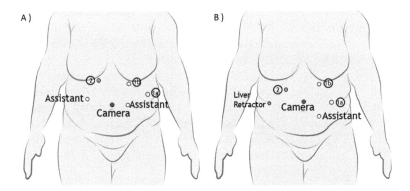

**Fig. 10.4** Port placement for a completely robotic roux-en-y gastric bypass. (**a**) Mohr [5]. Port 1b in the left upper quadrant is an optional addition if unable to reach Angle of His with Port 1a in left mid-abdomen. Arm 1 is redocked between small bowel and foregut portions of the operation. (**b**) Hubens [1]. Arm 1 is redocked between small bowel and foregut portions of the operation from Port 1a to Port 1b

patient's nose or mouth is the endotracheal tube and prevents unintentional incorporation of a nasogastric tube or esophageal temperature probe in the staple line. A stapler and two reloads are used to create a 15–30 mL pouch. A serosa-to-serosa

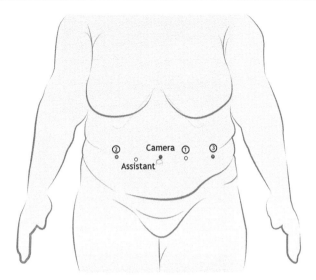

**Fig. 10.5** Port placement for a completely robotic roux-en-y gastric bypass using the da Vinci Xi robot. If stapling laparoscopically, the assistant port is 12 mm. If stapling robotically, Port 2 is a 12 mm port used to pass the stapler. If there is difficulty in reach with Port 1 and 3, the trocars can be advanced further into the patient

running absorbable suture is performed from the Roux limb to the pouch as the second layer of the back wall of the anastomosis (Fig. 10.6). A 20 mm gastrotomy and an enterotomy are created. A hand-sewn gastrojejunostomy is performed in two layers usingabsorbable absorbable suture (Fig. 10.7). A leak test can be performed using a trans-anastomotic orogastric tube with diluted methylene blue and air or standard endoscope.

## Post-operative Care

Post-operative care includes early mobilization, full liquid diet with protein supplementation, multi-modal pain control including narcotics, acetaminophen, ketorolac, and gabapentin. When these are used in combination with the transversus abdominus plane block and total intravenous anesthesia, patients are usually ready for discharge on post-operative day 1.

Patients are called on post-operative day 2. Most bariatric patients who have difficulties will exhibit them in the first 3 days. The vast majority of complaints are due to dehydration and if identified, these patients can be rescued from an emergency room visit by this phone call. Any patient not tolerating liquids is asked to come to the office for intravenous rehydration.

Follow-up visits are scheduled in advance for 2 weeks, 4 weeks, 6 weeks, 3, 6, and 12 months post-op. Following this, visits are scheduled yearly.

**Fig. 10.6** Completion of the outer layer of the back wall of the gastrojejunostomy, approximating the pouch to the small bowel

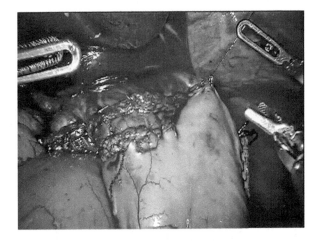

**Fig. 10.7** Final appearance of the two-layer hand-sewn gastrojejunostomy

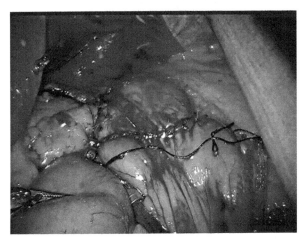

## Revisional Procedures

Revisional bariatric surgery always provides a challenge. Often the original operation was done by another surgeon and navigating the re-operative stomach can be difficult. However, in the era of failed adjustable gastric banding, more bariatric revisions are being done. Revisional surgery is known to be higher risk with a higher overall complication rate and an increased leak rate.

## Literature Supporting Robotic Revisional Bariatric Surgery

Very little data exist regarding robotic revisional bariatric surgery. In general, revision cases take longer than primary bariatric surgery, approximately 3 h [26, 27]. Forty-three patients in the literature underwent robotic bariatric revisional surgery.

Of these, no patients had a leak and morbidity was lower for patient undergoing robotic revisions as compared to open revisions [26]. The authors attributed the low anastomotic leak rate to the hand-sewn anastomosis. Certainly the improved visualization and tissue manipulation provide a significant advantage in revisional procedures. In our experience, taller staplers should be used due to scarring and edema, and there are greater concerns for tissue ischemia. As such, "firefly" technology on the robot may help to confirm tissue perfusion in select circumstances. Our most common revisions using the robot involve conversion of sleeves to bypass, typically in the setting of refractory heartburn. In such circumstances, investigations to rule out missed hiatal hernia are imperative. We do not perform completion gastrectomy on the remainder of the stomach in these patients; however, we do offer routine drainage.

## Pre-operative Evaluation

Pre-operative evaluation for revisional bariatric surgery should begin with all the elements mentioned above for RRYGB. In addition, every effort should be made to delineate the anatomy of the primary bariatric surgery. This includes endoscopy, upper gastrointestinal fluoroscopy, CT scan, and obtaining outside operative reports. All of these will assist in operative planning and improve the chances of a successful procedure.

## Robotic Revisional Bariatric Surgery

### Adjustable Gastric Band to Roux-en-Y Gastric Bypass

The operation is commenced by dividing the band tubing at the peritoneum. The adhesions over the band are divided using cautery until the band buckle is exposed. Newer models of the band can easily be unbuckled by pulling up on the buckle tab. Older models of the band usually need to be incised at the buckle in order to release them. Gentle but firm traction on the band in the direction of the right foot of the patient will allow the band to be removed from around the stomach. The band is then carefully inspected, looking for any black or brown discoloration of the band. If present, this indicates band erosion into the stomach and this must be addressed prior to continuing the operation.

The most difficult portion of the operation is undoing the gastric wrap. In an adjustable gastric banding, a portion of the fundus is sutured to the cardia to keep the band in place and prevent slipping. This is known as the gastric wrap. Most commonly, this is performed using non-absorbable suture material such as braided polyester. This material is rarely visible at the time of reoperation. Instead, the assistant provides lateral traction on the left side of the prior gastric band tunnel. Blunt dissection then reveals the scar plane of the prior wrap. Cold sharp division of this plane is then commenced, always favoring fundus over the cardia. This helps prevent gastrotomies in the new gastric pouch which could be problematic. Conversely, gastrotomies in the fundus of the future remnant stomach are easily repaired. Visualization of sutures along the division plane is confirmatory of being in the correct plane. The wrap is completely undone when the diaphragm is reached. Alternatively, the wrap can be undone using a stapler along the line between the fundus and cardia.

Next the gastric pouch is created. The path of the band determines the difficulty of this task. Most commonly, the angle of His is densely adherent to the diaphragm with capsule of the band in this area. Depending on the path of the band, the lesser sac may contain dense adhesions from the stomach to the retroperitoneum. Care must be taken not to injure the pancreas. A pouch is fashioned in a way that allows the future gastrojejunostomy to be positioned distal to the prior band site. Once the pouch is created, a leak test is performed at this time to determine if any gastrotomies were made during dissection. Only at this point is the small bowel work commenced. In revisions, the stomach portion is usually performed before the small bowel work so as to allow abortion of the case if needed. The remainder of the RRYGB is performed as described above. The decision to leave a drain is at the discretion of the operating surgeon. The case finishes with removal of the port.

## Vertical Banded Gastroplasty to Roux-en-Y Gastric Bypass

Vertical banded gastroplasty (VBG) was popularized in the 1980s, prior to the advent of laparoscopy. There are two components to this operation. First, the stomach was stapled, but not divided, from the incisura to the Angle of His. Then, a band was placed around the stomach at the inferior portion of this new pouch. The band was usually silastic or mesh.

Silastic bands can be identified on CT scan and are easily removed at the time of surgery. Mesh provides a greater challenge. Because of intense inflammatory reaction, removing the mesh from around the stomach can be difficult. Often the mesh is ingrained such that removing it requires stripping the serosa of the stomach. An alternate method of approaching the VBG with mesh is to place a stent in the area. The stent acts to erode the mesh through the stomach over the course of several weeks. After this, the mesh and the stent can be retrieved endoscopically prior to surgery. This circumvents the challenging dissection and presents the surgeon with an untraumatized stomach in the location of the future gastrojejunostomy.

The operation usually begins with an extensive lysis of adhesions to reach the stomach as most procedures were performed as open operations. Then, the anatomy of the prior operation is explored. Frequently, intraoperative endoscopy is useful to identify the location of the staple line and the band. The band is removed and a bougie is introduced to create the pouch. The pouch must be smaller in width than the previous VBG. The staple line on the remnant stomach is then excised to prevent necrosis of the stomach between the new pouch staple line and the old pouch staple line. Firefly on the robot can be used to assess tissue perfusion. In the event that the lesser sac cannot be entered via the pars flaccida or lesser curve due to scarring, it may be prudent to enter on the greater curve lower on the stomach and work toward this space for pouch definition. The remainder of the operation is as described above.

## Post-operative Care

Care following revisional surgery is much as it is in primary surgery. Often, we are more liberal about obtaining an upper gastrointestinal fluoroscopy study on the first day after surgery because of concern for leaks. Patients tend to stay in the hospital for 1 or 2 days longer after revisional surgery. Outpatient care and follow-up is similar to RRYGB.

## References

1. Hubens G, Balliu L, Ruppert M, Gypen B, Van Tu T, Vaneerdeweg W. Roux-en-Y gastric bypass procedure performed with the da Vinci robot system: is it worth it? Surg Endosc. 2008;22(7):1690–6.
2. Schauer P, Ikramuddin S, Hamad G, Gourash W. The learning curve for laparoscopic Roux-en-Y gastric bypass is 100 cases. Surg Endosc. 2003;17(2):212–5.
3. Oliak D, Ballantyne GH, Weber P, Wasielewski A, Davies RJ, Schmidt HJ. Laparoscopic Roux-en-Y gastric bypass: defining the learning curve. Surg Endosc. 2003;17(3):405–8.
4. Horgan S, Vanuno D. Robots in laparoscopic surgery. J Laparoendosc Adv Surg Tech A. 2001;11(6):415–9.
5. Mohr CJ, Nadzam GS, Curet MJ. Totally robotic Roux-en-Y gastric bypass. Arch Surg. 2005;140:779–86.
6. Scozzari G, Rebecchi F, Millo P, Rocchietto S, Allieta R, Morino M. Robot-assisted gastrojejunal anastomosis does not improve the results of the laparoscopic Roux-en-Y gastric bypass. Surg Endosc. 2011;25(2):597–603.
7. Myers SR, McGuirl J, Wang J. Robot-assisted versus laparoscopic gastric bypass: comparison of short-term outcomes. Obes Surg. 2013;23(4):467–73.
8. Tieu K, Allison N, Snyder B, Wilson T, Toder M, Wilson E. Robotic-assisted Roux-en-Y gastric bypass: update from 2 high-volume centers. Surg Obes Relat Dis. 2013;9(2):284–8.
9. Ayloo SM, Addeo P, Shah G, Sbrana F, Giulianotti PC. Robot-assisted hybrid laparoscopic Roux-en-Y gastric bypass: surgical technique and early outcomes. J Laparoendosc Adv Surg Tech A. 2010;20(10):847–50.
10. Ayloo SM, Addeo P, Buchs NC, Shah G, Giulianotti PC. Robot-assisted versus laparoscopic Roux-en-Y gastric bypass: is there a difference in outcomes? World J Surg. 2011;35(3):637–42.
11. Moser F, Horgan S. Robotically assisted bariatric surgery. Am J Surg. 2004;188(4A Suppl):38S–44S.
12. Parini U, Fabozzi M, Brachet Contul R, Millo P, Loffredo A, Allieta R, et al. Laparoscopic gastric bypass performed with the da Vinci Intuitive Robotic System: preliminary experience. Surg Endosc. 2006;20(12):1851–7.
13. Yu SC, Clapp BL, Lee MJ, Albrecht WC, Scarborough TK, Wilson EB. Robotic assistance provides excellent outcomes during the learning curve for laparoscopic Roux-en-Y gastric bypass: results from 100 robotic-assisted gastric bypasses. Am J Surg. 2006;192(6):746–9.
14. Park CW, Lam EC, Walsh TM, Karimoto M, Ma AT, Koo M, et al. Robotic-assisted Roux-en-Y gastric bypass performed in a community hospital setting: the future of bariatric surgery? Surg Endosc. 2011;25(10):3312–21.

15. Deng J, Lourie D. 100 Robotic-Assisted Laparoscopic Gastric Bypasses at a Community Hospital. Am Surg. 2008;74(10):1022–5.
16. Hagen ME, Pugin F, Chassot G, Huber O, Buchs N, Iranmanesh P, et al. Reducing cost of surgery by avoiding complications: the model of robotic Roux-en-Y gastric bypass. Obes Surg. 2012;22(1):52–61.
17. Sanchez BR, Mohr CJ, Morton JM, Safadi BY, Alami RS, Curet MJ. Comparison of totally robotic laparoscopic Roux-en-Y gastric bypass and traditional laparoscopic Roux-en-Y gastric bypass. Surg Obes Relat Dis. 2005;1(6):549–54.
18. Lawson EH, Curet MJ, Sanchez BR, Schuster R, Berguer R. Postural ergonomics during robotic and laparoscopic gastric bypass surgery: a pilot project. J Robot Surg. 2007;1(1):61–7.
19. Higa KD, Boone KB, Ho T. Complications of the laparoscopic Roux-en-Y gastric bypass: 1,040 patients—what have we learned? Obes Surg. 2000;10(6):509–13.
20. Higa KD, Boone KB, Ho T, Davies OG. Laparoscopic Roux-en-Y gastric bypass for morbid obesity: technique and preliminary results of our first 400 patients. Arch Surg. 2000;135(9):1029–33. discussion 33-4
21. Matthews BD, Sing RF, DeLegge MH, Ponsky JL, Heniford BT. Initial results with a stapled gastrojejunostomy for the laparoscopic isolated roux-en-Y gastric bypass. Am J Surg. 2000;179(6):476–81.
22. Nguyen NT, Goldman C, Rosenquist CJ, Arango A, Cole CJ, Lee SJ, et al. Laparoscopic versus open gastric bypass: a randomized study of outcomes, quality of life, and costs. Ann Surg. 2001;234(3):279–89. discussion 89-91
23. Mohr CJ, Nadzam GS, Alami RS, Sanchez BR, Curet MJ. Totally robotic laparoscopic Roux-en-Y gastric bypass: results from 75 patients. Obes Surg. 2006;16:690–6.
24. Van Nieuwenhove Y, Dambrauskas Z, Campillo-Soto A, van Dielen F, Wiezer R, Janssen I, et al. Preoperative very low-calorie diet and operative outcome after laparoscopic gastric bypass: a randomized multicenter study. Arch Surg. 2011;146(11):1300–5.
25. Hausel J, Nygren J, Lagerkranser M, Hellstrom PM, Hammarqvist F, Almstrom C, et al. A carbohydrate-rich drink reduces preoperative discomfort in elective surgery patients. Anesth Analg. 2001;93(5):1344–50.
26. Buchs NC, Pugin F, Azagury DE, Huber O, Chassot G, Morel P. Robotic revisional bariatric surgery: a comparative study with laparoscopic and open surgery. Int J Med Robot. 2014;10(2):213–7.
27. Bindal V, Gonzalez-Heredia R, Elli EF. Outcomes of robot-assisted Roux-en-Y gastric bypass as a reoperative bariatric procedure. Obes Surg. 2015;25(10):1810–5.

# Masters Program Colon Pathway: Robotic Right Hemicolectomy

11

Martin R. Weiser

Complete surgical resection is the cornerstone of the treatment of primary colon cancer. Adequate resection involves removal of the involved segment of the large bowel, mesentery, and associated vascular supply to completely excise the locoregional lymphatics at risk for containing metastatic disease. Although dependent on multiple variables, pathologic assessment of 12 lymph nodes is standard for determining the stage [1]. Minimally invasive colectomy is now widely used for primary colon cancer. Compared with open surgery patients, patients treated with minimally invasive approaches have faster recovery, less pain, and similar perioperative and oncologic outcomes. Among minimally invasive approaches, robotic surgery has emerged as a modality that provides improved optics and dexterity compared to straight laparoscopic surgery. The choice of technique depends on surgeon expertise and experience along with patient- and tumor-related factors.

## Indications

Indications for right colectomy in a fit patient include invasive cancers or noninvasive neoplastic lesions that are not amenable to colonoscopic removal. Patients who have undergone a polypectomy for a malignancy are candidates for a colectomy if margins are not cleared or there is a significant risk of nodal metastases. The risk of metastases to regional lymph nodes is related to features such as poor differentiation, vascular or lymphatic invasion, and extension below the submucosa [2]. Generally, the presence of one or more of these features is an indication for resection.

M.R. Weiser, M.D. (✉)
Department of Surgery, Memorial Sloan Kettering Cancer Center,
1275 York Ave, New York, NY 10065, USA
e-mail: weiser1@mskcc.org

© Springer International Publishing AG 2018
A.D. Patel, D. Oleynikov (eds.), *The SAGES Manual of Robotic Surgery*,
The SAGES University Masters Program Series, DOI 10.1007/978-3-319-51362-1_11

An extended right colectomy is indicated for lesions located in the proximal to mid-transverse colon, synchronous ascending and transverse colon cancers, and multiple adenomas, which may or may not be part of a genetic syndrome. Extended right hemicolectomy proceeds similarly to a standard right hemicolectomy with ligation of the middle colic pedicle at its origin. Anastomosis is created between the terminal ileum and distal transverse colon or descending colon, depending on vascular supply.

The decision to proceed with open or robotic colectomy depends on many factors including the surgeon's expertise and experience. There are no absolute contraindications for robotic colon cancer surgery. However, intestinal obstruction, large lesions, fistulizing tumors, or history of multiple previous abdominal surgeries can pose challenges for surgeons who are not experienced with the robotic approach. In the end, the surgical approach should be chosen with the goals of maximizing the chance of a margin-negative resection, limiting complications, and optimizing recovery.

## Preparation

Patient evaluation prior to surgery includes a complete history and physical examination, family history, routine laboratory analysis including carcinoembryonic antigen, and radiographic staging. Radiologic staging includes CT of the chest, abdomen, and pelvis with oral and intravenous contrast. MRI and PET are used selectively if an abnormality noted on a CT scan needs further definition and would change surgical management. Patients should undergo a full colonic evaluation, with histologic analysis of the colon lesion, prior to initiation of treatment. Preoperative medical consultation for risk stratification is obtained based on the patient's history, including geriatric evaluation for fragile patients and those older than 75 years.

Patients are started on a clear diet the day prior to surgery, and the intestine is purged with a polyethylene glycol–based agent. Oral antibiotics are prescribed for the day prior to surgery. The benefits of mechanical bowel preparation with oral antibiotics have recently been reported. In a study involving over 8400 patients from the National Surgical Quality Improvement Program targeted colectomy dataset, patients receiving mechanical bowel preparation with oral antibiotics had lower rates of surgical-site infection, anastomotic leak, and postoperative ileus than other patients [3].

Prophylaxis against thromboembolism includes preoperative subcutaneous heparin, intraoperative sequential compression devices, postoperative low molecular–weight heparin, and early ambulation. The incorporation of modified Surgical Care Improvement Project (SCIP) measures is essential, including normothermia, glucose control, appropriate hair removal, and suitable use of intravenous antibiotics, including administration prior to incision, re-dosing during the procedure, and discontinuation postoperatively.

Enhanced recovery pathways [4] are followed for patient management, with preoperative counseling on early ambulation and discharge once tolerating diet and passing flatus. Patients are given a clear liquid diet the morning of surgery with a complex carbohydrate drink including electrolytes and minerals. In the preoperative care unit, patients are given gabapentin, diclofenac, and alvimopan. Transverse abdominis plane (TAP) anesthetic blocks and goal-directed intraoperative fluid management are utilized, along with ketamine infusions, minimal opioids, and standardized antiemetics.

## Surgical Technique Using the da Vinci Xi Platform

With arms padded and tucked, the patient is positioned supine on a nonskid cushioned pad. The da Vinci Xi robot is positioned on the patient's right side. The bedside operating assistant stands on the patient's left side, and the scrub technician and instrument table are positioned on the left side. The robot will eventually be docked perpendicular to the operating room table. Figure 11.1 shows an overhead view of the recommended configuration. This setup and the following techniques can also be applied to the Si platform.

The Veress technique is utilized to establish pneumoperitoneum. Palmer's point, 3 cm below the left subcostal border in the midclavicular line, is generally chosen for Veress needle insertion. A five-port approach is employed: four robotic ports and an accessory port. The umbilical port is placed first. Ports are generally placed midline or to the left of the midline. There is slight variation depending on whether intracorporeal stapling is planned (Fig. 11.2). For intracorporeal anastomosis, a robotic or laparoscopic stapler is introduced via a larger, 12- to 15-mm, supraumbilical port that is later extended to become the extraction site. For extracorporeal anastomosis, the specimen is generally extracted via the supraumbilical port site.

Prior to robotic docking, the bed is tilted left side down with slight Trendelenburg positioning. The peritoneal cavity is inspected, and the omentum and the transverse

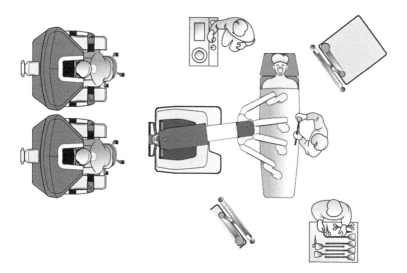

**Fig. 11.1**  Recommended configuration of the operating room

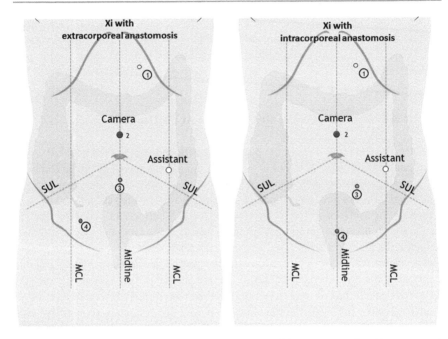

**Fig. 11.2** Port placement for robotic right hemicolectomy with extracorporeal and intracorporeal anastomosis. The 8-mm robotic and ports 5-mm accessory port are indicated

colon are placed cephalad over the liver tip. The small intestine is positioned to the left abdomen, exposing the ileocolic pedicle.

The robotic cart approaches from the right, perpendicular to the bed. When docking, automatic targeting by focusing the camera on anatomy ensures proper arm alignment to maximize the range of motion and limits arm collision. A robotic 0° endoscope is inserted into the #2, supraumbilical port. Arm 1 is typically paired with monopolar curved scissors or the robotic vessel sealer. Arm 3 is paired with the fenestrated bipolar instrument, and arm 4 is paired with the Cadiere grasper. A 5-mm assistant port accommodates the suction irrigator or laparoscopic bowel grasper controlled by the bedside assistant during the procedure. For obese patients, a second 5-mm assist port can be utilized to facilitate exposure to the base of the mesentery.

Using a medial-to-lateral approach, the terminal ileum/cecum is retracted with arm 4 to the right lower quadrant, elevating and placing tension on the ileocolic pedicle. This maneuver exposes the vascular pedicle for dissection (Fig. 11.3). With the fenestrated bipolar grasper in arm 3 and the bipolar scissor in arm 1, the peritoneum below the ileocolic pedicle is incised. Using arms 1 and 3 in a scissoring fashion, submesenteric dissection is initiated just below the level of the duodenum. Dissection continues exposing the retroperitoneal structures including duodenum, Gerota's fascia, gonadal vessels, and ureter (Fig. 11.4). The dissection continues laterally to the abdominal wall, inferiorly to the level of the sacral promontory, and superiorly exposing the duodenum and head of pancreas.

**Fig. 11.3** The initial step is placing the terminal ileum and cecum under tension to allow identification and incision of the peritoneum below the ileocolic pedicle. ©2016, Memorial Sloan Kettering Cancer Center

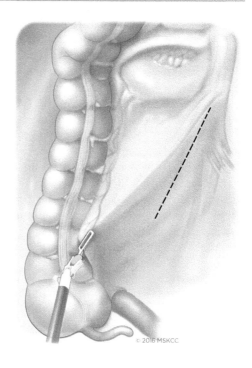

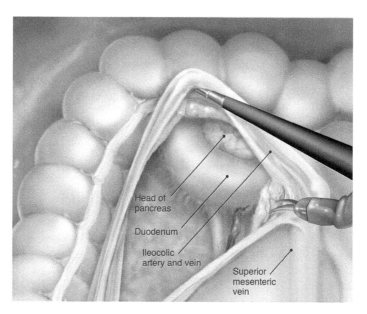

**Fig. 11.4** Medial-to-lateral dissection of the mesentery off the retroperitoneum, including the duodenum and the head of the pancreas. ©2016, Memorial Sloan Kettering Cancer Center

Once the right colon mesentery is dissected off the retroperitoneum, the vascular pedicles are dissected, ligated, and divided. Dissecting the anterior wall of the superior mesenteric vein inferior to the ileocolic vein facilitates total mesocolic excision and high pedicle ligation. Wristed instruments expedite this dissection. The ileocolic vein and artery, which courses over the vein, are ligated and divided sequentially, maintaining an intact mesocolon envelope. The middle colic pedicles are then addressed. The bedside assistant provides anterior and cephalad retraction on the transverse colon mesentery, exposing the middle colic pedicle. Dissection continues along the superior mesenteric vein to the level of the middle colic vein. Again, the artery is lateral. The right branch of the middle colic pedicle is ligated and divided in a standard right colectomy. The right colic pedicle is generally not encountered, as it is most commonly a branch of the ileocolic pedicle. On occasion, however, there is a right colic vein with a separate takeoff from the superior mesenteric vein between the ileocolic and middle colic pedicles. For proximal transverse colon lesions, the base of the middle colic pedicle is ligated and divided, and the gastrocolic vein (gastrocolic trunk of Henle) is divided for resection of the proximal omentum en bloc with the right colon. Finally, the mesentery is divided to the transverse colon.

Next, the omentum is dissected off the distal transverse colon with entry into the lesser sac. The omentum attached to the proximal transverse colon is generally resected and divided outside the gastroepiploic arcade. For proximal transverse colon lesions, the arcade is dissected with the specimen. Next, the transverse colon is placed on caudal tension, and the remaining omental and retroperitoneal (hepatic flexure) attachments are divided in a medial-to-lateral fashion. This dissection is facilitated by previous submesenteric dissection. The scissor or vessel sealer divides tissue, while arms 2 and 3 provide retraction and open the plane. Finally, the cecum, appendix, and terminal ileum are mobilized by dividing the peritoneal attachments in the right lower quadrant. Previous medial-to-lateral submesenteric dissection ensures that the ureter, kidney, and gonadal vessels remain in the retroperitoneum. The small bowel mesentery is freed to the level of the duodenum. Lastly, the terminal ileum mesentery is divided to the small bowel wall.

For extracorporeal anastomosis, a laparoscopic bowel grasper placed through the assistant port delivers the terminal ileum. The robot is then undocked and backed away from the table. The camera port incision is extended to a length sufficient for specimen extraction. A wound protector is placed, and the terminal ileum and right colon are delivered for resection and anastomosis. An anastomosis-in-continuity is created, generally in a stapled side-to-side, functional end-to-end–anastomosis manner (Fig. 11.5). After the procedure is completed, the base of the anastomosis is reinforced with suture and mesenteric defect is not closed. The wound protector is reapproximated, and insufflation allows for laparoscopic visualization of hemostasis and port removal. The fascia from the specimen retrieval site is irrigated and closed with interrupted absorbable monofilament sutures. The skin is reapproximated with absorbable skin sutures.

When intracorporeal anastomosis is employed, the terminal ileum and the transverse colon are divided with a laparoscopic or robotic stapler. An isoperistaltic, side-to-side anastomosis is fashioned. The distal terminal ileum is aligned with the transverse colon, an enterotomy and a colostomy are created, and the stapler is inserted and deployed. In general, the broader jaw of the robotic or laparoscopic stapler is inserted first into the colotomy, and then the ileum is brought over and the slimmer stapler jaw is inserted. The stapler is deployed, and the common enterotomy/colostomy is closed with intracorporeal interrupted or running suture. The suprapubic stapling port is enlarged (generally by creating a Pfannenstiel incision), and the specimen is extracted via a wound protector. The wound protector is then closed, insufflation is re-established, the abdomen is inspected for hemostasis, and ports are removed under direct visualization.

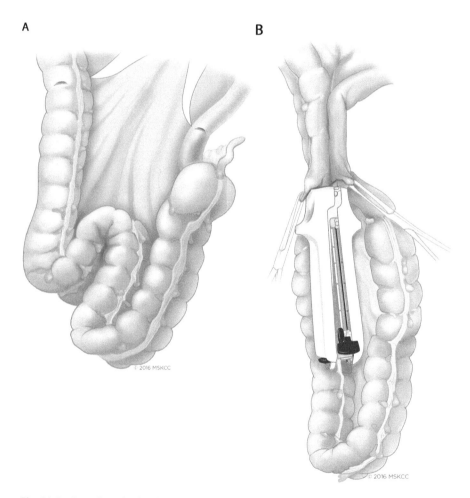

**Fig. 11.5** Once the colon has been mobilized and pedicles ligated, an anastomosis-in-continuity is fashioned. An enterotomy and a colostomy are then performed (**A**), the GIA 80 stapler is inserted and deployed (**B**), and the common enterotomy/colostomy is closed by deploying a TA90 stapler (**C**). ©2016, Memorial Sloan Kettering Cancer Center

C

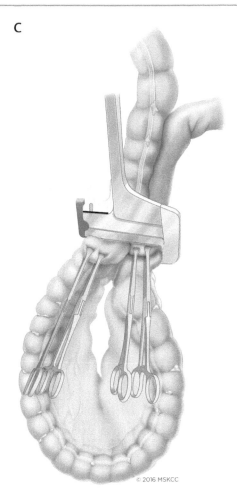

**Fig. 11.5** (continued)

## Lymphadenectomy

Complete mesocolic excision (CME), which includes dissection in the mesocolic plane with central vascular ligation, facilitates lymph node yield and possibly improves oncologic outcomes [5]. The goal is an anatomic resection with entire removal of the mesocolon along embryologic tissue planes. The surgical group in Erlangen, Germany, reported 5-year survival rates of >85% for patients undergoing CME [6]. This technique does require detailed knowledge of anatomical planes [7] and avoidance of any breaches of visceral fascial layers, which theoretically could lead to tumor cell contamination of the peritoneum and metastases. Additionally, work from Japan indicates that D3 lymphadenectomy along with CME may further improve outcomes. D3 lymphadenectomy consists of skeletonizing and ligating the vasculature flush with the origin of the involved vessels (e.g., ileocolic) followed by en bloc removal of the lymphatics along the lateral and ventral portion of superior mesenteric vein to Henle's gastrocolic trunk and final transection of the involved distal vasculature (e.g., right colic and right branch of middle colic vessels) at the respective origins [8].

## After the Surgery

Patients are given clear liquids in the recovery room and ambulate the day of surgery. Narcotics are minimized with liberal use of nonsteroidal anti-inflammatory medications. The diet is advanced to regular, and the Foley catheter is removed on postoperative day 1. The goal is to discharge on postoperative day 2 or 3.

With the use of Enhanced Recovery after Surgery (ERAS) protocols and perioperative care bundles, the rate of complications after right hemicolectomy is 5–10% [9]. Leak rates are 0.5–1% and can usually be managed with bowel rest, antibiotics, and possible percutaneous drainage if clinically necessary.

## Conclusion

Complete surgical resection of primary colon cancer is paramount for cure. Adequate resection entails the removal of the involved segment of bowel, mesentery, and associated vascular supply to completely excise the lymphatics. Precise surgical technique along with CME should allow for complete lymphadenectomy and evaluation of at least 12 lymph nodes for accurate staging. Robot-assisted surgery facilitates a complete anatomic resection by providing improved visualization, a stable camera platform, and a greater degree of freedom, thereby avoiding the mechanical limitations of laparoscopic surgical techniques.

## References

1. Chou JF, Row D, Gonen M, Liu YH, Schrag D, Weiser MR. Clinical and pathologic factors that predict lymph node yield from surgical specimens in colorectal cancer: a population-based study. Cancer. 2010;116(11):2560–70.
2. Haggitt RC, Reid BJ. Hereditary gastrointestinal polyposis syndromes. Am J Surg Pathol. 1986;10(12):871–87.
3. Kiran RP, Murray AC, Chiuzan C, Estrada D, Forde K. Combined preoperative mechanical bowel preparation with oral antibiotics significantly reduces surgical site infection, anastomotic leak, and ileus after colorectal surgery. Ann Surg. 2015;262(3):416–25, discussion 23-5
4. Vlug MS, Wind J, Hollmann MW, Ubbink DT, Cense HA, Engel AF, et al. Laparoscopy in combination with fast track multimodal management is the best perioperative strategy in patients undergoing colonic surgery: a randomized clinical trial (LAFA-study). Ann Surg. 2011;254(6):868–75.

5. West NP, Hohenberger W, Weber K, Perrakis A, Finan PJ, Quirke P. Complete mesocolic excision with central vascular ligation produces an oncologically superior specimen compared with standard surgery for carcinoma of the colon. J Clin Oncol. 2010;28(2):272–8.
6. Hohenberger W, Weber K, Matzel K, Papadopoulos T, Merkel S. Standardized surgery for colonic cancer: complete mesocolic excision and central ligation—technical notes and outcome. Colorectal Dis. 2009;11(4):354–64.
7. Acar HI, Comert A, Avsar A, Celik S, Kuzu MA. Dynamic article: surgical anatomical planes for complete mesocolic excision and applied vascular anatomy of the right colon. Dis Colon Rectum. 2014;57(10):1169–75.
8. Liang JT, Huang KC, Lai HS, Lee PH, Sun CT. Oncologic results of laparoscopic D3 lymphadenectomy for male sigmoid and upper rectal cancer with clinically positive lymph nodes. Ann Surg Oncol. 2007;14(7):1980–90.
9. Nelson G, Kiyang LN, Crumley ET, Chuck A, Nguyen T, Faris P, et al. Implementation of enhanced recovery after surgery (ERAS) across a provincial healthcare system: the ERAS Alberta colorectal surgery experience. World J Surg. 2016;40(5):1092–103.

# Masters Program Colon Pathway: Robotic Low Anterior Resection

12

## Seth Alan Rosen

## Abbreviations

| | |
|---|---|
| A# | Assistant port number |
| ACOSOG | American College of Surgeons Oncology Group trial |
| ALaCaRT | Australasian Laparoscopic Cancer of the Rectum trial |
| $CO_2$ | Carbon dioxide |
| COLOR | Colon carcinoma laparoscopic or open resection trial |
| COREAN | Comparison of open versus laparoscopic surgery for mid or low rectal cancer after neoadjuvant chemoradiotherapy trial |
| CRM | Circumferential resection margin |
| CUSUM | Cumulative sum analysis |
| DRM | Distal resection margin |
| EBL | Estimated blood loss |
| EEA | End-to-end anastomosis |
| ICG | Indocyanine green |
| IMA | Inferior mesenteric artery |
| IMV | Inferior mesenteric vein |
| LapLAR | Laparoscopic low anterior resection |
| LAR | Low anterior resection |
| LLQ | Left lower quadrant |
| LMQ | Left middle quadrant |
| LOS | Length of stay |

**Electronic supplementary material:** The online version of this chapter (doi: 10.1007/978-3-319-51362-1_12) contains supplementary material, which is available to authorized users. Videos can also be accessed at http://link.springer.com/chapter/10.1007/978-3-319-51362-1_12.

S.A. Rosen, M.D. (✉)
Department of Colorectal Surgery, Emory University,
6335 Hospital Parkway, Suite 112, Johns Creek, GA 30097, USA
e-mail: seth.rosen@emoryhealthcare.org

© Springer International Publishing AG 2018 151
A.D. Patel, D. Oleynikov (eds.), *The SAGES Manual of Robotic Surgery*,
The SAGES University Masters Program Series, DOI 10.1007/978-3-319-51362-1_12

| LUQ | Left upper quadrant |
| MRC-CLASICC II | Medical Research Council Conventional versus laparoscopic-assisted surgery in colorectal cancer trial |
| NIR | Near-infrared |
| OpenLAR | Open low anterior resection |
| P# | Port number |
| PILLAR II | Perfusion assessment in laparoscopic left-sided/anterior resection trial |
| R# | Robotic arm number |
| RA-CUSUM | Risk-adjusted cumulative sum analysis |
| RLQ | Right lower quadrant |
| RobLAR | Robotic low anterior resection |
| ROLARR | Robotic-assisted versus laparoscopic resection for rectal cancer trial |
| RUQ | Right upper quadrant |
| TME | Total mesorectal excision |

## Background

Low anterior resection refers to a proctectomy which includes: (1) mobilization of the rectum off the anterior attachments to the sacrum; (2) dissection of the lateral stalks from the pelvic sidewall; (3) development of a plane between the rectum and the anterior pelvic organs; and (4) an anastomosis created distal to the peritoneal reflection. Common indications for LAR include the surgical treatment of rectal cancer, larger rectal polyps, diverticular disease, and Crohn's disease. Although first described in 1991 [1] and despite the well-known advantages of minimally invasive surgery, LapLAR has not become widely performed. Twenty years after its initial description, LAR was still performed predominantly via open technique (60.7% Open LAR, 33.5% LapLAR, 5.9% RobLAR) [2].

## Laparoscopic Low Anterior Resection

A steep learning curve has been described for LapLAR [3–9] typically requiring 30–70 cases. Barriers to performing laparoscopic proctectomy include two-dimensional visualization while working in a three-dimensional field, tremor amplification at the tips of 30 cm instruments, fulcrum effect at the port site, poor surgeon ergonomics, unstable image, impaired ability to effectively retract and counter-retract, limited degrees of mobility of the surgical instruments (i.e., 4), and difficulty with intra-corporeal suturing due to all of the above. Resulting frustrations with LapLAR include prolonged operative times due to tedious and cumbersome dissections [10–12], high conversion rates [11–13], positional injuries for the operating surgeon [14], and perhaps "cutting corners" during some procedures in attempts not to convert.

Acceptance of LapLAR for rectal cancer is supported by the COREAN, COLOR, MRC-CLASICC II, ACOGSOG Z6051, and ALaCaRT trials [15–19]. Feasibility and safety have been demonstrated, with short-term complications and long-term outcomes, including oncologic outcomes, comparable to open surgery. Unfortunately, these trials and others have shown high conversion rates (10–34%) for LapLAR [15–20]. Conversion from laparoscopic to open surgery can be associated with longer operative times, increased intraoperative complications, higher postoperative morbidity rates, longer hospital stay, and possibly higher long-term recurrence rates [21–26]. Additionally, large controlled series of LapLAR for rectal cancer have demonstrated alarming rates of circumferential margin involvement [27–29].

## Rationale for Robotic Low Anterior Resection

Recent data demonstrate that RobLAR is increasingly being used to perform proctectomy, with year-over-year growth of over 30% between 2013 and 2015 [30]. Benefits of the da Vinci platform include high-definition 3D images with tenfold magnification, motion filtering to decrease tremor, surgeon-controlled camera on a stable platform, a third operating arm controlled by the surgeon and "wristed" instrumentation (7 degrees of freedom). Additionally, the master and slave system allows improved ergonomics for the surgeon. During RobLAR, the da Vinci platform is particularly useful for fine dissection of the inferior mesenteric vessels, sharp dissection in Heald's plane while working in the narrow, bony pelvis, identification of the ureters and gonadal vessels, preservation of the autonomic nerves, ultralow dissection and intra-corporeal suturing [31, 32]. Because RobLAR offers superior visualization, exposure and maneuverability in the confined spaces of the bony pelvis, it may increase the feasibility of minimally invasive proctectomy for more patients, decreasing the conversion rate to open surgery [20, 33–35].

## Data for Robotic Low Anterior Resection

Since 2010, a number of studies, analyzing data from over 1000 patients, have been published about RobLAR. Operative times range from 180 to 396 min (mean 293 min) with longer times often represented by ultralow dissections, including intersphincteric resections, with coloanal anastomosis [36]. Mean estimated blood loss (EBL) is 111.5 ml (range 0–232 ml), conversion to open surgery occurs in 0–9.5% of patients, postoperative complications in 10–41% (mean 20%) of patients, including anastomotic leaks in 6.4% (range 0–13.6%), urinary or sexual dysfunction in 5.5–37%, and mortality in 0–3.4% [2, 31, 32, 37–39]. In terms of oncologic outcomes, the mean number of excised lymph nodes is 16.2 (range 10.3–20.6), distal resection margin (DRM) length ranges from 1.4 to 4 cm (mean 2.75 cm), positive circumferential margin (CRM) rates range from 0 to 7.5% (mean 6.8%), local recurrence ranges from 2.5% to 3.2% with 5-year disease-free survival documented as 81.9% [2, 39, 40].

Although many of these outcomes compare equally to LapLAR and OpenLAR, there are some notable differences. In a systematic review of the literature, Mak et al. compared 1062 patients who underwent RobLAR with 706 patients who underwent LapLAR [31]. This meta-analysis demonstrated much higher conversion rates for LapLAR (1.8–22%) than RobLAR (0–8%). The most common reasons for conversion in both groups included obesity, difficulty anatomy, bulky tumor, narrow pelvis, adhesions from prior surgery, equipment malfunction, and intra-operative complications. In the same meta-analysis, two studies found a statistically significant higher rate of EBL in the LapLAR group compared to the RobLAR group [41, 42]. Although overall morbidity was similar between the groups, sexual and urinary dysfunction was higher in the LapLAR group than the RobLAR group (3–57% vs. 0–37%). In addition, median length of stay (LOS) was shorter in the RobLAR group than the LapLAR group (7.1 vs. 9.6 days). Although similar results were seen in terms of CRM positivity, DRM length, lymph node sampling, and local recurrence, two studies comparing TME quality found RobLAR to be superior [41, 43].

Speicher et al. retrospectively reviewed the National Cancer Data Base, including 1912 LapLAR patients and 956 RobLAR patients. Similar to Mak et al., the outcomes regarding lymph node sampling, positive margins, readmission rates, and 30-day mortality were similar, but a difference in conversion rates was noted (RobLAR 9.5% vs. LapLAR 16.4%) [2].

A recent meta-analysis of eight studies revealed a lower positive CRM rate in RobLAR than in LapLAR [20]. Distal surgical margins were longer in the RobLAR group when compared with the LapLAR group, suggesting that superior vision and dexterity with the robotic system may translate to better pathologic outcomes [44]. Ghezzi et al. compared 65 patients undergoing RobLAR with 109 patients undergoing OpenLAR, and found significant differences in CRM positivity (0% in RobLAR vs. 1.8% in OpenLAR), while performing more ultralow dissections with coloanal anastomosis in the RobLAR group (16.9% vs. 1.8%) [45].

Numerous studies have demonstrated better quality of TME with RobLAR [31, 34, 46]. Quality of TME is likely a better surrogate of quality of dissection than CRM, which may be influenced by tumor stage and location in relation to the fascia propria of the rectum [20].

## Patient Selection

When considering which patients are appropriate for RobLAR, the surgeon should review all pertinent history. Robotic-assisted surgery, like laparoscopy, may involve prolonged intra-abdominal carbon dioxide insufflation and Trendelenburg position, which may be problematic in patients with morbid obesity, poor pulmonary compliance, or limited cardiac reserve. A history of prior abdominal surgery may suggest the presence of adhesions preventing standard placement of trocars, whereas a history of prior pelvic surgery or radiation therapy may alert one to a more challenging pelvic dissection. Any prior bowel surgery, such as intestinal bypass or colectomy, should be noted by the surgeon contemplating RobLAR. These issues, as well as coagulopathy, general bowel habits, sphincter function, and urinary and sexual function should be considered preoperatively. The surgeon should perform a complete physical examination, including rigid proctosigmoidoscopy and complete colonoscopy. Radiologic imaging should be reviewed as well, with particular attention to pathology involving adjacent structures, including small intestine, bladder, vagina, prostate, seminal vesicles, iliac vessels, and ureters. The potential need for other robotically trained surgical specialists should be part of preoperative planning.

## Surgeon Learning Curve

The surgeon who is new to RobLAR is advised to appreciate the learning curve and plan accordingly. Using cumulative sum method (CUSUM) and risk-adjusted cumulative sum method (RA-CUSUM), multiple authors have evaluated their own experiences with RobLAR [44, 47–50]. There are classically three phases to the surgeon's learning curve: the initial learning curve (15–40 cases), the competent period (next 30–50 cases), and the challenging period (after 70–80 cases). During phase 1, the surgeon will undertake less complicated procedures, should expect longer operating times and higher conversion rates, but should see no increased short-term complications. In phase 2, the surgeon gains more comfort with the technology and will often see console times, total operating times, and conversion rates decrease. It is during phase 3 that the surgeon broadens the inclusion criteria to include more complex pathology, morbidly obese patients, post-radiation cancers, lower dissections in the pelvis, and combined procedures with other surgeons. Operating times may plateau or temporarily increase during this phase. There certainly can be overlap between the phases, depending on the surgeon, prior open and laparoscopic surgery experience, operating room personnel ability, and practice composition.

The surgeon needs to be knowledgeable about the robotic system and facile with complicated robotic instruments. This includes docking of the patient cart, installing the instruments, and safely controlling the instruments from the surgeon's console [48]. Bokhari et al. evaluated their own experience and concluded that the learning curve entails the surgeon's mastery of three important and unique facets of robotic technology: (1) overcoming the loss of tensile and tactile feedback by recognizing visual cues with regard to tension and manipulation of tissues; (2) conceptualizing the spatial relationships of robotic instruments outside the active field of view; and (3) mentally visualizing the spatial relationships of the robotic arms and cart while operating at the console [47]. There is potential for external clashing of robotic arms, and instruments outside the camera's view have to be located properly without causing iatrogenic injuries. Also, the techniques of retracting and dissecting are different than with laparoscopic instruments. As a prerequisite for RobLAR, the surgeon needs thorough knowledge of pelvic anatomy, be able to identify the correct avascular plane as well as the autonomic nerves, and must observe the principles of Dr. Heald [48].

## Overcoming the Learning Curve

RobLAR can be divided into the following steps: (1) dissection of the lateral attachments of the left and sigmoid colon (and possible splenic flexure mobilization); (2) pelvic dissection with total or partial mesorectal excision; (3) inferior mesenteric artery (IMA) dissection and ligation; (4) distal transection and proximal transection of the bowel; (5) anastomosis. During the initial phase of his learning curve, the surgeon is advised to use robotic-assisted techniques for some of these steps and either laparoscopic or open modalities to complete other steps. The surgeon should set goals regarding which steps will be done robotic-assisted, with time limits and specific hard stops established prior to the operation. Over time, the surgeon can expect to convert from performing a hybrid procedure to a totally robotic procedure. During the surgeon's early experience (i.e., 5–15 cases), it is advised to limit console time to a maximum of 60–90 min, as visual, mental and physical fatigue unique to working at the surgeon console may be expected.

During the initial phase, it is extremely valuable to gain experience with various robotic instruments and modalities in order to appreciate the strengths and weaknesses of these different technologies. Understanding the abilities and limitations of da Vinci instrumentation in regard to visibility, haptic feedback, degrees of freedom at instrument tip, forces generated, and potential hazards takes dedicated time. For example, dissecting with the Monopolar Curved Scissors is often more efficient than the Monopolar Cautery Hook, but is more likely to cause irksome bleeding. The EndoWrist One Vessel Sealer can be quite efficient for safely transecting mesocolic and mesorectal vessels, but can also result in fusing planes, whereas a monopolar device is more suited to opening embryologic planes. In regard to visualization, most procedures can be completed with a 0° camera, but the 30° camera can be invaluable when trying to see over the splenic flexure (down position) or behind the rectum (up position). When considering port placement and position, it is helpful to recognize that some RobLARs will be easily achieved with single-docking, while others will benefit from double-docking, and these decisions may be planned preoperatively and modified intra-operatively. In a similar vein, sometimes a second assistant port is more helpful than the third robotic arm, and at times "port-jumping" and/or "port-nesting" may be beneficial for a specific portion of the procedure. Port-jumping refers to relocating a robotic arm from one port to another, or even swapping a robotic arm for an assistant instrument. Port nesting refers to placement of a 5 mm or 8 mm port in a 12 mm port, so as to use the same port for different technologies during separate phases of a procedure.

As the surgeon moves into the competent phase, the indications will expand, for example, from diverticulitis to diverticulitis complicated by fistula or abscess. Performing combined cases with urologists and gynecologists with compromised port placements also occurs during the competent phase. Lastly, the surgeon may add robotic-assisted intra-corporeal anastomosis to the armamentarium.

Throughout the process, the surgeon is strongly encouraged to record, view, and critique his own videos. Reviewing videos will highlight inefficiencies with utilizing the third arm for retraction and dissection, problems arising from poor port placement, issues from suboptimal instrument choices, and opportunities for development and modification of techniques. Opportunities exist for formal video review from surgical societies and educational entities.

The experience of one young surgeon with a single year of laparoscopic experience is illustrative. Byrn et al. reviewed their own progression during their first 85 robotic-assisted rectal dissections. Operative times improved from 267 min to 224 min, direct hospital costs decreased from $17,349 to $13,680, number of lymph nodes excised increased from 11.8 to 20 per patient, while LOS decreased from 8.3 to 5.9 days [51].

## Room Set-up and Patient Positioning

Fig. 12.1 demonstrates a typical operating room set-up for RobLAR. The patient is positioned on the operating table with buttocks hanging slightly off the edge of the bed so as to allow access to the anus. The lower extremities are secured in adjustable stirrups, thighs at approximately 180° angle with the torso, with attention to positioning of the feet and knees so as to avoid any nerve compression. It is helpful to use either a foam mattress (author preference *Prime Medical Trendelenburg OR Table Pad STP100*), a sandbag, a safety strap across the patient's chest and/or shoulder bolsters to prevent patient movement during steep Trendelenburg positioning. Both upper extremities are tucked and padded alongside the torso with careful attention to wrist and finger position and protection. An upper body warming system (author preference

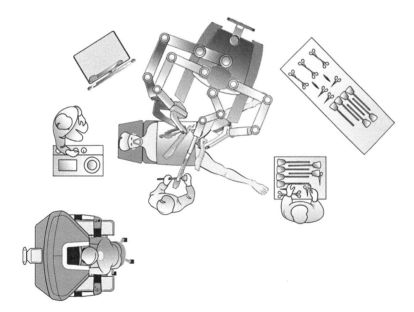

**Fig. 12.1** Room set-up for anterior resection via single docking. Patient in Trendelenburg position, with right side of patient rotated downward

3M™ Bair Paws™ Flex) is recommended to maintain normothermia. Orogastric tube decompression and bladder catheterization are standard. Anesthesia personnel and cart are located at the head of the table. The left side of the patient will need to be accessible for the robotic patient cart. During the laparoscopic portion of the procedure, monitors for both the surgeon and surgical assistant are useful.

## Laparoscopic Phase

A 12 mm × 130 mm Applied Kii® balloon blunt tip system (author preference) is placed in the right middle quadrant using an open technique, lateral to the rectus sheath, a 0° laparoscope is introduced, and the abdomen is explored. Some authors prefer midline camera placement for aesthetic benefit, but in this author's experience, camera proximity to the root of the IMA may be an issue during medial-to-lateral dissection if the port is placed midline. If an ileostomy is likely, this location can be used for the camera port. Before any further port placement, it is useful to identify the location of intra-abdominal adhesions, the extent of colon redundancy, splenic flexure position, and the location and extent of the pathology to be addressed. Advantages and disadvantages of medial-to-lateral and lateral-to-medial dissection are considered based on the patient's anatomy and pathology. The patient is placed in Trendelenburg position with the right side of the patient tilted toward the floor. The goal is for the abdominal contents to clear out of the pelvis allowing the medial aspect of the rectosigmoid mesentery to become visible and accessible.

## Port Placement

Ports are placed according to Fig. 12.2, with minor adjustments based on the findings of the laparoscopic exploration. This port placement is intended for a single-dock procedure. Port 1 (P1) is placed in the right lower quadrant (RLQ), more cephalad for lower pelvic cases and more lateral for rectosigmoid pathology. Using an 8 mm port nested in a 12 mm port allows use of both standard instrumentation and the da Vinci EndoWrist Stapler. Placement of P2 in the right upper quadrant (RUQ) enables it to be useful both during the pelvic dissection and mobilization of the left colon including the splenic flexure. Placement of P3 in the left middle quadrant (LMQ) allows it to be useful primarily during the pelvic phase, but if placed medial enough (i.e., midclavicular line), it will also be useful during sigmoid colon mobilization. The assistant port (A1) is placed lateral to the camera port, along the right anterior axillary line. Modifications to this set-up include:

1. Double-dock procedure: add an 8 mm P4 in the LLQ. P1, P2, and P4 are used for robot arm 1 (R1), R2, and R3 during splenic flexure mobilization, with R3 on the same side of the patient cart as R1; an assistant port (A1) is located along the right anterior axillary line; during the pelvic phase, R3 is flipped around to the same side of the patient cart as R2 and used via P3. The patient cart is docked over the LUQ for splenic flexure mobilization, with the patient in reverse

**Fig. 12.2** Port placement for sigmoid or upper rectal pathology, single-docking

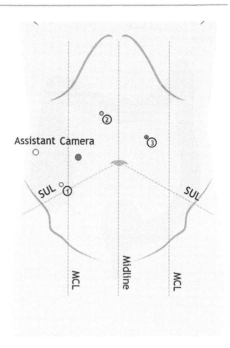

Trendelenburg position; it is docked over the left lower quadrant (LLQ) for the pelvic phase, with the patient now in Trendelenburg position.

2. Similar to 1, but during the pelvic dissection R1, R2, and R3 are used in P1, P3, and P4. The assistant may use ports A1 and P2 during the pelvic dissection [52].
3. Similar to 1, but P5 is in a midline suprapubic position; R3 is utilized via P5 for splenic flexure mobilization; during the pelvic phase, P2 is used as a second assistant port, and P1, P3, and P4 are used for the pelvic dissection with R1, R2, and R3. P5 is incorporated into the extraction site (Fig. 12.3).
4. Similar to 1, but no re-docking of the patient cart is performed ("flip arm technique") [53].
5. Similar to 1, but R2 and R3 are switched (R2 in P3 and R3 in P2).

Again, taking a few moments to laparoscopically assess at the beginning of the procedure will allow the surgeon to modify port placement according to the specifics of the patient's anatomy, to plan single or double-docking, medial or lateral approach, and consider other potential operative issues before docking and sitting down at the surgeon's console.

## Docking of Patient Cart

For single-docking RobLAR, the patient cart is docked over the left lower corner of the operating room table, with the legs of the patient cart straddling the corner of the table. For lower pathology, the patient cart is parallel to the patient's left lower

**Fig. 12.3** Port placement
for lower rectal pathology,
double-docking

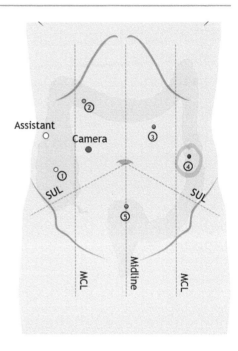

extremity; for higher pathology, an angle more perpendicular to the patient's body is preferred. For double-docking, the splenic flexure mobilization is best achieved with the patient in reverse-Trendelenburg and docking at a 45° angle over the patient's left shoulder.

## Instrument Selection

Many surgeons prefer to dissect with the Monopolar Curved Scissors via R1P1, while others utilize ether a Monopolar Cautery Hook or Spatula. The scissors is quite efficient at opening the peritoneum, dissecting around vessels, developing avascular planes along the line of Toldt, developing the "golden plane" posterior to the rectum, and incising Waldeyer's and Denonvilliers' fascia. In addition to dissecting with the tip of the scissors, the flexed heel is excellent for providing exposure in an atraumatic fashion.

At times, the monopolar instrument can be swapped for the da Vinci EndoWrist One Vessel Sealer, which is particularly useful for blunt dissection and ligation of mesenteric vessels in obese patients. The vessel sealer uses bipolar energy (radiofrequency) and compression force to weld tissues together and seal. It has a 20 mm jaw length with 16 mm of sealing surface and 13 mm of cut length. It has computer-controlled closing pressure, minimal thermal spread of 1–2 mm, >600 mm HG burst pressure and independent seal and cut functions [54]. When needed, one can remove the 8 mm trocar nesting in the 12 mm sleeve, enabling P1 to be used for the da Vinci EndoWrist Stapler. The EndoWrist Stapler's "smart-clamp technology" takes a series of measurements and provides audio and visual feedback prior to firing. If the stapler detects inadequate jaw closure for a proper "B-staple form", firing is prevented and the surgeon is obligated to open and re-clamp the tissue until appropriate parameters for safe transection are met [55]. Data is lacking, but early experience suggests this may help surgeons avoid forcing a stapling that should not occur. The Fenestrated Bipolar Forceps is used via R2P2 and the Cadiere via R3P3. The EndoWrist One Suction/Irrigator and/or EndoWrist Grasping Retractor may be helpful, particularly during the pelvic dissection. At times it is helpful for the assist to suction and the surgeon to use an arm to retract, whereas in other circumstances, the reverse is true - the approach should be individualized to the particular situation, and creative thinking and flexibility is required from the surgeon. Appropriate instrument selection and attentiveness are critical to avoiding bowel injury during the procedure. Whereas Fenestrated Bipolar Forceps and Cadiere Forceps are considered safe for grasping the colon and small bowel, the ProGrasp™ closes with a higher compression force which increases the risk of serosal injury.

*→ Tip up Fenestrated Grasper*

A standard disposable 5 mm port is often used as A1, although a 12 mm port allows the assistant surgeon to utilize laparoscopic endostaplers available from Covidien or Ethicon. Another option, which this author prefers, is to use the AirSeal system (available in 5 mm, 8 mm and 12 mm), which maintains stable pneumoperitoneum and efficient smoke evacuation, including during proctotomy or vaginotomy.

## Dissection of Lateral Attachments and Pelvic Dissection

First, the surgeon uses the Fenestrated Bipolar Forceps and the assistant uses an atraumatic bowel grasper (author preference Epix laparoscopic grasper) to retract the left colon and sigmoid colon medially. Dissection along the Line of Toldt is carried out proximally up to the splenic flexure and distally to the upper 1/3 of the rectum, being careful to identify and preserve the left ureter. Fine dissection is possible with the Monopolar Curved Scissors. When significant progress has been made, the Cadiere is used to retract the rectosigmoid anteriorly and laterally so as to put the medial peritoneum on tension. The peritoneum is incised with the Monopolar Curved Scissors, which allows $CO_2$ insufflation to enter the retroperitoneum and reveal the plane between the mesorectal fascia and presacral fascia. This avascular plane is sharply dissected with the Monopolar Curved Scissors (see Video 12.1). Posterior mobilization of the rectum is performed with the scissors and bipolar forceps using the "Saturday Night Fever" move (described below). The inferior hypogastric nerves and, distally, the pelvic nerve plexus are identified and preserved. Dissection proceeds until retraction is no longer sufficient, then the right lateral attachments are divided in a similar fashion. During this phase of the procedure, it is helpful to bring the third arm posterior to the rectum and use it to push the rectum anteriorly. It is now easy to continue dissecting in the posterior plane, down to the levator muscles if needed. Final attachments along the right side and right posterolateral aspect may be divided in the low pelvis with the same exposure. Throughout this phase, the assist should evacuate smoke, suction bleeding, and/or provide atraumatic retraction.

Next, the surgical assistant uses an atraumatic grasper to pull the rectum cephalad and right, the Cadiere is used for lateral wall counter-traction or to assist with pushing the rectum to the right, and the surgeon dissects down the left side using the scissors and bipolar forceps. As progress is made, the Cadiere is shifted to provide anterior counter-traction by pushing up and out on the vagina (or seminal vesicles), enabling completion of the dissection from the left posterior pelvis to the left anterior plane. Lastly, the assistant retracts the rectum cephalad and posterior, while the surgeon dissects anteriorly, connecting the two lateral dissections. Again, the Cadiere is used to provide counter-traction by pushing the anterior pelvic organs "up and out". When transecting the mesorectum, the scissors is quite useful for scoring the mesorectal envelope and dissecting around mesorectal vessels, while the bipolar forceps and vessel sealer are efficient for transecting the vessels.

Division of the large intestine can be achieved with standard laparoscopic stapling devices, of which there are multiple vendors, lengths, staple-heights, and handle systems. The da Vinci EndoWrist Stapler is preferred by some surgeons as it allows precise placement and fine adjustments to be in the hands of the operating surgeon. The EndoWrist Stapler offers 108° of lateral articulation and 54° of vertical articulation. At the time of this writing, staple loads of 45 mm length are available with two options for staple height: A blue load is 3.5 mm open and 1.5 mm closed, while a green load is 4.3 mm open and 2.0 mm closed. At times, two or three "fires" are required to completely transect the rectum, a change in practice for many surgeons accustomed to striving for a single staple line with no junctions. Although there are data that suggest increased complications at the anastomosis may occur with numerous firings of laparoscopic stapler [56], no clinical data exist regarding outcomes after multiple fires of the EndoWrist Stapler.

## IMA Dissection   *Anterior traction sigmoid colon → Tip UP Grasper*

This step may be accomplished before dissection of the lateral attachments or the pelvic dissection, or as part of either of those steps. The Cadiere is used to retract the rectosigmoid anteriorly and laterally, exposing the IMA at its origin from the aorta. Monopolar Curved Scissors and Fenestrated Bipolar Forceps (or Maryland Bipolar Forceps) are now used to dissect the mesocolic tissues around the base of the IMA. The left ureter and aortic hypogastric nerve plexus are clearly visualized and protected during this dissection due to the superior image afforded by the da Vinci system. The IMA is divided with a Large Clip Applier or EndoWrist Stapler, and medial to lateral dissection may proceed up to the inferior border of the pancreas (see Video 12.2).

*cut 1cm from origin* ←

## Medial to Lateral Dissection of Left Colon and Splenic Flexure Mobilization

The surgical assistant can retract the colon superiorly (anteriorly) by positioning an instrument posterior to the mesocolon and lifting. The inferior mesenteric vein (IMV) is selectively transected close to the fourth portion of the duodenum, with either the Large Clip Applier, vessel sealer, or bipolar forceps. Dissection continues medial to lateral until the left colon is free from the retroperitoneum. The left ureter and gonadal vessels are identified and preserved. Although this author finds complete mobilization is needed in fewer than 20% of these procedures, if further mobilization of the splenic flexure is required, re-docking over the LUQ with the patient in reverse Trendelenburg is helpful with repositioning of the robotic arms according to any of the appropriate set-ups described above. The omentum is retracted by rolling it over the transverse colon, allowing its weight to fall cephalad, thus exposing the correct plane. The scissors or vessel sealer can be used to develop a plane between the transverse colon and the omentum. During this phase the assistant retracts caudad on the colon while the surgeon uses the bipolar forceps for micro-retractions of the omentum. The omentum is completely separated from the transverse colon, followed by division of the splenocolic and renocolic ligaments ensuring complete splenic flexure mobilization.

When adequate mobilization for a tension-free anastomosis has been achieved, an appropriate proximal transection point is chosen. Using scissors, a window is created adjacent to the colon wall, the EndoWrist Stapler is used to divide the bowel and either the bipolar forceps or vessel sealer may be used to harvest the remaining mesocolic vessels.

The specimen is delivered through a low midline or Pfannensteil incision, and the anastomosis is performed via hand-assisted, laparoscopic-assisted, or mini-laparotomy techniques.

## Surgical Tips

From the author's personal experience, the following tips are provided:

- During medial-to-lateral dissection and/or posterior pelvic dissection, the "Saturday Night Fever" move is invaluable: with fingers clenched in the master control, push up and away with the left hand, followed by the right hand coming underneath with a similar move; the left hand is now rolling over the right and toward the surgeon's body as the right hand moves up and away; the left hand completes the circle by coming under the right hand (ala John Travolta on the dance floor). The goal is to use the heel of each flexed instrument tip to push tissue up and away, exposing the avascular plane, and then use the Monopolar Curved Scissors to incise through the fine, wispy tissue. This move is repeated and significant progress is made.
- Use the sides and heels of flexed instruments to push into tissues, rather than the jaws of instruments to grasp tissues. This will provide excellent retraction with minimal trauma to the bowel or its mesentery.
- Zoom in. Many laparoscopic surgeons "use the robot to do laparoscopy". The visual field from the surgeon's cart is different than the view of open or laparoscopic surgery. Zooming in physically or digitally, changing camera angle, or swapping to a 30° camera often enables safer, finer dissection. It takes experience to fully appreciate and utilize the capabilities of the platform. A common error is to accept inadequate visualization.

- Learn from collisions. When you have internal or external collisions, this is an opportunity to evaluate your patient cart placement, port placement, and operative technique. Notice when and where in the procedure collisions occur, stand up, and walk over to the patient cart to visualize the issues with arm positions and port placement. This is instrumental when modifying port placement and arm position during future operations.
- Be able to troubleshoot. Cap leak, "instrument not recognized", "energy device not working", insufflation failure, power outage, motor pack malfunction, and "hard shutdown" will occur. Be familiar with these situations and how to remedy them.

## Modifications of Approach

### Natural Orifice Extraction

Some surgeons use an open rectal stump or colotomy for specimen removal, rather than an elongated port incision or alternative extraction site on the abdomen. Potential benefits include limiting incisional issues such as pain, infection, hematoma, and hernia. Removal of the specimen trans-vaginally is safe and feasible [57].

### Robotic Purse-String

Prasad et al. described a "robotic purse-string technique" as an alternative to the commonly practiced double-stapling technique [58]. The laparoscopic double-stapled technique is hindered by its reliance on laparoscopic staplers which usually result in angled staple lines (because of fulcrum effect) and often require multiple firings to completely transect the rectum. An irregular staple line creates potential anastomotic issues due to areas of ischemia. Additionally, laparoscopic stapling often results in "dog ears" on both corners of the resected margin, resulting in an uneven, irregular DRM and a distal donut not representing the real distal margin. Robotic surgery enables controlled, right-angled transection of the rectum even in the low pelvis and straightforward intra-corporeal suturing (i.e., creation of a purse-string under direct vision) [58]. Potential sites of weakness and ischemia resulting from standard double-stapled technique common in laparoscopic surgery may be avoided.

### Robotic-Assisted Anastomosis

Prior to proximal transection of the bowel, one option is to create a colotomy just proximal to the pathology and place the anvil of an EEA (end-to-end anastomosis) stapler in the colon. The anvil is milked proximally in the colon and the proximal stapling is performed at the planned location (distal to the anvil). A new colotomy is created to allow protrusion of the anvil stalk and a purse-string is performed around this colotomy via robotic-assisted suturing. EEA anastomosis is performed in the standard fashion.

## Indocyanine Green Fluorescence (Firefly™)

This technology allows surgeons to view high-resolution near-infrared (NIR) images of blood flow in vessels, as well as tissue perfusion in real-time. The endoscopes are available in 8.5 mm and 12 mm sizes, with both 0° and 30° tips. Indocyanine green (ICG) is a water-soluble dye with a peak spectral absorption of 800 nm and a half-life of 3–5 min which can bind to plasma proteins and emit infrared signals when excited by laser light [59]. It is administered by anesthesia personnel through a peripheral vein, typically at a dose of 2.5–5 mg. It can be used in colorectal procedures to identify mid-sacral vessels during rectopexy, to distinguish areas of well-perfused bowel from areas of ischemic bowel, to identify collateral arteries and the Arc of Riolan in the "IMV critical zone" [60] and to identify the ureters during retroperitoneal dissection.

Jafari et al. examined the use of ICG for evaluating anastomotic perfusion issues during robotic surgery [61]. Although the study included a small number of patients, 18.8% underwent a revision in the location of the anastomosis after evaluation with Firefly™ and none of these patients experienced postoperative anastomotic failure. Further, the leak rate in the control group (18%) was triple the leak rate in the ICG group. The authors concluded that "the use of ICG fluorescence to delineate the perfusion of colorectal anastomosis may result in relatively frequent revision of the bowel transection point" and that this may ultimately lead to a decreased rate of anastomotic leaks [61].

The PILLAR II study was a prospective multicenter feasibility trial looking at 139 patients who underwent LAR or left colectomy [62]. Fluorescence angiography changed surgical plans in 8% of patients. Anastomotic leak rate was an enviable 1.45%. No leaks were seen in the 11 patients who had a change in surgical plan based on intra-operative perfusion assessment. The authors concluded that the use of fluorescence angiography may: (1) result in revisions of bowel transection point; (2) can provide confirmation of a well-perfused anastomosis; (3) may decrease the rates of anastomotic leak and thereby improve patient outcomes [62].

Both of these studies demonstrate that hypoperfused bowel may appear normal in standard (white) light mode. It is hypothesized that this technology can improve upon the naked eye's ability to detect areas of poor blood supply. Rather than relying on experience, active bleeding from the resection margin, palpable pulse in the mesentery, or pale appearance of the bowel, ICG viewed with NIR may be a more informative alternative.

## Intraoperative Challenges

### Inadequate Reach for Tension-Free Anastomosis

Splenic flexure mobilization is often utilized during open and laparoscopic surgery to ensure a tension-free anastomosis in the pelvis. Although low pelvic dissection is challenging via open or laparoscopic approach, splenic flexure mobilization includes well-defined risks of injury to the spleen, pancreas, and left mesocolic vessels. With the set-up for RobLAR, the exposure and retraction is quite conducive to continued pelvic dissection down to the levator muscles. In fact, the surgeon who has spent his career blindly dissecting and using "feel" to find the correct planes during the distal dissection for low proctectomy will be pleasantly presented with a stable, magnified, high-definition image of the distal pelvis while performing posterior, anterior, and lateral dissections. Mobilization of the rectum will often provide the length needed for a tension-free anastomosis. In the author's experience of over 100 RobLARs, complete splenic flexure mobilization is required less than 20% of the time, typically for distal rectal anastomosis.

When complete mobilization of the splenic flexure is proving difficult, the following maneuvers may be helpful: Convert to a 30° downward camera to improve visualization over the colon; add a second assistant port either in the right abdomen or suprapubic region (i.e., proposed extraction site) enabling your assistant to triangulate with two instruments; re-dock over the patient's LUQ with the patient in reverse Trendelenburg and use a LLQ port for R3.

## Unable to Maintain Exposure During Pelvic Dissection

Large, bulky mesorectal tissue in a small male pelvis, radiation fibrosis, large tumor, abscess/phlegmon, enlarged uterus or fibroid uterus, and floppy bladder are all issues that may prevent the assistant and surgeon from achieving or maintaining adequate exposure. Helpful moves include the following: a 5 mm trocar in the suprapubic position for the surgical assistant to pull up on the uterus, bladder or rectum; a Keith needle to suture through the offending structure and pull up via an extracorporeal hemostat; the Large Grasping Retractor (Graptor™) used as a "V" posterior to the rectum, pushing anteriorly and superiorly. Exposure issues should be handled with "robot-think", not open or laparoscopic techniques. For example, with open or laparoscopic rectal surgery, often the goal is to set up a stable exposure and work for many minutes at a time. With RobLAR, the pelvic dissection is often achieved efficiently with multiple, short micro-retractions (10–20 s) that expose a few centimeters of working area at a time, visualized with a camera tip located just a few centimeters from the area of dissection. A change of mindset is often helpful, as is patience. Using the third arm is critical during the pelvic dissection as it enables you to lock the rectum in a retracted position (i.e., up against the anterior abdominal wall) and then proceed as described above with micro-maneuvers and fine adjustments using the other two working arms. Switching to the 30° upward camera can be helpful when positioning the tip of the camera deep in the pelvis, anterior to the downward-sloping sacrum, with the camera now pointing toward the back of the mesorectum.

## Proximal Transection Point for Diverticulitis

When operating for sigmoid diverticulitis, the distal transection point should be on the upper third of the rectum, or below the most distal inflammation, whichever is lower, so as to minimize the risk of recurrence. The proximal transection point should be on the left colon where the colon "looks and feels normal", that is, proximal to any hypertrophy of the muscularis or inflammatory changes of the colon or mesentery. Although most surgeons are comfortable making this assessment via open approach with direct palpation, many are unclear on how to assess with the limited haptic feedback of laparoscopy or robotic-assisted surgery. In many of these situations, a hand-port is helpful when deciding the location of proximal transection.

## Ureter Identification    *2.5mg ICG i̇ 10mL ⟶ 5-10ml @ ureter*

In the presence of phlegmon or abscess, in the post-radiated pelvis, or in re-operative pelvic surgery, identification and protection of the ureters is of paramount importance. Many surgeons favor ureteral stents to assist with ureter identification. In the author's experience, ureteral stent use is dramatically decreased by the use of robotic-assisted surgery, as the tenfold magnification dramatically improves visualization. In rare situations, Firefly™ may be beneficial.

## Difficult Stapling Angles in the Low Pelvis

It is helpful to place P1 in a location that will allow for passage of the EndoWrist Stapler medial to the right pelvic wall and below the sacral promontory without difficulty. Placing P1 slightly cephalad and medial is often helpful. At times, the stapler head will easily accommodate for transverse stapling (hinge on right, mouth to left), but the surgeon may need to staple in the anterior–posterior or posterior–anterior direction. Two or even three staple loads may be required to transect larger rectums.

## Author's Experience

From January 2014 to February 2016, the author performed 111 pelvic dissections, including low anterior resection, abdominal perineal resection, and sigmoid resection with rectopexy. Of these 111 patients, 100 were scheduled as robotic-assisted (90.1%), of which 91 were completed using robotic-assisted technique (9% conversion rate) (Figs. 12.4, 12.5, and 12.6). Sixteen percent (16/100) were preoperatively

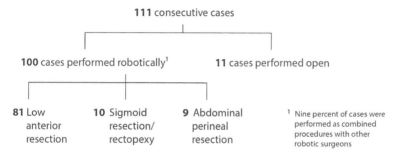

**Fig. 12.4**  Breakdown of surgery performed from 01/14 to 02/16

## Breakdown of 100 Robotic Procedures

*General data*

|  | mean | range |
|---|---|---|
| Age (years) | 59.9 | 18-91 |
| BMI (kg/m²) | 28.5 | 18-48 |
| Length of stay (days) | 4 | 2-36 |
| OR time (minutes) | 179 | 114-265 |
| Prior surgery [1] (# procedures) | 0.8 | 0-5 |

*Case breakdown*

| | |
|---|---|
| Low anterior resection | 81 |
| Sigmoid resection/rectopexy | 10 |
| Abdominal perineal resection | 9 |

**Indications for Surgery [2]**

| | |
|---|---|
| Rectal cancer | 42 |
| Diverticular disease | 39 |
| Rectal prolapse | 8 |
| Rectal polyp | 6 |
| Other | 5 |

[1] Most common procedures (Appendectomy, Cholecystectomy, C-section, Gastric bypass, Total abdominal hysterectomy)

[2] Pre-Operative diagnosis includes abscess and/or fistula in 16% of patients

**Fig. 12.5** Baseline characteristics

## Conversion Rate                                                                       9 %

*Reason for conversion* (#)

| | | | |
|---|---|---|---|
| Abscess and/or fistula | 3 | Redo low anterior resection, hostile pelvis | 1 |
| Anastomotic stapler failure | 1 | Sacral invasion | 1 |
| Obesity/prior TRAM[1] prevented insufflation | 1 | Second pathology found in separate location | 1 |
| Pathology involving small bowel and phlegmon | 1 | [1] Transverse rectus abdominus musculocutaneous flap | |

**Fig. 12.6** Conversion data

**Fig. 12.7** Readmission data

| **Readmission Rate** | 15% |
|---|---|
| *Reason for readmission* | (#) |
| Acute renal failure or dehydration | 8 |
| Abscess/deep infection | 3 |
| Small bowel obstruction | 2 |
| Myocardial infarction | 1 |
| Uroma | 1 |

diagnosed with abscess or fistula related to the primary colorectal pathology, and 9% (9/100) were part of a multi-organ resection. Mean operative time was 179 min (range 114–265 min), median LOS was 4 days (range 2–36 days) and readmission was required in 15% (15/100) of patients, most commonly due to dehydration related to high-output ileostomy (Fig. 12.7). Three anastomotic leaks (3%) were

**Post-Operative Complications (#)**

| | | | |
|---|---|---|---|
| Ileus | 13 | Sexual/urinary dysfunction | 3 |
| Wound infection | 7 | Myocardial infarction/atrial fibrillation | 2 |
| Abscess/deep surgical site infection | 3 | Reoperation | 2[1] |
| Acute renal failure or dehydration | 3 | Ureter injury | 2[2] |
| Anatstomotic leak | 3 | Death | 1 |
| Pneumonia | 3 | Urinary tract infection | 1 |
| Small bowel obstruction | 3 | [1] For small bowel obstruction    [2] Combined procedures with other surgeons | |

**Fig. 12.8** Postoperative complications

**Fig. 12.9** Oncologic data

**Oncologic Data**

| | mean | range |
|---|---|---|
| Total patients | | 42 |
| Received pre-operative radiation therapy | | 21 |
| Lymph nodes | 15.8 | 6-30 |
| Positive circumferential margin | | 2/42 |
| Positive distal margin | | 0/42 |

diagnosed, either clinically or by radiologic testing, and two ureteral injuries (2%) occurred during multi-organ resections performed with co-surgeons from gynecology and urology (Fig. 12.8). In regard to oncologic outcomes, 50% (20/40) of patients with rectal cancer had received preoperative radiation therapy, a mean of 15 lymph nodes were retrieved during pathologic review, and two specimens revealed positive CRMs (3.4%). Both occurrences of positive CRM involved T4 lesions, one involving the sacrum and one involving the vagina, and both were positive despite conversion to open technique. No DRMs were positive (Fig. 12.9).

## Discussion

After two decades of experience, conversion rates for LapLAR still range from 12.2 to 34%, while early in the robotic colorectal surgery experience, RobLAR conversion rates are 0–9.5% [45]. According to the MRC CLASICC trial, the primary reasons for conversion during LapLAR were tumor fixation, uncertainty of tumor clearance, obesity, anatomic issues, and tumor inaccessibility [17]. In the ROLARR trial, there was only a trend toward fewer conversions with RobLAR (12.3 vs. 8.1%, $p > 0.05$). However, the median number of robotic operations performed by surgeons in the ROLARR trial was only 25, suggesting many were still in the early or middle phase of their learning curve. Despite this, subgroup analysis in the ROLARR trial showed benefit of RobLAR over LapLAR in male and/or obese patients, and during lower pelvic dissections [63]. These outcomes confirm what many surgeons find in their own experience; enhanced imaging, superior ability to retract in an atraumatic fashion, finer instrument movement, and a stable working platform enable the surgeon to complete more challenging operations in a minimally invasive fashion.

In regard to oncologic dissection, concerns exist regarding the ability of most surgeons to routinely achieve negative CRM during LapLAR, with high positive CRM rates reported in the literature. Many authors have found not only lower CRM rate with RobLAR, but truly superior TME specimens [13, 31, 41, 45]. Lymph node retrieval and local recurrence rates for RobLAR are similar to LapLAR and OpenLAR, but longer DRMs and higher likelihood of sphincter preservation are seen by surgeons using the da Vinci platform [13, 39, 64–70].

Other documented benefits to RobLAR include decreased blood loss, improved sexual and urinary function, shorter LOS, and higher patient satisfaction. The superior hypogastric plexus and the pelvic splanchnic nerves are common sites of nerve damage leading to sexual dysfunction. In the MRC CLASICC trial, sexual dysfunction was reported in 41% of men treated with LapLAR compared to 23% of men treated with OpenLAR [71]. It is likely that the robotic dissection around the IMA pedicle is a critical step if these functional outcomes are compared between robotic and laparoscopic rectal resections. Recent studies have suggested decreased postoperative sexual and urinary dysfunction after RobLAR [71–73].

Ubiquitously, the criticism of robotic-assisted surgery focuses on cost and operative time. Analysis of the learning curve of many surgeons demonstrates that within 20–50 procedures, operating times can be expected to approach that of OpenLAR and/or LapLAR. Equally, as with much new technology, cost can be expected to decrease as economies of scale and free-market forces exert their influence. Perhaps, on the other hand, the increased cost and time is "the price to be paid in order to provide our patients with surgery of the highest quality and to achieve better results" [45].

The newest version of the da Vinci platform, the Xi, also addresses many of the limitations of the prior technology. Efficient multi-quadrant operations with single-docking, universal ports for instruments and cameras, and synchronization of operating table (TruSystem® 7000dV OR Table) and patient cart movement are a few of the advantages provided by the Xi.

## Conclusions

Minimally invasive surgery offers many benefits to the patient undergoing LAR. Despite its introduction over two decades ago, LapLAR has not become the standard approach due to many of the limitations of laparoscopic technique, which are amplified in the deep, bony pelvis. RobLAR offers a quantum leap forward in visualization, retraction and fine maneuverability, and as a result is rapidly gaining acceptance by colon and rectal surgeons throughout the world.

Although proven safe and feasible through numerous published reports, comparison to OpenLAR and LapLAR demonstrates limited vision. The da Vinci system creates a computer interface between the patient and surgeon, allowing not just substitution for, but rather expansion beyond the human eye and hand. Imaging is not simply magnified and high-definition, it may also include dynamic immunofluorescence, dynamic ultrasound, and perhaps other "molecular" imaging in the future. Instruments smaller and more precise than the surgeon's hand offer the promise of higher quality surgery with fewer complications, and may alter the management of colorectal diseases. Extended pelvic nodal dissection, "total mesocolic excision", sentinel lymph node dissection, and hybrid minimally invasive procedures combining transanal and transabdominal approaches are not new concepts, but are now being seriously pursued as technology catches up with our collective imagination.

## References

1. Jacobs M, Verdeja JC, Goldstein HS. Minimally invasive colon resection (laparoscopic colectomy). Surg Laparosc Endosc. 1991;1(3):144–50.
2. Speicher PJ, Englum BR, Ganapathi AM, Nussbaum DP, Mantyh CR, Migaly J. Robotic low anterior resection for rectal cancer: a national perspective on short-term oncologic outcomes. Ann Surg. 2015;262(6):1040–5.
3. Bege T, Lelong B, Esterni B, Turrini O, Guiramand J, Francon D, et al. The learning curve for the laparoscopic approach to conservative mesorectal excision for rectal cancer: lessons drawn from a single institution's experience. Ann Surg. 2010;251(2):249–53.
4. Dincler S, Koller MT, Steurer J, Bachmann LM, Christen D, Buchmann P. Multidimensional analysis of learning curves in laparoscopic sigmoid resection: eight-year results. Dis Colon Rectum. 2003;46(10):1371–8. discussion 8-9
5. Ito M, Sugito M, Kobayashi A, Nishizawa Y, Tsunoda Y, Saito N. Influence of learning curve on short-term results after laparoscopic resection for rectal cancer. Surg Endosc. 2009;23(2):403–8.
6. Kayano H, Okuda J, Tanaka K, Kondo K, Tanigawa N. Evaluation of the learning curve in laparoscopic low anterior resection for rectal cancer. Surg Endosc. 2011;25(9):2972–9.
7. Park IJ, Choi GS, Lim KH, Kang BM, Jun SH. Multidimensional analysis of the learning curve for laparoscopic resection in rectal cancer. J Gastrointest Surg. 2009;13(2):275–81.
8. Schlachta CM, Mamazza J, Seshadri PA, Cadeddu M, Gregoire R, Poulin EC. Defining a learning curve for laparoscopic colorectal resections. Dis Colon Rectum. 2001;44(2):217–22.
9. Son GM, Kim JG, Lee JC, Suh YJ, Cho HM, Lee YS, et al. Multidimensional analysis of the learning curve for laparoscopic rectal cancer surgery. J Laparoendosc Adv Surg Tech A. 2010;20(7):609–17.
10. deSouza AL, Prasad LM, Ricci J, Park JJ, Marecik SJ, Zimmern A, et al. A comparison of open and robotic total mesorectal excision for rectal adenocarcinoma. Dis Colon Rectum. 2011;54(3):275–82.
11. Krane MK, Fichera A. Laparoscopic rectal cancer surgery: where do we stand? World J Gastroenterol. 2012;18(46):6747–55.
12. Toda S, Kuroyanagi H. Laparoscopic surgery for rectal cancer: current status and future perspective. Asian J Endosc Surg. 2014;7(1):2–10.
13. deSouza AL, Prasad LM, Marecik SJ, Blumetti J, Park JJ, Zimmern A, et al. Total mesorectal excision for rectal cancer: the potential advantage of robotic assistance. Dis Colon Rectum. 2010;53(12):1611–7.

14. Miller K, Benden M, Pickens A, Shipp E, Zheng Q. Ergonomics principles associated with laparoscopic surgeon injury/illness. Hum Factors. 2012;54(6):1087–92.
15. Bonjer HJ, Deijen CL, Haglind E. A Randomized Trial of Laparoscopic versus Open Surgery for Rectal Cancer. N Engl J Med. 2015;373(2):194.
16. Fleshman J, Branda M, Sargent DJ, Boller AM, George V, Abbas M, et al. Effect of laparoscopic-assisted resection vs open resection of stage II or III rectal cancer on pathologic outcomes: the ACOSOG Z6051 randomized clinical trial. JAMA. 2015;314(13):1346–55.
17. Green BL, Marshall HC, Collinson F, Quirke P, Guillou P, Jayne DG, et al. Long-term follow-up of the Medical Research Council CLASICC trial of conventional versus laparoscopically assisted resection in colorectal cancer. Br J Surg. 2013;100(1):75–82.
18. Jeong SY, Park JW, Nam BH, Kim S, Kang SB, Lim SB, et al. Open versus laparoscopic surgery for mid-rectal or low-rectal cancer after neoadjuvant chemoradiotherapy (COREAN trial): survival outcomes of an open-label, non-inferiority, randomised controlled trial. Lancet Oncol. 2014;15(7):767–74.
19. Stevenson AR, Solomon MJ, Lumley JW, Hewett P, Clouston AD, Gebski VJ, et al. Effect of laparoscopic-assisted resection vs open resection on pathological outcomes in rectal cancer: the ALaCaRT randomized clinical trial. JAMA. 2015;314(13):1356–63.
20. Formisano G, Marano A, Bianchi PP, Spinoglio G. Challenges with robotic low anterior resection. Minerva Chir. 2015;70(5):341–54.
21. Agha A, Furst A, Iesalnieks I, Fichtner-Feigl S, Ghali N, Krenz D, et al. Conversion rate in 300 laparoscopic rectal resections and its influence on morbidity and oncological outcome. Int J Color Dis. 2008;23(4):409–17.
22. Law WL, Lee YM, Choi HK, Seto CL, Ho JW. Laparoscopic and open anterior resection for upper and mid rectal cancer: an evaluation of outcomes. Dis Colon Rectum. 2006;49(8):1108–15.
23. Pugliese R, Di Lernia S, Sansonna F, Scandroglio I, Maggioni D, Ferrari GC, et al. Results of laparoscopic anterior resection for rectal adenocarcinoma: retrospective analysis of 157 cases. Am J Surg. 2008;195(2):233–8.
24. Rottoli M, Bona S, Rosati R, Elmore U, Bianchi PP, Spinelli A, et al. Laparoscopic rectal resection for cancer: effects of conversion on short-term outcome and survival. Ann Surg Oncol. 2009;16(5):1279–86.
25. Slim K, Pezet D, Riff Y, Clark E, Chipponi J. High morbidity rate after converted laparoscopic colorectal surgery. Br J Surg. 1995;82(10):1406–8.
26. Yamamoto S, Fukunaga M, Miyajima N, Okuda J, Konishi F, Watanabe M. Impact of conversion on surgical outcomes after laparoscopic operation for rectal carcinoma: a retrospective study of 1,073 patients. J Am Coll Surg. 2009;208(3):383–9.
27. Guillou PJ, Quirke P, Thorpe H, Walker J, Jayne DG, Smith AM, et al. Short-term endpoints of conventional versus laparoscopic-assisted surgery in patients with colorectal cancer (MRC CLASICC trial): multicentre, randomised controlled trial. Lancet. 2005;365(9472):1718–26.
28. Jayne DG, Guillou PJ, Thorpe H, Quirke P, Copeland J, Smith AM, et al. Randomized trial of laparoscopic-assisted resection of colorectal carcinoma: 3-year results of the UK MRC CLASICC Trial Group. J Clin Oncol. 2007;25(21):3061–8.
29. Scheidbach H, Rose J, Huegel O, Yildirim C, Kockerling F. Results of laparoscopic treatment of rectal cancer: analysis of 520 patients. Tech Coloproctol. 2004;8(Suppl 1):s22–4.
30. daVinci Rectal Resections in US 2015: Quarterly Procedure Evolution [Graph]2015.
31. Mak TW, Lee JF, Futaba K, Hon SS, Ngo DK, Ng SS. Robotic surgery for rectal cancer: a systematic review of current practice. World J Gastrointest Oncol. 2014;6(6):184–93.
32. Papanikolaou IG. Robotic surgery for colorectal cancer: systematic review of the literature. Surg Laparosc Endosc Percutan Tech. 2014;24(6):478–83.
33. Ortiz-Oshiro E, Sanchez-Egido I, Moreno-Sierra J, Perez CF, Diaz JS, Fernandez-Represa JA. Robotic assistance may reduce conversion to open in rectal carcinoma laparoscopic surgery: systematic review and meta-analysis. Int J Med Robot. 2012;8(3):360–70.
34. Trastulli S, Farinella E, Cirocchi R, Cavaliere D, Avenia N, Sciannameo F, et al. Robotic resection compared with laparoscopic rectal resection for cancer: systematic review and meta-analysis of short-term outcome. Color Dis. 2012;14(4):e134–56.

35. Xiong B, Ma L, Huang W, Zhao Q, Cheng Y, Liu J. Robotic versus laparoscopic total meso-rectal excision for rectal cancer: a meta-analysis of eight studies. J Gastrointest Surg. 2015;19(3):516–26.
36. Baek SJ, Al-Asari S, Jeong DH, Hur H, Min BS, Baik SH, et al. Robotic versus laparoscopic coloanal anastomosis with or without intersphincteric resection for rectal cancer. Surg Endosc. 2013;27(11):4157–63.
37. Alecu L, Stanciulea O, Poesina D, Tomulescu V, Vasilescu C, Popescu I. Robotically per-formed total mesorectal excision for rectal cancer. Chirurgia (Bucur). 2015;110(2):137–43.
38. Biffi R, Luca F, Pozzi S, Cenciarelli S, Valvo M, Sonzogni A, et al. Operative blood loss and use of blood products after full robotic and conventional low anterior resection with total mesorectal excision for treatment of rectal cancer. J Robot Surg. 2011;5(2):101–7.
39. Park EJ, Cho MS, Baek SJ, Hur H, Min BS, Baik SH, et al. Long-term oncologic outcomes of robotic low anterior resection for rectal cancer: a comparative study with laparoscopic surgery. Ann Surg. 2015;261(1):129–37.
40. Sun Y, Xu H, Li Z, Han J, Song W, Wang J, et al. Robotic versus laparoscopic low anterior resection for rectal cancer: a meta-analysis. World J Surg Oncol. 2016;14(1):61.
41. Erguner I, Aytac E, Boler DE, Atalar B, Baca B, Karahasanoglu T, et al. What have we gained by performing robotic rectal resection? Evaluation of 64 consecutive patients who underwent laparoscopic or robotic low anterior resection for rectal adenocarcinoma. Surg Laparosc Endosc Percutan Tech. 2013;23(3):316–9.
42. Shin JY. Comparison of short-term surgical outcomes between a robotic colectomy and a lapa-roscopic colectomy during early experience. J Korean Soc Coloproctol. 2012;28(1):19–26.
43. Baik SH, Kwon HY, Kim JS, Hur H, Sohn SK, Cho CH, et al. Robotic versus laparoscopic low anterior resection of rectal cancer: short-term outcome of a prospective comparative study. Ann Surg Oncol. 2009;16(6):1480–7.
44. Kim YW, Lee HM, Kim NK, Min BS, Lee KY. The learning curve for robot-assisted total meso-rectal excision for rectal cancer. Surg Laparosc Endosc Percutan Tech. 2012;22(5):400–5.
45. Ghezzi TL, Luca F, Valvo M, Corleta OC, Zuccaro M, Cenciarelli S, et al. Robotic versus open total mesorectal excision for rectal cancer: comparative study of short and long-term out-comes. Eur J Surg Oncol. 2014;40(9):1072–9.
46. Memon S, Heriot AG, Murphy DG, Bressel M, Lynch AC. Robotic versus laparoscopic proc-tectomy for rectal cancer: a meta-analysis. Ann Surg Oncol. 2012;19(7):2095–101.
47. Bokhari MB, Patel CB, Ramos-Valadez DI, Ragupathi M, Haas EM. Learning curve for robotic-assisted laparoscopic colorectal surgery. Surg Endosc. 2011;25(3):855–60.
48. Foo CC, Law WL. The learning curve of robotic-assisted low rectal resection of a novice rectal surgeon. World J Surg. 2016;40(2):456–62.
49. Park EJ, Kim CW, Cho MS, Baik SH, Kim DW, Min BS, et al. Multidimensional analyses of the learning curve of robotic low anterior resection for rectal cancer: 3-phase learning process comparison. Surg Endosc. 2014;28(10):2821–31.
50. Park EJ, Kim CW, Cho MS, Kim DW, Min BS, Baik SH, et al. Is the learning curve of robotic low anterior resection shorter than laparoscopic low anterior resection for rectal cancer?: a comparative analysis of clinicopathologic outcomes between robotic and laparoscopic surger-ies. Medicine (Baltimore). 2014;93(25):e109.
51. Byrn JC, Hrabe JE, Charlton ME. An initial experience with 85 consecutive robotic-assisted rectal dissections: improved operating times and lower costs with experience. Surg Endosc. 2014;28(11):3101–7.
52. Choi DJ, Kim SH, Lee PJ, Kim J, Woo SU. Single-stage totally robotic dissection for rectal cancer surgery: technique and short-term outcome in 50 consecutive patients. Dis Colon Rectum. 2009;52(11):1824–30.
53. Obias V, Sanchez C, Nam A, Montenegro G, Makhoul R. Totally robotic single-position 'flip' arm technique for splenic flexure mobilizations and low anterior resections. Int J Med Robot. 2011;7(2):123–6.
54. EndoWrist One Vessel Sealer. In: Surgical I, editor. p. 1–2.
55. New da Vinci EndoWrist Stapler Takes Robotic-Assisted Surgery to the Next Level. [Intuitive Internal White Paper]. In press.

56. Kawada K, Hasegawa S, Hida K, Hirai K, Okoshi K, Nomura A, et al. Risk factors for anastomotic leakage after laparoscopic low anterior resection with DST anastomosis. Surg Endosc. 2014;28(10):2988–95.
57. Choi GS, Park IJ, Kang BM, Lim KH, Jun SH. A novel approach of robotic-assisted anterior resection with transanal or transvaginal retrieval of the specimen for colorectal cancer. Surg Endosc. 2009;23(12):2831–5.
58. Prasad LM. deSouza AL, Marecik SJ, Park JJ, Abcarian H. Robotic pursestring technique in low anterior resection. Dis Colon Rectum. 2010;53(2):230–4.
59. [This page was last modified on 1 November 2015, at 23:31.]. Available from https://en.wikipedia.org/wiki/Indocyanine_green.
60. Asari SA, Cho MS, Kim NK. Safe anastomosis in laparoscopic and robotic low anterior resection for rectal cancer: a narrative review and outcomes study from an expert tertiary center. Eur J Surg Oncol. 2015;41(2):175–85.
61. Jafari MD, Lee KH, Halabi WJ, Mills SD, Carmichael JC, Stamos MJ, et al. The use of indocyanine green fluorescence to assess anastomotic perfusion during robotic assisted laparoscopic rectal surgery. Surg Endosc. 2013;27(8):3003–8.
62. Jafari MD, Wexner SD, Martz JE, McLemore EC, Margolin DA, Sherwinter DA, et al. Perfusion assessment in laparoscopic left-sided/anterior resection (PILLAR II): a multi-institutional study. J Am Coll Surg. 2015;220(1):82–92. e1
63. https://www.fascrs.org/video/results-robotic-vs-laparoscopic-resection-rectal-cancer-rolarr-study-2015.
64. Baek SJ, Kim CH, Cho MS, Bae SU, Hur H, Min BS, et al. Robotic surgery for rectal cancer can overcome difficulties associated with pelvic anatomy. Surg Endosc. 2015;29(6):1419–24.
65. Buchs NC. Robotic technology: optimizing the outcomes in rectal cancer? World J Clin Oncol. 2015;6(3):22–4.
66. Cho MS, Baek SJ, Hur H, Min BS, Baik SH, Lee KY, et al. Short and long-term outcomes of robotic versus laparoscopic total mesorectal excision for rectal cancer: a case-matched retrospective study. Medicine (Baltimore). 2015;94(11):e522.
67. Kim CN, Bae SU, Lee SG, Yang SH, Hyun IG, Jang JH, et al. Clinical and oncologic outcomes of totally robotic total mesorectal excision for rectal cancer: initial results in a center for minimally invasive surgery. Int J Color Dis. 2016;31(4):843–52.
68. Kwak JM, Kim SH. Robotic surgery for rectal cancer: an update in 2015. Cancer Res Treat. 2016;48(2):427–35.
69. Ng KH, Lim YK, Ho KS, Ooi BS, Eu KW. Robotic-assisted surgery for low rectal dissection: from better views to better outcome. Singap Med J. 2009;50(8):763–7.
70. Pai A, Marecik SJ, Park JJ, Melich G, Sulo S, Prasad LM. Oncologic and clinicopathologic outcomes of robot-assisted total mesorectal excision for rectal cancer. Dis Colon Rectum. 2015;58(7):659–67.
71. Brown SR, Mathew R, Keding A, Marshall HC, Brown JM, Jayne DG. The impact of postoperative complications on long-term quality of life after curative colorectal cancer surgery. Ann Surg. 2014;259(5):916–23.
72. Jayne DG, Brown JM, Thorpe H, Walker J, Quirke P, Guillou PJ. Bladder and sexual function following resection for rectal cancer in a randomized clinical trial of laparoscopic versus open technique. Br J Surg. 2005;92(9):1124–32.
73. Kim JY, Kim NK, Lee KY, Hur H, Min BS, Kim JH. A comparative study of voiding and sexual function after total mesorectal excision with autonomic nerve preservation for rectal cancer: laparoscopic versus robotic surgery. Ann Surg Oncol. 2012;19(8):2485–93.

# Masters Program Colon Pathway: Robotic Left Hemicolectomy and Total Colectomy

**13**

Shanglei Liu, Cristina Harnsberger, Simone Langness, and Sonia Ramamoorthy

## Introduction

While the majority of colon resections are still performed with a traditional open approach, the use of minimally invasive approaches (i.e., laparoscopic, laparoscopic-assisted or robotic) in colorectal procedures has gain popularity over the last decade [1]. The advantages of enhanced recovery resulting in decreased length of hospital stay, decreased post-operative pain, and earlier return of bowel function have stimulated surgeon interest in using a minimally invasive approach to treat colorectal disease [2]. Robotic techniques are newer but not yet as widespread as its laparoscopic counterpart. However, it offers significant advantages over traditional laparoscopy including improved visualization, increased range of motion, decreased physiologic tremor, improved ergonomics, and the ability to use more than two instruments simultaneously [3, 4]. Furthermore, the robot provides the only integrated single platform minimal invasive device that includes automatic staplers, energy devices, and florescent-guided imaging.

However, these advantages come at the cost of the loss of tactile feedback, increased equipment expenses, and the need for specialized training. Although there are proposed advantages of robotic surgery over laparoscopic procedures when operating in obese patients or those with narrow pelvises, these advantages are less true in trans-abdominal colectomy.

S. Liu, M.D. (✉) • C. Harnsberger, M.D. • S. Langness, M.D.
Department of Surgery, University of California, San Diego, Healthcare Systems, 9300 Campus Point Dr, La Jolla, CA 92037, USA
e-mail: s5liu@ucsd.edu; charnsberger@ucsd.edu; slangness@ucsd.edu

S. Ramamoorthy, M.D.
Department of Colorectal Surgery, University of California, San Diego, Healthcare Systems, 9300 Campus Point Dr, La Jolla, CA 92037, USA
e-mail: sramamoorthy@mail.ucsd.edu

© Springer International Publishing AG 2018
A.D. Patel, D. Oleynikov (eds.), *The SAGES Manual of Robotic Surgery*,
The SAGES University Masters Program Series, DOI 10.1007/978-3-319-51362-1_13

While the majority of attention to the use of robotics in colorectal surgery has been dedicated to rectal cancer and dissection within the narrow pelvis, it is important to highlight its role in other procedures such as robotic colectomy. Techniques for robotic total abdominal colectomy (TAC) and left colectomy (LC) will be discussed in this chapter. Because this is a relatively new area of surgery for the robotic platform and the gap in versatility between newer generations of the robotic platform, there is not yet a defined consensus on trocar placement and surgical algorism. Thus, variations from the technique we present here may exist in clinical practice depending on the institution. The procedures described in this chapter are adapted for the DaVinci® (Sunnyvale, California, USA) Xi model robotic platform.

## Indications

The indications for TAC and LC can be broadly categorized into two groups: those conditions resulting from primary lesions, and those due to secondary lesions [5]. Primary lesions leading to an indication for LC or TAC include colon cancer and polyp disease. Diffuse adenomatosis of the colon is most commonly seen in the form of the inherited familial adenomatous polyposis (FAP) syndrome. This is managed by TAC as the lifetime risk of carcinoma development is nearly 100%. Additionally, hereditary non-polyposis colorectal cancer (HNPCC), or Lynch syndrome, is another primary lesion that can be managed with total colectomy, as the risk of metachronous colon cancer is high if segmental colectomy is performed [6].

Secondary lesions that may require total colectomy include inflammatory bowel disease (IBD), pseudomembranous colitis, and motility disorders. Ulcerative colitis with bloody stool that is refractory to medical management, or chronic ulcerative colitis with complications or dysplasia are indications for total colectomy. Crohn's disease that is refractory to medical therapy has multi-segment colonic involvement, or with neoplastic transformation can be managed with total colectomy, although the indications for colonic preservation are not clearly defined [7, 8]. Pseudomembranous colitis resulting from Clostridium difficile infection that is not responsive to medical management or causes toxic megacolon is treated with TAC. The motility disorder characterized by weak muscular activity of the colon such as the case of colonic inertia that is refractory to medical management should be managed with TAC as well [9].

In the case of any of the above indications for TAC, the patient should also be a suitable candidate for minimally invasive surgery. Surgical emergency, physiologically instability, or highly complex diseases are often contraindications to most minimal invasive approaches including robotics. Obesity, however, is not a contraindication to minimally invasive surgery. Though conversion rates are higher than they would be in the non-obese, robotics has been considered the optimal technical approach in this patient population due to the ability to perform intracorporeal anastomosis and vessel ligation [10].

Initial pilot studies demonstrated the success of robotic colectomy when performed for a variety of benign indications, such as diverticular disease, complications of diverticular disease (colovesiclar fistula, etc.) and colonoscopically unresectable polyps [3, 11]. However, there remained concerns for the application of minimally invasive surgery to oncologic resections relating to the adequacy of the lymph node retrieval, margins of excision, and the adherence to other strict oncologic surgical principals. The CLASSICC trial compared pathologic specimens of patients randomized to either open or laparoscopic approaches for segmental colectomy and found equivalent lymph node retrieval and surgical margins [12]. The subsequent COST trial from the United States investigated overall and disease-free survival between these methods and, similarly, found no difference between the techniques used [13]. While robotic-specific data are less rigorously studied, there appears to be sufficient evidence to demonstrate an oncologically acceptable resection for colorectal malignancy with a robotic approach [4]. Furthermore, with the improved dexterity and visualization of the robotic approach, it stands to reason that robotics may offer a more thorough mesocolic resection than perhaps laparoscopic or open surgery. Table 13.1 is a literature review of publications in the last 5 years with studies whose evaluation included TAC, RC (Right Colectomy), or LC. Total number of robotic cases evaluated, rates of conversion, average node identified per case, 30-day mortality, operative time, and anastomotic leaks are identified.

## Procedure: Sigmoid and Left Colectomy

The following is a description of general technique for the robotic left and/or sigmoid colectomy. This particular technique is adapted for the DaVinci® Xi robotic surgery platform. First, the patient is positioned in either supine or lithotomy position and secured to allow for steep right-tilt and reverse Trendelenburg [3, 4, 11, 19, 23]. Operating room setup and patient positioning is illustrated in Fig. 13.1.

Trocar placement for the sigmoid colectomy is seen in Fig 13.2a. This is similar to the set up for robotic LAR with some flexibility built in based on the need to mobilize more proximally or distally, depending on the location of the pathology. Traditionally, with the Si there was a need to have the ports at least 10 cm apart to avoid collisions, however with the Xi ports can be placed closer with less risk of collision. Additionally, ports are placed in a more linear arrangement for maximal access to the whole hemi-abdomen. Initial entry and pneumoperitoneum is usually obtained at the umbilicus by following the umbilical stalk under direct visualization. The lowest trocar in the right lower quadrant is 12 mm in size to allow for either a robotic or laparoscopic stapler. The rest of the robotic ports should be 8 mm in size. The left subcostal port may be moved more inferior laterally to accommodate for the ribs in the costal margin. If a laparoscopic assistant is available, then a 5 mm laparoscopic port can be placed in the upper right quadrant.

For a left colectomy, the trocar placement is similar to sigmoid colectomy except all the ports are placed midline or just off midline to avoid the falciform ligament

**Table 13.1** Recent literature review of robotic colectomy cases

| Year | Author | N | Surgery | Convert to open | Lymph nodes | 30-day mortality | Operative time (min) | Leak |
|---|---|---|---|---|---|---|---|---|
| 2015 | Lujan [14] | 58 | RC | 0 | 20.7 | 0 | 193.2 (console time) | 1 (1.7%) |
| 2015 | Trastulli [15] | 102 | RC | 4 (3.9%) | 20.3 | 0 | 287.4 | 3 (2.9%) |
| 2014 | Casillas [16] | 68 | LC | 4 (5.8%) | 14 | 0 | 188 | 0 |
| 2014 | Casillas [16] | 52 | RC | 4 (7.7%) | 26 | 0 | 143 | 0 |
| 2013 | Morpurgo [17] | 48 | RC | n/a | 26 | 0 | 266 | 0 |
| 2013 | Helvind [18] | 101 | RC, LC, TAC | 5 (5.0%) | 23.36 | 1 (1%) | 165.8 (console time) | 5 (5%) |
| 2013 | Shin [19] | 30 | RC, LAR | 0 | 18.4 | 0 | 371.8 | 1 (3.3%) |
| 2012 | DeSouza [20] | 40 | RC | 1 (2.5%) | n/a | 0 | 158.9 | 0 |
| 2012[a] | Park [21] | 35 | RC | 0 | n/a | 0 | 65 (minutes more than lap) | 1 (2.9%) |
| 2012 | Deutsch [11] | 61 | LC, LAR, AR | 2 (3.3%) | 10 | 0 | 203 (console time) | 1 (1.6%) |
| 2012 | Deutsch [11] | 18 | RC | 2 (11%) | 21.1 | 1 (5.6%) | 134.7 (console time) | 1 (5.6%) |
| 2011 | Luca [22] | 33 | RC | 0 | 26.6 | 0 | 191.7 | 0 |
| 2011 | Huettner [3] | 102 | RC, SC | 5 (4.9%) | N/a | 0 | 126.6 (console time) | 1 (1%) |

Note: *AR* anterior resection, *LAR* low anterior resection, *SC* sigmoid colectomy
[a]Randomized controlled trial

(Fig. 13.2b). Once again the most inferior non-assistant port is 12 mm in size to allow for passage of the stapler.

The dissection can follow standard surgical approaches using either a medial to lateral or lateral to medial approach depending on the surgeon's preference, the patient's body habitus, or the disease process. The steps of these procedures are well described and our approaches are detailed below. The new integrated robotic energy device, stapler, and fluorescent imaging capabilities have proven most useful for performing colectomy.

## Medial to Lateral

1. Place patient in Trendelenberg position with left side up
2. Sweep away any small bowel that is overlying the mesentery
3. Identify the inferior mesenteric artery (IMA) and tent it up toward the anterior abdominal wall

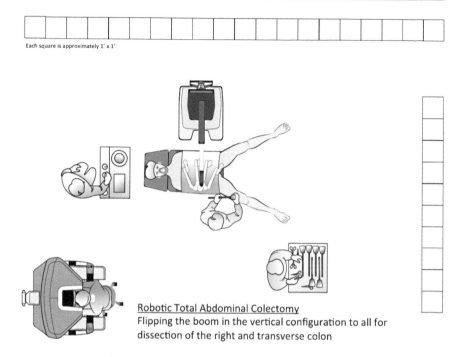

Each square is approximately 1′ x 1′

Robotic Total Abdominal Colectomy
Flipping the boom in the vertical configuration to all for
dissection of the right and transverse colon

**Fig. 13.1**  Robotic setup of the DaVinci® Xi for robotic sigmoid and left colectomy

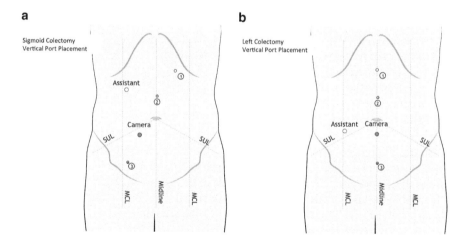

**Fig. 13.2**  (**a**) Trocar placement for sigmoid colectomy, (**b**) trocar placement for left hemicolectomy

4. Score the mesentery on either side of the IMA
5. Identify the left ureter prior to ligating the IMA
6. Ligate the IMA and further open the medial to lateral plane using light cautery
   and gentle spreading superiorly toward splenic flexure, laterally toward the
   peritoneal reflection and inferiorly toward the sacral promontory

7. Identify the proximal and distal points of transection
8. Release the renocolic attachments
9. Mobilize the transverse colon, IMV and omentum proximally as needed.
10. Transect the bowel
11. Exteriorize the transected bowel and perform intra- or extracorporeal anastomosis
12. Perform a leak test

## Lateral to Medial

1. Place patient in Trendelenberg position with left side up
2. Sweep away any small bowel that is overlying the mesentery
3. Retract the sigmoid and left colon medially to expose the White line of Toldt (peritoneal reflection).
4. Open the peritoneal reflection at the rectosigmoid junction and mobilize up to the splenic flexure
5. Identify the left ureter
6. Spread gently in a lateral to medial fashion and release the renocolic and splenocolic attachments
7. Mobilize the transverse colon, IMV and omentum proximally as needed
8. Identify the IMA and tent it up toward the anterior abdominal wall
9. Score the mesentery on either side of the IMA
10. Ligate the IMA and further open the medial to lateral plane using light cautery and gentle spreading superiorly toward splenic flexure, laterally toward the peritoneal reflection and inferiorly toward the sacral promontory
11. Identify the proximal and distal points of transection
12. Transect the bowel
13. Exteriorize the transected bowel and perform intra- or extracorporeal anastomosis
14. Perform a leak test

During the procedure, the mesorectum is divided by a robotic bipolar energy sealer or an ultrasonic dissector. Either a laparoscopic or robotic linear stapler is used to divide the proximal and distal borders of the specimen. The resected colon is removed through either enlarging the umbilical incision or creating a new Pfannenstiel incision. The anastomosis can either be accomplished with an intra- or extracorporeal approach, which is described in a separate section later.

## Procedure: Total Abdominal Colectomy

The technique for total abdominal colectomy involves adding a right hemicolectomy (RC) to the LC procedure described above. The usage of newer robotic surgery platforms allows for easy redocking of instruments for a right-sided abdominal operation with minimal impact on operative time. The robotic right hemicolectomy is well described by several authors with minor variation with respect to port placement and order of dissection [3, 4, 11, 19, 21, 23–25]. The patient is positioned in either supine or lithotomy position and care is taken to secure the legs and chest to allow for steep table tilt and Trendelburg maneuvers. For technique using prior Si model, please refer to our previously published chapter [26].

## Vertical Approach

One approach to this operation is the vertical trocar placement. This is very similar to the LC port placement described prior except having the assistant port at low midline (Fig. 13.3a). When using this trocar placement, the LC dissection is typically performed first followed by switching the robotic boom 180° to perform the right side dissection (Fig. 13.4). This is followed by retrocecal mobilization, which can be performed medially to laterally. We advocate for completing the division of the lateral attachments as the final step before stapling as this can stabilize the specimen within the abdominal cavity during the operation. Vascular control of the ileocolic pedicle and right border of the superior mesenteric artery is obtained next. Finally, the colon is freed and the ileum is divided with either a laparoscopic or a robotic linear stapler. An anastomosis can be created either intra- or extracorporeally.

## Horizontal Approach

The other approach is the horizontal trocar placement approach (Fig. 13.3b). In this case, the inferior and pelvis dissection of both the left and right colon is performed

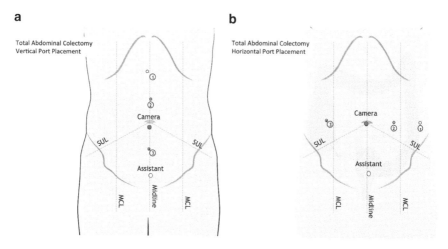

**Fig. 13.3** (**a**) Vertical trocar placement configuration for total abdominal colectomy, (**b**) Horizontal trocar placement configuration for total abdominal colectomy

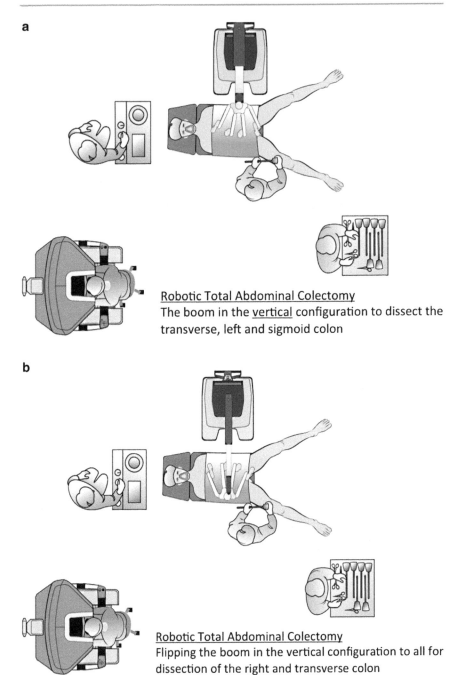

**a**

Robotic Total Abdominal Colectomy
The boom in the <u>vertical</u> configuration to dissect the transverse, left and sigmoid colon

**b**

Robotic Total Abdominal Colectomy
Flipping the boom in the vertical configuration to all for dissection of the right and transverse colon

**Fig. 13.4** (**a**, **b**) Utilization of the robotic boom in vertical trocar configuration

first followed by switching the boom to perform the superior dissection. This trocar placement is made possible on the newer robotic platform due to the increased versatility of the boom positioning. In this case, the 12 mm stapler entry port is often placed in the lower right quadrant but can be just as easily switched to the mirror port on the patient's left depending on the dominant hand preference of the surgeon. This trocar configuration is often useful when performing a staged TAC with J-pouch as the same trocar scars can be utilized in the J-pouch creation. In this configuration, the superior dissection of both sides of the colon and the transverse colon dissection are performed first. Then, the robotic boom can be rotated for the inferior dissection and stapling (Fig. 13.5). Anastomosis can be created if necessary and the specimen can be removed either through a new Pfannenstiel incision or through the enlargement of the umbilical trocar site.

## Intracorporeal Anastomosis

The option of intracorporeal anastomosis that the robotic approach provides has certain distinct advantages and disadvantages. Perhaps the greatest advantage is that the risk of mesenteric twisting is virtually eliminated and the anastomosis is less likely to be undue tension. Additionally, the surgeon is better able to choose an optimal location for the anastomosis. At least two studies report statistically smaller incisions as a result of the intracorporeal anastomosis technique [4, 23, 25]. In regards to the integrity of the anastomosis, it appears to be equivalent to extracorporeal techniques in mean leak pressure and number of sutures placed [5]. If the intracorporeal anastomosis is to be performed by an EEA™ style of stapler, the anvil can be introduced into the proximal bowel through a variety of techniques. The most common of which involves placement of the anvil into the abdomen by enlarging one of the trocars or utilizing the incision for specimen extraction. An additional incision is made at the bowel close to the anastomosis through which the anvil is placed intraluminally for deployment.

The primary drawback to intracorporeal anastomosis is that it takes longer to perform. However, it is important to note that the technique of intracorporeal suturing is relatively new. The continued innovation of instrument design along with mastery of technique should lead to improvements in performance time in the future. Of interest, the use of robotic technology to perform intracorporeal anastomosis may be more intuitive than a laparoscopic approach due to improved ergonomics, more natural needle motion, superior visualization, and an easier learning curve. Lujan et al. found that medical students new to both laparoscopic and robotic intracorporeal suture techniques made fewer errors within the robot group compared to the laparoscopic [25].

## Laparoscopic Comparison

The majority of the published research to date is focused on the feasibility of robotic segmental colectomy as well as a comparison to either open or laparoscopic techniques. In most categories, robotic and laparoscopic right or sigmoid colectomies have

a

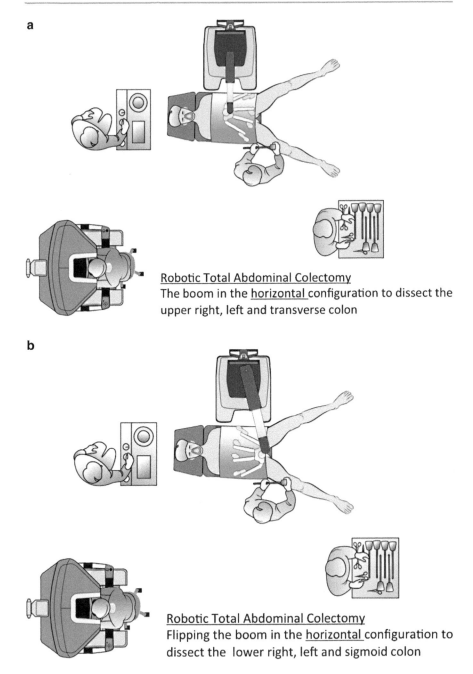

Robotic Total Abdominal Colectomy
The boom in the horizontal configuration to dissect the
upper right, left and transverse colon

b

Robotic Total Abdominal Colectomy
Flipping the boom in the horizontal configuration to
dissect the lower right, left and sigmoid colon

**Fig. 13.5** (**a**, **b**) Utilization of the robotic boom in horizontal trocar configuration

equivalent results, including estimated blood loss, conversion rates, and overall mortality. Individual investigators have reported comparable results in post-operative measures such as time to return of bowel function, total length of stay, and post-operative pain, with neither technique offering a distinct advantage [6–8, 11, 19, 21, 23, 25]. National database review shows similar results to the single surgeon experiences in most categories. Two national database reviews found robotic colectomies having increased operative time by about 50 min and decreased length of stay by 0.5–1 day with no clear differences in other surgical outcomes and morbidities [27, 28].

The most striking difference between the techniques is operative time and cost. In a meta-analysis of robotic versus laparoscopic approach, the robotic approach took on average 40 min longer to complete and cost approximately $800US more, although there is a wide range of results published [6–8, 11, 19, 21, 23, 25]. While more recent papers demonstrate an overall decrease in robotic operation time, suggesting that the learning curve has yet to plateau, the majority of the increased surgical time appears to come from the robotic set-up and docking, which may change in the future as the robotic technology advances.

There is a substantial cost burden for the initial investment of the robot as well as for ongoing maintenance, none of which is calculated into the cost comparisons of laparoscopic colectomies [13]. While both operative and total hospital costs are elevated in robotic approaches, the majority of the cost burden comes from the operating room [23]. The robotic equipment is consistently more expensive than the laparoscopic counterparts, there is a shelf life of ten operations for the robotic instruments and, with longer operative times, the personnel and operating room running time expenses are higher. This has been cited as the biggest drawback of a robotic approach, with nearly 75% of surgeons polled in a survey indicating that the system price is not financially feasible in their practices [6]. This will become even more important as the focus on healthcare costs takes center stage.

## Future Directions

While longer operating times and higher costs are certainly drawbacks to a robotic approach, it is important to consider that this is a relatively new technology and, is therefore, burdened with a learning curve and new product expenses that all new technology and techniques are susceptible [25]. Studies investigating the learning curve in robotic surgery attempt to better predict how much influence more training will have on operative outcomes and length of time. There appears to be a steeper learning curve with respect to the robotic system over traditional laparoscopy, perhaps due to the more intuitive and better ergonomics offered by the robotic [6, 19]. Schlachta et al. suggest that the learning curve plateau for laparoscopic colectomies is between 55 and 70 cases, whereas robotics may be closer to 15–25 cases [10]. Furthermore, the majority of research compiled on laparoscopic versus robotic colectomy is based on procedures performed by highly trained minimally invasive surgeons who are likely to have maximally optimized their laparoscopic skills as opposed to their newly developed robotic skills.

The training required to develop the skills of minimally invasive surgery lends itself more easily to a robotic approach than traditional laparoscopy, predominantly due to the availability of dual controls. Residents and trainees are able to perform surgery with an identical view as the instructor and with the capability of the instructor taking control at any time. Several studies comment on the increased level of resident involvement in robotic colectomies versus more traditional techniques [29]. Furthermore, this can be extended into the field of telerobotics and telementoring, where a trainee may be able to have the same advantage of close mentorship despite being in geographically separated regions [30].

Lastly, the application of robotics to more simple procedures in colorectal surgery, such as segmental resections, allows the surgeons an opportunity to familiarize themselves with the robotic equipment and techniques in vivo prior to graduating to more challenging procedures, such as low anterior resections [11]. While there continues to be debate regarding the utility and/or superiority of robotic segmental colectomies, it clearly can be viewed as a safe alternative approach to open or laparoscopic techniques that may have advantages beyond the traditionally measured outcomes.

## References

1. Kaiser AM. Evolution and future of laparoscopic colorectal surgery. World J Gastroenterol. 2014;20(41):15119–24.
2. Kim CW, Kim CH, Baik SH. Outcomes of robotic-assisted colorectal surgery compared with laparoscopic and open surgery: a systematic review. J Gastrointest Surg. 2014;18(4):816–30.
3. Huettner F, Pacheco PE, Crawford DL. One hundred and two consecutive robotic-assisted minimally invasive colectomies—an outcome and technical update. J Gastrointest Surg. 2011;15(7):1195–204.
4. Annibale AD, Pernazza G, Morpurgo E, Monsellato I, Pende V, Lucandri G, et al. Robotic right colon resection: evaluation of first 50 consecutive cases for malignant disease. Ann Surg Oncol. 2010;17(11):2856–62.
5. Stefanidis D, Wang ÆF, Korndorffer ÆJR, Dunne JB, Scott DJ. Robotic assistance improves intracorporeal suturing performance and safety in the operating room while decreasing operator workload. Surg Endosc. 2010;24(2):377–82.
6. Hanly EJ, Talamini MA. Robotic abdominal surgery. Am J Surg. 2004;188:19–26.
7. Zimmern A, Prasad L. Robotic colon and rectal surgery: a series of 131 cases. World J Surg. 2010;34(8):1954–8.
8. Delaney C, Lynch A, Senagore A, Fazio V. Comparison of robotically performed and traditional laparoscopic colorectal surgery. Dis Colon Rectum. 2003;46(12):1633–9.
9. Bokhari MB, Patel CB, Haas EM. Learning curve for robotic-assisted laparoscopic colorectal surgery. Surg Endosc. 2011;25(3):855–60.
10. Schlachta C, Mamazza J, Seshadri P, Cadeddu M, Gregoire R, Poulin E. Defining a learning curve for laparoscopic colorectal resections. Dis Colon Rectum. 2001;44(2):217–22.
11. Deutsch GB, Anantha S, Zemon H, Klein JDS, Denoto G. Robotic vs. laparoscopic colorectal surgery: an institutional experience. Surg Endosc. 2012;26(4):956–63.
12. Aloia T. Impact of laparoscopic resection for colorectal cancer on operative outcomes and survival. Ann Surg. 2007;246(2):338–41.

13. Fleshman J, Sargent DJ, Green E, Anvari M. Laparoscopic colectomy for cancer is not inferior to open surgery based on 5-year data from the COST study group trial. Ann Surg. 2007;246(4):655–64.

14. Lujan HJ, Molano A, Burgos A, Rivera B, Plasencia G. Robotic right colectomy with intracorporeal anastomosis: experience with 52 consecutive cases. J Laparoendosc Adv Surg Tech A. 2015;25(2):117–22.

15. Trastulli S, Coratti A, Guarino S, Piagnerelli R, Annecchiarico M, Coratti F, et al. Robotic right colectomy with intracorporeal anastomosis compared with laparoscopic right colectomy with extracorporeal and intracorporeal anastomosis: a retrospective multicentre study. Surg Endosc. 2015;29(6):1512–21. doi:10.1007/s00464-014-3835-9.

16. Casillas MA, Leichtle SW, Wahl WL, Lampman RM, Welch KB, Wellock T, et al. Improved perioperative and short-term outcomes of robotic versus conventional laparoscopic colorectal operations. Am J Surg. 2014;208(1):33–40. doi:10.1016/j.amjsurg.2013.08.028.

17. Morpurgo E, Contardo T, Molaro R, Zerbinati A, Orsini C, D'Annibale A. Robotic-assisted intracorporeal anastomosis versus extracorporeal anastomosis in laparoscopic right hemicolectomy for cancer: a case control study. J Laparoendosc Adv Surg Tech A. 2013;23(5):414–7. doi:10.1089/lap.2012.0404.

18. Helvind NM, Eriksen JR, Mogensen A, Tas B, Olsen J, Bundgaard M, et al. No differences in short-term morbidity and mortality after robot-assisted laparoscopic versus laparoscopic resection for colonic cancer: a case-control study of 263 patients (Surg Endosc 2013). Surg Endosc. 2013;27(10):3940.

19. Shin JY. Coloproctology comparison of short-term surgical outcomes between a robotic colectomy and a laparoscopic colectomy during early experience. J Korean Soc Coloproctol. 2012;28(1):19–26.

20. De Souza A, Prasad L, Park J, Marecik S, Blumeitti J, Abcarian H. Robotic assistance in right hemicolectomy: is there a role? Dis Colon Rectum. 2010;53(7):1000–6.

21. Park JS, Choi GS, Park SY, Kim HJ, Ryuk JP. Randomized clinical trial of robot-assisted versus standard laparoscopic right colectomy. Br J Surg. 2012;99(9):1219–26.

22. Luca F, Ghezzi TL, Valvo M, Cenciarelli S, Radice D, Crosta C, et al. Surgical and pathological outcomes after right hemicolectomy: case-matched study comparing robotic and open surgery. Int J Med Robot. 2011;7:298–303.

23. Rawlings AL, Woodland JH, Vegunta RK, Crawford DL. Robotic versus laparoscopic colectomy. Surg Endosc. 2007;21:1701–8.

24. Yu H, He Y, Ni Y, Wang Y, Lu N, Li H. PORP vs. TORP: a meta-analysis. Eur Arch Otorhinolaryngol. 2013;270(12):3005–17.

25. Lujan H, Maciel V, Romero R, Plasencia G. Laparoscopic versus robotic right colectomy: a single surgeon's experience. J Robot Surg. 2013;7(2):95–102.

26. Harnsberger C, Cajas L, Oh SY, Ramamoorthy S. Robotic-assisted total abdominal colectomy. In: Ross HM, SWL L, Champagne BJ, Pigazzi A, Rivadeneira DE, editors. Robotic approaches to colon and rectal surgery. Cham: Springer; 2015. p. 149–55.

27. Miller PE, Dao H, Paluvoi N, Bailey M, Margolin D, Shah N, et al. Comparison of 30-day postoperative outcomes after laparoscopic vs robotic colectomy. J Am Coll Surg. 2016;223(2):369–73. doi:10.1016/j.jamcollsurg.2016.03.041.

28. Dolejs SC, Waters JA, Ceppa EP, Zarzaur BL. Laparoscopic versus robotic colectomy: a national surgical quality improvement project analysis. Surg Endosc. 2016; doi:10.1007/s00464-016-5239-5.

29. Marecik SJ, Prasad LM, Park JJ, et al. Evaluation of midlevel and upper-level residents performing their first robotic-sutured intestinal anastomosis. Am J Surg. 2008;195:333–8.

30. Weber P, Merola S, Wasielewski A, Ballantyne G. Telerobotic-assisted laparoscopic right and sigmoid colectomies for benign disease. Dis Colon Rectum. 2002;45(12):1689–94.

# Part II
# System Details

# 14

Arinbjorn Jonsson and Ankit D. Patel

The origins of modern surgical robotics can be traced, as with many other technologies, to the military. In the mid-1980s, a team of researchers at NASA began a collaboration with robotics experts at the Stanford Research Institute (SRI). The goal was to combine two emerging technologies, virtual reality and robotic telemanipulation, to deliver a virtual surgeon interface that could effectively bring the surgeon to the patient. The surgeon would have control over robotic arms equipped with enhanced dexterity to perform complex open surgical procedures.

The collaborative effort of NASA and SRI, called the Green Telepresence Surgery project, piqued the interest of the military and in 1992 the Pentagon began funding under the Advanced Research Projects Agency (ARPA). The military had a vision of carrying an injured soldier into a vehicle equipped with robotic surgical equipment and allow a surgeon to perform damage control surgery remotely from a mobile army surgical hospital (MASH) unit. Testing on the prototype proved promising in animal models and by 1996, the SRI team demonstrated that damage control surgeries could be performed remotely from over a 5 km distance [1]. As combat scenarios changed from the field to cities in the 1990s, the system was never able to be fully implemented. However, it laid the groundwork for the emerging field of surgical robotics and telesurgery.

At this time, a parallel development was emerging and having a more immediate impact in general surgery. The laparoscopic cholecystectomy, first performed by Mouret in 1987 and presented at the international stage by Jacques Perissat in 1989, led to an explosion in minimally invasive surgery. However, there were drawbacks

A. Jonsson, M.D • A.D. Patel, M.D., F.A.C.S (✉)
Department of General & Gastrointestinal Surgery, Emory University School of Medicine, Atlanta, GA, USA
e-mail: apatel7@emory.edu

© Springer International Publishing AG 2018
A.D. Patel, D. Oleynikov (eds.), *The SAGES Manual of Robotic Surgery*,
The SAGES University Masters Program Series, DOI 10.1007/978-3-319-51362-1_14

including higher costs, high learning curve, diminished visualization and exposure, and impaired dexterity.

One side project funded by ARPA sought to bring robotic technology to laparoscopy. The Automated Endoscopic System for Optimal Positioning (AESOP) was developed by Yulun Wang at the University of California, at Santa Barbara [2]. This voice-controlled camera allowed the surgeon to perform a laparoscopic procedure without the need for an assistant or camera holder. In 1993, The AESOP became the first FDA-approved robotic device for general surgery. It would later become a part of the Zeus surgical system (Computer Motion Inc., Santa Barbara, CA) which was released in 1997 and carried a similar platform to the modern da Vinci.

In 1995, Dr. Frederick Moll acquired the license of the SRI's Green Telepresence Surgery program and founded Intuitive Surgical (Mountain View, CA), initially a company of only five engineers [3]. The group changed the focus away from open procedures and used the new technology to address some of the pitfalls of conventional laparoscopy. The project was extensively redesigned over the next few years and morphed into the modern da Vinci surgical system. This was approved by the FDA for use as an assist device for laparoscopic procedures in 1997. That same year, Cadiere and Himpens performed the first robotic cholecystectomy in Belgium [4]. The initial prototype, called the MONA, used a two-arm robot and special 3D goggles for the surgeon to use while looking at a monitor.

Now in clinical use and with surgeon feedback, the new da Vinci surgical system underwent a rapid evolution. The console became equipped with the familiar binocular surgeon interface and demonstrated the improved dexterity for intracorporeal suturing. Within one year, the da Vinci had been used to perform more complex surgeries including Nissen fundoplication and coronary artery bypass. By 2001, the da Vinci was FDA approved for thoracoscopic surgery and prostate surgery.

Also in 2001, in a remarkable demonstration of the possibilities of telesurgery, Jacques Marescaux performed the first transatlantic cholecystectomy from New York City on a patient in Strasbourg, France [5]. By 2005, surgeons in Canada established the first telesurgery program, performing dozens of operations in remote hospitals in the north from a central facility over 400 km away [6].

In 2015, there were 700,000 robotic surgeries performed worldwide [7]. Today, in the United States, 85% of all prostatectomies are performed with robotic assistance [8]. Industry experts expect the rapid growth to continue, forecasting the 3-billion-dollar-a-year industry to grow to 21 billion by 2021 [7].

While the da Vinci surgical system remains the only device on the market, industry powerhouses have taken notice. Start-ups, industry giants like Medtronic, and even tech giants like Google are all developing their own robotic surgical systems. They will have to contend with Intuitive's nearly 15 years of market monopoly and their newest system, the Xi, released in 2014 and equipped with a markedly improved docking platform and camera versatility.

The future of robotic surgery is limited only by the human imagination. NASA is planning to send surgical robots to the International Space Station. Robots equipped with artificial intelligence are being trained to perform complex surgical tasks without direct human control. By incorporating cross-sectional imaging into the computer, robotics can aide in more precise dissection of difficult tumors. With a bevy of new high tech devices about to hit the market, there is no doubt that the size and scope of robotic surgery will continue to grow.

**Acknowledgement** This work is supported in part by the Foundation for Surgical Fellowships.

## References

1. Lanfranco AR, Castellanos AE, Desai JP, et al. Robotic surgery: a current perpective. Ann Surg. 2004;239:14–21.
2. Rosen J, Hannaford B, Satava RM. Surgical robotics: systems applications, and visions. Berlin: Springer; 2011.
3. Satava RM. Surgical robotics: the early chronicles: a personal historical perspective. Surg Laparosc Endosc Percutan Tech. 2002;12:6–16.
4. Himpens J, Leman G, Cadiere GB. Telesurgical laparoscopic cholecystectomy. Surg Endosc. 1998;12:1091.
5. Marescaux J, Leroy J, Gagner M, et al. Transatlantic robot-assisted telesurgery. Nature. 2001;413:379–80.
6. Anvari M, McKinley C, Stein H. Establishment of the World's first telerobotic remote surgical service: for provision of advanced laparoscopic surgery in a rural community. Ann Surg. 2005;241(3):460–4.
7. Curtiss ET. Surgical robots: market shares, strategy, and forecasts, worldwide, 2015 to 2021. Winter Green Research, Inc: Lexington, MA; 2015.
8. Oberlin DT, Flum AS, Lai JD, Meeks JJ. The effect of minimally invasive prostatectomy on practice patterns of American Urologists. J Urologic Onc. 2016;34(6):255e1–5.

Nathaniel Lytle

## Introduction

Though many individuals, companies, and research institutes have been involved with the development and conception of robotic surgical systems, the currently available robotic platforms come from Intuitive Surgical, Inc. Founded in 1995, Intuitive launched the da Vinci Surgical System in 1999 and was the first system cleared by the FDA for general laparoscopic use [1]. Other companies, such as Titan Medical, Medtronic, and TransEnterix, are currently developing other robotic surgical platforms, but at the time of this writing, the only FDA approved and commercially available robotic system is Intuitive's da Vinci system. Therefore, this chapter will focus on the currently available da Vinci models, Si and Xi, as well as highlight the Single-Site platform.

The da Vinci Surgical System is a robotic surgical platform that allows the surgeon to control robotic arms that use precision instruments through small incisions to perform complex surgical tasks. This is achieved by the use of four key mechanical components of the robotic system. These components (surgeon console, patient-side cart, EndoWrist instruments, and the vision cart) are present in both da Vinci robot models though there are some aspects that are different between the models.

The surgeon console is the operating console that is used to manipulate the robotic arms and instruments (Fig. 15.1). It consists of the display, the wrist support with master controls, and the foot pedal platform. The surgeon is ergonomically seated and can adjust the display, wrist support, and foot pedal platform to a comfortable position. The display provides a three-dimensional (3D), high-definition (HD) view of the operative field. It also provides a heads-up display of

N. Lytle, M.D. (✉)
General Surgery, MIS/Bariatrics, Kaiser Permanente, Southeast Permanente Medical Group, Atlanta, GA, USA
e-mail: nathaniel.w.lytle@kp.org; nathan.lytle@gmail.com

© Springer International Publishing AG 2018                                                    195
A.D. Patel, D. Oleynikov (eds.), *The SAGES Manual of Robotic Surgery*,
The SAGES University Masters Program Series, DOI 10.1007/978-3-319-51362-1_15

**Fig.15.1** Surgeon console illustrating the display (**a**), wrist support with master controls (**b**), and foot pedal platform (**c**). ©2016 Intuitive Surgical, Inc.

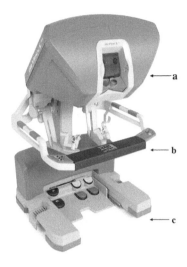

the types of instruments being used, type of energy connected, as well as orientation of the camera. The wrist support, with the master controls, allows seamless translation of hand, wrist, and finger movements into real-time movements of the surgical instruments. The thumb, first, and second fingers are used to manipulate the controls while the wrists are supported by a padded support. The foot pedal platform gives control of the camera and energy devices to the surgeon. Using the left foot, the surgeon can control camera positioning, orientation, and focus. The right foot pedals control energy devices that are connected to the robotic instruments. Both fast and slow energy applications are available depending on the energy device used.

The patient-side cart supports the three or four robotic arms that carry out the surgeon's commands. The arms are attached to a center post that is positioned over the patient with the use of the rolling platform to guide positioning. Once the patient-side cart is in proper position, the arms are docked to trocars that have been placed through the patient's abdominal wall. The docking process then allows the robotic arms to move around fixed pivot points to decrease trauma to the patient's abdominal wall. One arm is used to hold the camera, and the other arms are used to control different types of instruments based on the operation performed.

The EndoWrist instruments allow the surgeon's hand and wrist movements to be replicated at the instrument tips. They are designed with seven degrees of motion that give even more mobility than the human wrist. There are a wide range of instruments available designed for specific tasks, such as dissecting, suturing, grasping, cutting, and coagulating. There are also specialized devices like an ultrasonic scalpel, vessel sealer, and stapler.

The last common component of the da Vinci surgical system is the vision cart. This cart is equipped with a 3D HD image-processing unit that sends the image from the laparoscope to the surgeon console and to a large viewing monitor for the assistant. The monitor is a widescreen 2D image of what the surgeon is seeing at the console. It also provides onscreen indicators of energy being used, types of instruments inserted, and other feedback data. The monitor also provides tools to allow proper setup and configuration of the laparoscope by the OR team.

The following sections will go into depth about these four main components of the da Vinci surgical system and focus on key differences between the currently available models. The Single-Site platform will also be addressed and how it is integrated into the current da Vinci models.

## da Vinci Si Model

The da Vinci Si Model, from Intuitive Surgical, was launched in April 2009 as an advancement from the prior S Model. Three key features of da Vinci surgical systems (3D HD vision, EndoWrist instrumentation, and surgeon console ergonomics) were maintained, but improved upon for this model. Several features where added to this model over the prior. The Si Model allows dual-console capability, enhanced high-definition 3D vision, updated user interface, and OR integration capabilities.

The dual-console option (Fig. 15.2) with the Si Model has allowed improved robotic training and collaboration. Each surgeon sits at a separate console and visualizes the same operative view though the endoscope. Two modes can be used. The teaching mode allows the student surgeon to visualize the movements of the mentoring surgeon and then can be given control of the same instruments at any time. This allows real-time feedback for the trainee, improved safety for the patient, and

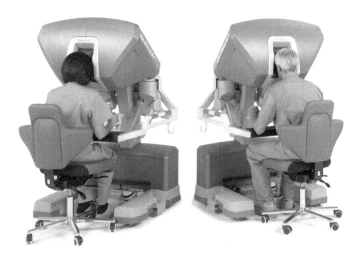

**Fig. 15.2** Dual console. ©2016 Intuitive Surgical, Inc.

improves operative times over teaching on a single console [2, 3]. The collaborative mode allows two surgeons to operate at the same time. One surgeon will perform the primary operation, while the assistant surgeon performs retraction or counter-traction. This mode allows all working arms to be used in concert.

The enhancement of the optics and console display of the Si Model is another improvement from the prior model. The 3D image now has enhanced HD, giving the surgeon the ability to see anatomic structures with more natural colors, up to 10× magnification, and with more clarity than before. 3D visualization has been shown to improve surgeon skill and efficiency at performing certain tasks when compared to traditional 2D visualization from a standard laparoscope [4]. This 3D view and image enhancement provide a superior advantage over standard laparos-copy in terms of anatomic visualization of the operative field.

Intuitive Surgical made improvements to the surgeon interface with the robotic system with the Si Model as well. In addition to the enhancement of the visual reso-lution provided to the surgeon, a few more modifications were made. Improved ergonomic settings of the surgeon console allow adjustment of the display, wrist board, and footswitch panel. The display position can be modified in four different parameters to allow the surgeon to find the most ergonomic position for his or her neck and upper back. An integrated surgeon control interface on the wrist board gives control of the video, audio, and system settings to the surgeon. The settings are then stored with a unique user profile so that the individualized settings can be recalled for future cases.

Control of the robotic arms and EndoWrist instruments has been enhanced with the Si Model. The master controllers allow precise, dexterous control using scaling algorithms that enable adjustments of hand to instrument movement ratios. These adjustments and scaling provide precise, fluid motion while elimi-nating the natural twitch of the human hand. The foot pedal platform enables full control of the camera, instrument swapping, and energy. Different types of energy can be utilized depending on the instrument types used and the pedals that are pushed. The foot pedal platform is also scalable to support future advancements in robotic instrumentation.

As with any new technology, adoption into the OR setting can be difficult, inef-ficient, and time consuming. This leads to longer OR times, higher cost, and less efficient use of resources. To address these concerns, the Si Model has enhance-ments that focus on OR efficiency, ease of use, and simple time saving setup. First, the 3D HD camera head is more lightweight, with integrated controls for focus, illumination, and scope setup. This allows one person to fully prepare the camera once it is connected. The patient-side cart is motor driven to help facilitate a quicker and more controlled dock (Fig. 15.3). The robotic arm drapes are a one-piece system with built-in instrument adapter to allow more efficient draping of the patient cart. The communication lines for the three components (vision cart, patient cart, and surgeon console) have been designed to allow one-step cable connections, which again will save time and allow quick and efficient setup in the OR. The Si Model is a robust option for robotic surgery and is currently the most used model by da Vinci.

**Fig. 15.3** Patient Cart of
the da Vinci Si Model.
©2016 Intuitive Surgical,
Inc.

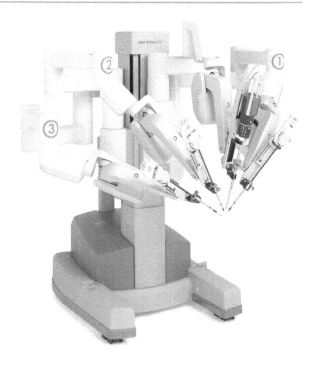

## da Vinci Model Xi

The fourth generation of the da Vinci surgical system was FDA approved on April 1, 2014, and unveiled at the annual SAGES meeting in Salt Lake City, UT. This model was met with much anticipation due to the expected advancements in technology that would lead to a more efficient setup, greater adaptability to multi-quadrant operations, and simplified use. Moving from the Si to the Xi Model, Intuitive made improvements to all core technologies of the surgical system resulting in a system that is more advanced but also scalable to future innovations.

First, the view at the surgeon console was upgraded with new heads-up displays that can orient the surgeon to instruments out of the field of vision, decreasing unwanted contact of the instruments with surrounding structures (Fig. 15.4). The same 3D HD magnified image remains as the hallmark of the improved visualization gained with robotic surgery. The same ergonomic adjustments to the display, wrist board, and foot pedal platform are maintained. The control screen on the wrist board now allows further functionality in regard to controlling the more advanced laparoscope, such as the ability to flip from a 30° downward view to a 30° upward view with the touch of a button. The majority of the changes for the Xi model come in the patient-side cart and vision cart.

The patient-side cart was redesigned into a lighter, more mobile, and easier to position platform (Fig. 15.5). The robotic arms are now placed on a boom system that can be extended out over the patient and rotated so that docking the patient-side

**Fig. 15.4** Surgeon
Console for da Vinci Xi
Model. ©2016 Intuitive
Surgical, Inc.

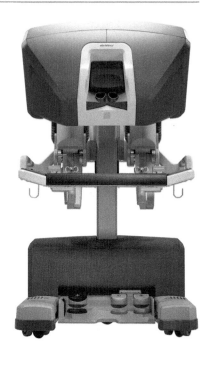

**Fig. 15.5** da Vinci Xi
patient-side cart. ©2016
Intuitive Surgical, Inc.

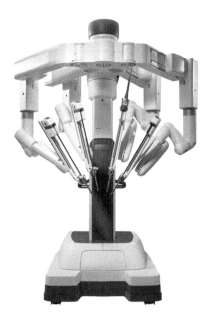

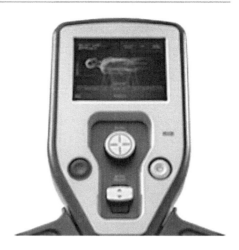

**Fig. 15.6**  da Vinci Xi patient-side cart interface with one-button setup and targeting system. ©2016 Intuitive Surgical, Inc.

cart can be done from any side or angle of the patient. This allows full access to the patient for the operative staff, ease of setup, and improved mobility to allow four-quadrant access without having to reposition the patient. This advancement has added more flexibility and ease when performing highly complex operations in multi-quadrants. In addition to placing the robotic arms on a boom, the arms themselves have been redesigned. The arms are lighter, thinner, and allow a longer reach with more range of motion. This again allows simplified and safer multi-quadrant surgery, as well as a more flexible port placement. Another innovation that was added to simplify the patient-side cart is a one-button setup (Fig. 15.6). This provides a guided walkthrough with voice assistance to help the OR staff safely and efficiently place the patient-side cart into position. Once the patient-side cart has been placed into position, the camera can be attached to any arm, pointed at the target anatomy, and the targeting system will arrange the boom and remainder of the robot arms for most efficient configuration for the operation being performed. This allows quick, optimal setup of the robotic arms.

The vision cart and laparoscope have had major advancements as well. The laparoscope from prior models came in multiple components that needed to be assembled and configured correctly for optimal picture quality. The camera head was relatively heavy and needed to be draped for the case. The Xi endoscope now is an integrated handheld design that needs no calibration, white balancing, focusing, or draping, allowing time-saving setup and simplicity (Fig. 15.7). Firefly Fluorescence imaging has also been added as a standard feature to the laparoscopes. With the use of injectable indocyanine green (ICG) and Firefly imaging technology, tissue perfusion, lymph node identification, and visualization of biliary structures can be performed with a simple toggle of the clutch button on the surgeon master controller. The use of Firefly technology is an advancing area of research in the fields of foregut, colorectal, oncologic, and biliary surgery [5–7]. The laparoscope is now an 8 mm scope, which allows it to be placed through any robotically docked trocar. This provides increased flexibility for visualizing the operative field. The vision cart also received improvements (Fig. 15.8). The mounted screen is now larger and wider, with touchscreen capabilities for a better picture and more functionality for

**Fig. 15.7** da Vinci Xi
laparoscope. ©2016
Intuitive Surgical, Inc.

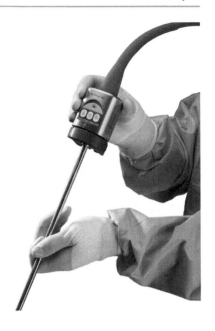

**Fig. 15.8** Vision cart for
da Vinci Xi Model. ©2016
Intuitive Surgical, Inc.

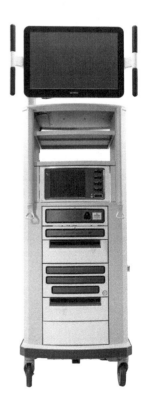

the assistant and OR staff. The vision cart also has integrated energy for EndoWrist instruments that are capable of delivering energy. The generator manages mono and bipolar energy by setting the desired tissue effect.

The Xi Model was designed with future advancements in mind. This platform is constructed to allow seamless integration of future innovations. Therefore, as new instruments, simulators, and software upgrades are developed, they can easily be added to the current surgical system.

## da Vinci Single-Site Platform

Single-site laparoscopic surgery continues to be a viable option for certain procedures and surgeons. When it was first introduced, there was a wave of attempts to incorporate the technique into broad use due to early studies showing better cosmetic outcomes and faster recovery [8, 9]. Without larger scale studies, these conclusions still need to be proven. Nevertheless, interest and advancement of the technique remain. Laparoscopic single-site procedures have significant obstacles, mostly due to instrument clashes, inferior retraction of the operative field, and surgeon fatigue and discomfort due to poor body positioning and increased strain on instruments. Using the da Vinci Single-Site platform can eliminate the majority of these shortcomings [10]. The platform was initially designed for the Si Model, but recently has been validated for use with the Xi Model as well. The platform uses a specifically designed port, curved cannulas that cross within the port, software that reassigns the surgeon's hands to the corresponding robotic arms, and semi-rigid instruments that follow the curve of the cannulas (Fig. 15.9).

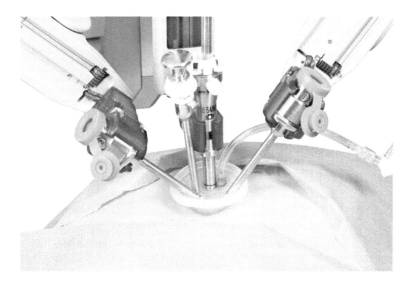

**Fig. 15.9** Docked position of the Single-Site platform. ©2016 Intuitive Surgical, Inc.

**Fig. 15.10** Single-Site setup showing port and crossing of curved cannulas. ©2016 Intuitive Surgical, Inc.

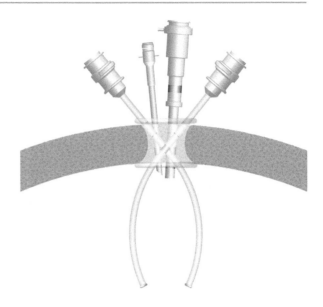

The da Vinci Single-Site Port consists of five lumens, providing access for two instruments, an 8 or 8.5 mm 3D HD laparoscope, a 5 or 10 mm accessory port, and the insufflation adaptor. The port is designed to fit through a 1.5 cm incision, usually at the umbilicus for best cosmetic results. Once the port is in place and pneumoperitoneum is achieved, two 5 mm curved instrument cannulas are introduced into the field. The cannulas cross each other to optimize triangulation and minimize external instrument collisions, as well as allowing better range of motion and decreasing instrument crowding at the target anatomy (Fig. 15.10). With these improvements, robotic single-site surgery is now more comfortable, flexible, and adaptable to a growing number of procedures.

## Non-FDA-Approved Systems

Two other companies are developing and testing new robotic systems at this time. Titan Medical and TransEnterix are making major progress to commercially release their robotic platforms. Currently, Titan Medical is developing the SPORT Surgical System, which consists of a single incision robotic platform and a surgeon workstation with 3D HD visualization. It is pending FDA approval, and expected to be commercially available in late 2016 in Europe and in mid-2017 in the United States. This system is designed to expand robotic surgery to a broader field of surgery and surgery centers in a cost-effective manner [11]. TransEnterix is in development of the ALF-X Surgical Robotic System, as well as the SurgiBot System. The ALF-X system consists of a surgeon console that provides 3D HD visualization, camera control with eye tracking technology, and haptic feedback of the surgical instruments. It is a multiport platform that has separate robotic arm units, which replicate laparoscopic motion and port placement. The SurgiBot system comprises a patient-side cart, which allows single incision surgery with flexible instruments that are directly controlled by the surgeon in the sterile operative field. A 3D HD monitor provides the operative view with the use of 3D glasses. The company and products are still in the development phase with no advertised timetable for commercial release at this time [12].

## Conclusion

Robotic surgical systems have seen rapid growth, advancement, and adoption of use in the past 20 years, with only more options and innovations on the way. Currently, Intuitive Surgical leads the way in the development and implementation of robotic platforms. The available da Vinci Si and Xi Models, along with the Single-Site configuration, give surgeons safe, flexible, yet advanced options for minimally invasive procedures. 3D HD visualization, favorable surgeon ergonomics, and EndoWrist instrumentation are the core technologic advantages that robotic surgical systems provide. In addition to the da Vinci Models, there are other systems that are in development, which continue to push innovation, advancement, and adaptability of the field of robotic surgery.

## References

1. IntuitiveSurgical.com [Internet]. Sunnyvale (CA): Intuitive Surgical Inc; c2016 [cited 2016 Apr 20]. Available from: http://www.intuitivesurgical.com
2. Morgan M, Shakir NA, Garcia M, Ozayar A, Gahan JC, Friedlander J, et al. Single versus dual-console robot-assisted radical prostatectomy: impact on intraoperative and postoperative outcomes in a teaching institution. World J Urol. 33(6):781–6.
3. Smith AL, Erwin S, Krivak TC, Olawaiye AB, Chu T, Richard SD. Dual-console robotic surgery: a new teaching paradigm. J Robot Surg. 2013;7(2):113–8.
4. Chang L, Satava RM, Pellegrini CA, Sinanan MN. Robotic surgery: identifying the learning curve through objective measurement of skill. Surg Endosc. 2003;17(11):1744–8.
5. Hellan M, Spinoglio G, Pigazzi A, Lagares-Garcia JA. The influence of fluorescence imaging on the location of bowel transection during robotic left-sided colorectal surgery. Surg Endosc. 2014;28(5):1695–702.
6. Sarkaria IS, Bains MS, Finley DJ, Adusumilli PS, Huang J, Rusch VW, et al. Intraoperative near-infrared fluorescence imaging as an adjunct to robotic-assisted minimally invasive esophagectomy. Innovations. 2014;9(5):391–3.
7. Alander, J, et al. A review of indocyanine green fluorescent imaging in surgery. Int J Biomed Imaging. 2012; article 7.
8. Raman SR et al. Does transumbilical single incision laparoscopic adjustable gastric banding result in decreased pain medicine use? A case-matched study. Surg Obes Relat Dis. 7(2):129–33.
9. Chow A et al. Single-incision laparoscopic surgery for cholecystectomy: a retrospective comparison with 4-port laparoscopic cholecystectomy. Arch Surg. 145:1187–91.
10. Kroh M, El-Hayek K, Rosenblatt S, Chand B, Escobar P, Kaouk J, et al. First human surgery with a novel single-port robotic system: cholecystectomy using the da Vinci Single-Site platform. Surg Endosc. 2011 Nov;25:3566.
11. TitanMedicalInc.com [Internet]. Toronto, Canada: Titan Medical Inc; c2016 [cited 2016 Apr 20]. Available from: http://www.titanmedicalinc.com
12. TransEnterix.com [Internet]. Morrisville (NC): TransEnterix Inc; c2016 [cited 2016 Apr 20]. Available from: http://www.transenterix.com

# System Control Overview and Instruments

16

Jamil Luke Stetler

## Introduction

Science and technology have always been and will always be driving forces in the field of medicine. The evolution of surgery itself has been accelerated by advancements in technology as well. In our lifetime, we have seen the field of surgery grow from open to minimally invasive procedures. Within the last decade we have seen multiple advancements within the arena of minimally invasive surgery from standard laparoscopy to now robotic-assisted surgery. The catalyst for the development of these innovations has largely been to improve patient outcomes: improve recovery time, shorten hospital stays, decrease postoperative pain, decrease complications, etc.

With robotic surgery there have been additional benefits largely for the surgeon, including better visualization (3D), increased dexterity provided by wristed instruments, improved surgeon comfort, and improved ergonomics that may increase the surgeon's career. The advancements of robotic surgery in the field of minimally invasive surgery are not a revolution, but more of an evolution of the surgical techniques created by the founding surgeons of laparoscopy. Surgeons should use the robotic surgery tools to enhance their technique in order to provide patients with optimal outcomes. At the end of the day, the most important goal for a surgeon is to provide the technique that in their hands provides the best outcome they are capable of with the lowest risk for patient morbidity and mortality.

---

For more details on the Si and Xi platforms training modules at https://www.davincisurgerycommunity.com can be reviewed, login required.

All images were adapted from http://www.intuitivesurgical.com/products/instruments/with permission from Intuitive Surgical.

J.L. Stetler, B.S., M.D. (✉)
General Surgery, Emory University Hospital,
1365 Clifton Rd., NE., Atlanta, GA 30322, USA
e-mail: jstetle@emory.edu

© Springer International Publishing AG 2018
A.D. Patel, D. Oleynikov (eds.), *The SAGES Manual of Robotic Surgery*,
The SAGES University Masters Program Series, DOI 10.1007/978-3-319-51362-1_16

207

## da Vinci Systems

As discussed in the previous chapter, there are three iterations of the da Vinci system that have each seen incremental improvements. In this chapter, we will focus on the two newest and most commonly used versions, which are the Si and Xi systems. We will review the system components which include the Surgeon console, Patient cart, and vision cart (Fig. 16.1). We will also discuss the robotic instrumentation.

## Surgeon Console

The surgeon console is the control center for the robotic platform. From the surgeon console, the surgeon can control the endoscope and instruments by using the hand controls and footswitch panel. All actions taken by the surgeon at the console are relayed to the vision system for processing and sent to the patient cart for implementation. The surgeon console is made up of several components that are similar on the two latest versions of the robotic system (Si/Xi): stereoviewer, master controllers, touchpad, and the footswitch panel (Fig. 16.2). One of the added benefits of the surgeon console is that it can be paired with a second console to allow two surgeons to work simultaneously on the same patient (Fig. 16.3). This feature can be used to collaborate with other surgeons, for proctoring, and for teaching.

The stereoviewer provides a high definition 3D view of the surgical field that can be magnified up to 10× (Fig. 16.2). The stereoviewer is ergonomically designed to support the surgeons head and neck during surgical procedures. Additionally, the stereoviewer displays messages and icons to the user about the system status.

The master controllers use fingertip controls that allow the surgeon to control the endowristed instruments and endoscope (Fig. 16.4). They are also designed with ergonomics in mind to optimize the comfort of the surgeon. The surgeon's

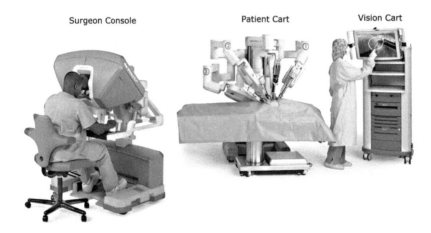

**Fig. 16.1** Surgeon console, patient cart, and vision cart

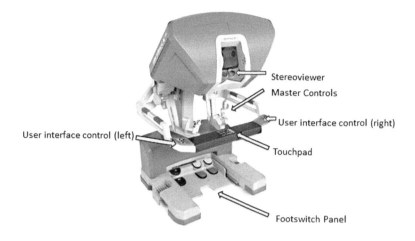

Fig. 16.2  Surgeon console — stereoviewer, master controls, touchpad, and footswitch panel

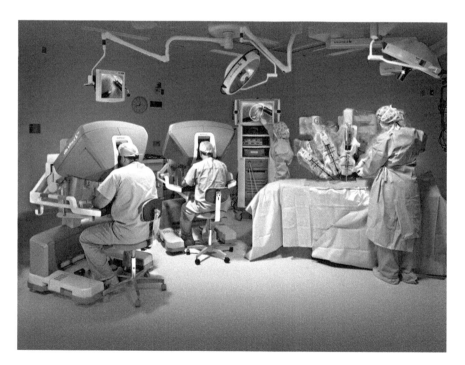

Fig. 16.3  Dual console

movements are instantaneously replicated at the patient cart while also filtering out potential hand tremors. With the addition of motion scaling the surgeon can fine tune the hand-to-instrument movement ratios to their choosing.

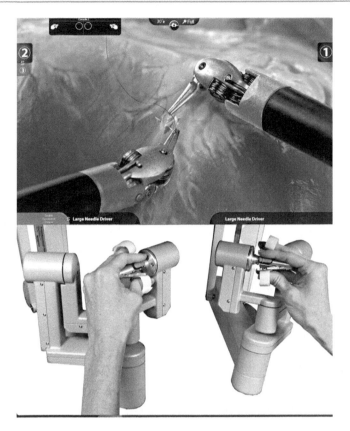

**Fig. 16.4** Master controls

The user interface controls are housed in pods on the left and right side of the surgeon console arm rest (Fig. 16.2). The left sided pod contains the ergonomic control levers that allow the surgeon to adjust the height and tilt of the stereoviewer, adjust the armrest up or down, and move the footswitch panel in or out. The user's unique settings can be saved and when the user logs into the system they are automatically recalled. The right sided pod contains the power button and emergency stop button.

A touch pad is located in the center of the surgeon console armrest (Fig. 16.2). The touchpad can be used by the surgeon to save and access their own user preferences and ergonomic settings. Again, when the surgeon logs into the system their system preferences and ergonomic settings will automatically be recalled. After logging in, a home screen will appear that gives the surgeon access to surgeon console controls and settings. Along the bottom of the screen, there are tabs for accessing video, audio, and utility preferences. The video tab gives the surgeon the ability to adjust brightness, make advanced video adjustments, modify camera and endoscope setup, and access display preferences. The audio tab allows for volume adjustments and/or muting the surgeon console microphone. The utility tab allows entry into account management, inventory management, event logs, and control

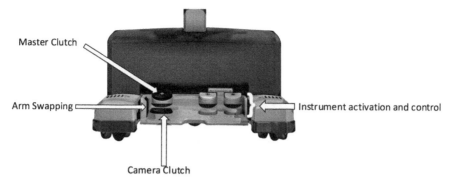

**Fig. 16.5** Footswitch panel components

preferences; scaling, finger clutch, TilePro QuickClick, haptic zoom, master associations. There are also three quick settings buttons down the middle of the touchpad that contain settings for scope angle, zoom level in the stereoviewer, and motion scaling.

Lastly, the footswitch panel is used by the surgeon for robotic arm swapping, master clutching, cameral control, and instrument activation and control (Fig. 16.5). The left lateral pedal allows the user to swap control of the instrument arms so the user can control a different instrument arm with one of their master controllers. This is done by tapping the pedal with the side of your foot. The left upper pedal is a master clutch pedal and can be used to decouple the masters from the controls of the instruments which allows the user to relocate the masters for improved comfort. The left lower pedal is the camera clutch and allows the user to control the focus and position of the endoscope. The right sided foot pedals are used for instrument activation and control. For example, the right sided foot pedals can be used by the surgeon to activate the coagulation function of a vessel sealer as well as the cutting function when necessary.

## Patient Cart Components

The patient cart is composed of several components. The setup joints position the robotic arms to optimize range of motion for the endowristed instruments and endoscope (Figs. 16.6 and 16.7). The instrument arms and the camera arm(s) on the Si and Xi systems interface with the robotic instruments and the camera assembly. The instrument and camera arms are draped for sterility and allow the surgeons and/or assistant to attach and adjust the robotic instruments and camera assembly at bedside. The instrument and camera arms also give the surgeon control over the robotic instruments and endoscope. The robotic arms use remote center technology, allowing the instruments and camera assembly to move around a fixed point in space. LEDs on top of the robotic arms provide feedback on the arm status to the surgeon/assistant.

The greatest difference between the Si and Xi systems lies with the patient cart (Figs. 16.6 and 16.7). One of the enhancements to the patient cart is the adjustable column and overhead boom. The boom is an adjustable support structure from

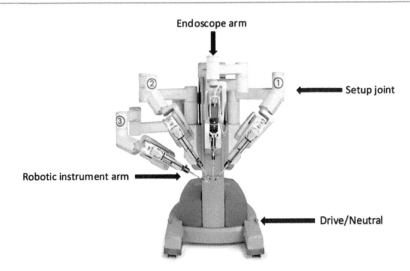

**Fig. 16.6** Si patient cart

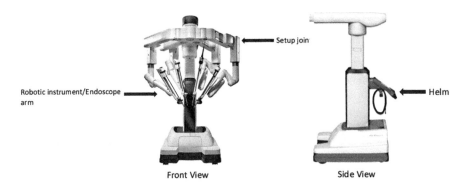

**Fig. 16.7** Xi patient cart

which the robotic arms are now attached. The boom allows easier docking, extended range of motion, as well as more flexibility with patient positioning. The docking process has also been enhanced with the use of a laser pointing system that helps direct arm placement. The arms on the Xi system are also smaller, lighter, and now universal, meaning the instruments and endoscopes can be used interchangeably in any of the robotic arms. Additional upgrades to the endoscope have also been made. The endoscope no longer needs calibration, white balance, or draping.

There are several differences in the patient cart drive controls between the Si and Xi systems. First, we will discuss the Si system. The shift switches and motor drive control the movement of the patient cart. The shift switches allow the patient cart to be moved manually (N) or with a motor drive (D) (Fig. 16.6). Manual mode is for moving the patient cart long distances, for example, moving the cart from OR to OR. Motor drive is designed to provide faster and easier docking and quick OR reconfiguration. Drive (D) is also used to set the patient cart brakes. An unsterile OR staff member will drive the patient cart into the desired location for docking. The Xi system's patient cart is moved using the helm (Fig. 16.7). The helm has a touch screen that is used for guided setup. The assistant will select the target anatomy as well as the cart position. Next, the deploy for docking icon is selected. The boom will simultaneously raise, pivot, extend, and rotate into position and audio feedback will notify the staff that deployment is complete. Once deployed the staff member will drive the cart into position over the patient using the helm. A laser-guiding system assists in positioning of the patient cart.

## Vision Cart Components

The Si system vision cart is composed of the CORE, illuminator, camera assembly, camera control unit, touch screen, and tank holder (Fig. 16.8). The endoscope provides a 3D, HD image of the surgical field. The video travels through the endoscope cable to the vision system. The vision system components process the video feed and send the feed to the touch screen monitor as well as the surgeon console 3D viewer. The CORE is the processing center for the robotic system. The system cables, auxiliary equipment, and AV connections are channeled through the CORE. The illuminator is the light source for the endoscope which is supplied via a single fiber optic cable. The front panel controls are used to power on the lamp as well as adjusting the light output. The camera assembly contains an integrated light guide cable for illuminating the surgical field and provides a 3D, HD view that can be magnified up to 10×. The camera control unit acquires and processes images from the camera assembly. A touch screen on the vision cart provides audio and

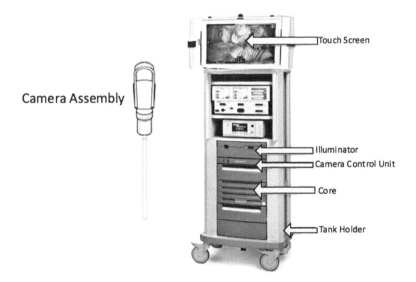

**Fig. 16.8** Si vision cart

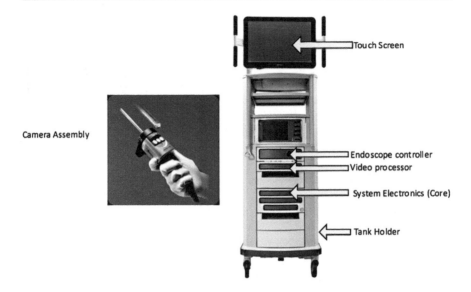

**Fig. 16.9** Xi vision cart

video controls patient side. Additionally, the touch screen is capable of telestration which can be used to guide the surgeon during a case. Lastly, the tank holder is housed on the vision cart for storing insufflation tanks.

The Xi system vision cart is similarly to the Si systems, but there are a few differences. The Xi system vision cart is composed of system electronics (CORE), endoscope controller, video processor, camera assembly, touch screen, and tank holder (Fig. 16.9). The systems electronics (CORE) on the Xi system also processes all the information from each system component. The endoscope cable is connected to the endoscope controller, which provides the light source for illuminating the surgical field. It also contains the electronics for the initial processing of the endoscopic video. The video processor contains a USB port that allows the staff to capture images from a procedure onto a flash drive. The camera assembly for the Xi system has an integrated design and does not require draping, focusing, white balance, or calibration. The touch screen again provides a view of the surgical field at the patient side. The touch screen also gives the OR staff the ability to adjust audio, video, and system settings controls as well as telestration capabilities.

## Robotic Endoscopes, Trocars, and Instruments

The robotic endoscope is a dual-channel laparoscope that generates a three-dimensional (3D) high definition image for the surgeon. The endoscopes come in 8.5 and 12 mm sizes as well as 0° and 30° angles. Additionally, da Vinci® now offers scopes with integrated fluorescence imaging, also known as Firefly, which can assist in identifying anatomy using near-infrared technology.

The abdominal cavity is accessed in the same fashion as laparoscopic surgery. Robotic reusable trocars are available from 5 to 13 mm sizes. The robotic endoscopes can be used with standard 12 mm laparoscopic ports or can be used with their respected robotic reusable trocars. The robotic instruments must be used with the robotic reusable trocar cannulas. Once the trocars are placed they can be docked with the patient cart. Once docked the endowristed instruments and endoscope can be inserted.

One of the greatest benefits afforded by the robotic surgery platform is the endowristed instruments. The endowristed instruments are designed to mimic the dexterity of the human wrist (Fig. 16.10). Most of the robotic instruments are designed with seven degrees of freedom (insertion, external pitch, external yaw, rotation, wristed pitch, wristed yaw, and grasp) and 90° of articulation which give the surgeon a tremendous range of motion. This is an advantage over standard laparoscopic instruments as it may lower the learning curve for surgeons performing complex minimally invasive tasks, and in some instances it allows the surgeon to perform tasks that may not be possible laparoscopically. The endowristed instruments provide the surgeons additional angles to approach dissections and to operate more precisely in confined spaces.

The robotic catalog of instruments is robust and has instrument offerings that parallel those in laparoscopy, offering tools for grasping, retracting, suturing, dissecting, dividing tissue, hemostasis, aspirating, clipping, as well as stapling. Some of the instruments can be paired with energy in order to perform electrosurgery, while the platform also offers its own vessel sealer. The most common sized instruments are 8 mm, but some of the robotic instruments come in 5 and 12 mm sizes as well. Unlike the majority of laparoscopic instruments, the robotic instruments do have a limited number of uses. The number of uses left on an instrument can be visualized at the surgeon console. Next, we will briefly review some of the more commonly utilized robotic instruments.

**Fig. 16.10** Endowristed instrument

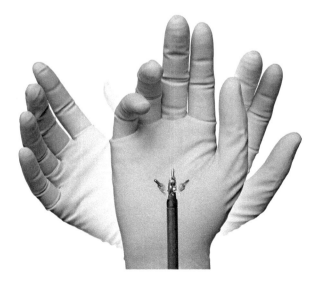

**Fig. 16.11** Cadiere grasper

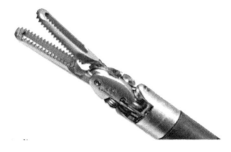

**Fig. 16.12** Double fenestrated grasper

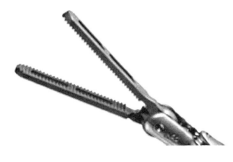

**Fig. 16.13** ProGrasp™

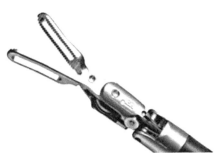

The robotic platform has a variety of grasping forceps that are designed for various tissue types. The Cadiere (Fig. 16.11) and Double fenestrated graspers (Fig. 16.12) can be utilized for grasping finer tissue like peritoneum and bowel. For denser or more fibrous tissue, a ProGrasp™ (Fig. 16.13) can be utilized as it has more grip strength. A traumatic grasper such as the Cobra (Fig. 16.14) is designed with teeth at the tip of its jaws that can be utilized for securing thicker tissue or organs that one plans on excising, for example, retracting the fundus of an inflamed and/or distended gallbladder.

There is also a variety of instruments for suturing. Two examples are the Mega™ needle driver (Fig. 16.15) and Mega SutureCut™ (Fig. 16.16). The Mega™ needle driver is used solely for suturing, while the Mega SutureCut™ has built in scissors in the heel of the instrument so that I can be used for suturing and cutting. This dual ability instruments advantage is that it may decrease the number of instrument exchanges during cases.

**Fig. 16.14**  Cobra grasper

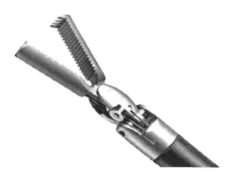

**Fig. 16.15**  Mega™ needle driver

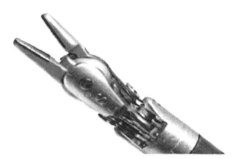

**Fig. 16.16**  Mega SutureCut™

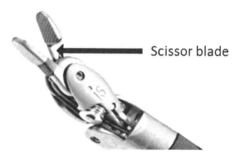

Scissor blade

For electrosurgery, there is an assortment of instruments that can be paired with energy. This includes monopolar instruments such as Hot Shears™ (Fig. 16.17) and the Permanent cautery hook (Fig. 16.18). Some examples of bipolar instruments are Maryland bipolar forceps (Fig. 16.19), PK® dissecting forceps (Fig. 16.20), Fenestrated bipolar forceps (Fig. 16.21), and the Vessel sealer (Fig. 16.22). For ultrasonic shears, the system also carries the Harmonic ACE® curved shears (Fig. 16.23).

Several specialty instruments also exist. Those most commonly used for general surgery procedures included the robotic suction/irrigator (Fig. 16.24) and clip appliers. The clip appliers come in small, medium-large, and large sizes. The small clip applier supports Weck HemoClip® small titanium clips (Fig. 16.25). The medium-large (Fig. 16.26) and large (Fig. 16.27) clip appliers utilize Weck Hem-o-lock medium-large and large polymer clips, respectively.

**Fig. 16.17** Hot Shears™

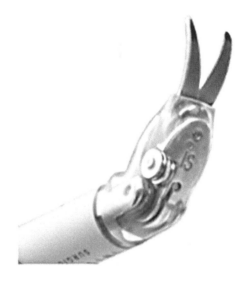

**Fig. 16.18** Permanent cautery hook

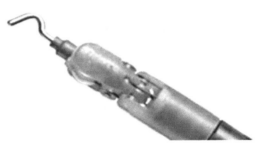

**Fig. 16.19** Maryland bipolar forceps

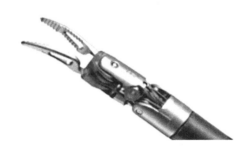

**Fig. 16.20** PK® dissecting forceps

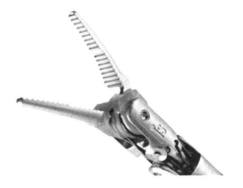

**Fig. 16.21**  Fenestrated
bipolar forceps

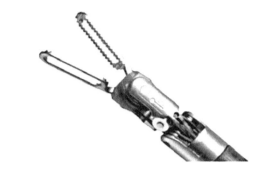

**Fig. 16.22**  Vessel sealer

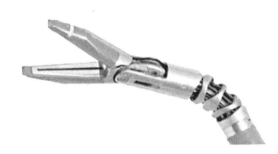

**Fig. 16.23**  Harmonic
ACE® curved shears

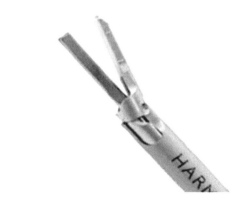

**Fig. 16.24**  Suction/
irrigator

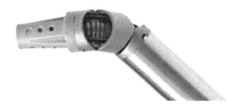

**Fig. 16.25** Small clip
applier

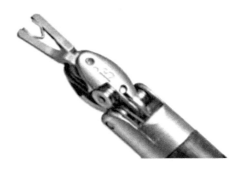

**Fig. 16.26** Medium-large
clip applier

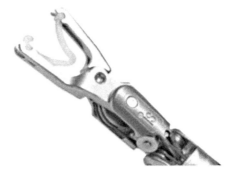

**Fig. 16.27** Large clip
applier

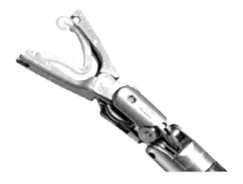

# Starting and Developing a Robotic Program

**17**

Lava Y. Patel and Ankit D. Patel

## Introduction

There are several views on how to develop and maintain a successful robotics program. Administration may support a program for marketing purposes or oppose one secondary to costs. Many surgeons support having a program for similar reasons, but may struggle to expand the program without further training or maintaining quality across specialties. The purpose of this chapter is not how to start a program, but to focus specifically on maintaining a successful program, especially with training and credentialing. These are the true cornerstones of maintaining quality and ultimately will lead to a successful robotics program. In addition, we will focus on training in an academic setting since the majority of graduating surgical residents and fellows are interested in robotics.

## Building a Robotic Program

The first major obstacle of starting a program is having a robotic system. Currently, only one commercial system is available in the United States, which is the da Vinci Surgical System (Intuitive Surgical). Per the company, over 3600 systems are around the world, with over 2/3 in the United States alone. Several promising platforms from Titan Medical, TransEnterix, Medtronic, and even Google are in the works or are close to acquiring FDA approval; however, it may be several years before they become mainstream and will have likely have their own unique issues.

L.Y. Patel, M.D. • A.D. Patel, M.D., F.A.C.S.(✉)
Department of General & Gastrointestinal Surgery, Emory University School of Medicine, Atlanta, GA, USA
e-mail: apatel7@emory.edu

© Springer International Publishing AG 2018
A.D. Patel, D. Oleynikov (eds.), *The SAGES Manual of Robotic Surgery*,
The SAGES University Masters Program Series, DOI 10.1007/978-3-319-51362-1_17

As a result, the foundation of a new program must be a solid business plan. The cost of one of the current systems can range from $1.5 to 2.4 million US depending on the type, functionality, or options included. Additionally, there are yearly maintenance contracts that average around $150,000 US. Instruments are disposable and can cost $200–500 US per use, on average. The costs add up quickly and will likely consume most if not all of a system's capital budget. Infrastructure may need to be updated to handle the size and weight of the system and its components. Staff members will need to be trained to handle the equipment, especially sterilization. At one of our local institutions that did not previously have a robotic system, the estimated cost for a new dual console Xi system with initial capital equipment was over $2.6 million US in the first year alone. That makes it nearly impossible for any single service line or department to ask for a new system; therefore, it is essential to have a multi-department and/or multi-surgeon approach when developing a plan for acquisition. Markets will vary across the country, but it is vital that there be adequate surgical volume that can be supported by a new system. Other aspects of a successful business plan should include the different types of new cases that could be accomplished with the robotic platform (more minimally invasive options), potential yearly case volume, and potential expansion into other services.

The most important part of any successful program is invested perioperative staff. This includes not only the surgeons, but also the first assistants, surgical scrub techs, operating room nurses, and anesthesia staff. It is also key to identify one or two people who can function as a coordinator to facilitate scheduling cases, help train and build a dedicated robotics team, and collect case data and metrics. This will eventually lead to improvements in efficiency, team-building, and case outcomes. The above holds true for all surgical cases, but is essential in robotics due to the nature of the specialized equipment and demands of the system.

## Training

The number of robotic-assisted general surgery cases being performed around the world, especially in the United States, continues to rise each year (Fig. 17.1) [1–3]. According to Intuitive Surgical, robot utilization in general surgery has seen significant growth over the past 5 years, being led by use in hernia repair and colorectal procedures [3].

A recent survey of current general surgery residents in the United States showed that more than 96% of respondents were training at an institution where a surgical robotic was available [4]. With continued interest and increase in surgical case volumes at these centers, training general surgery residents to use the robotic platform is necessary to keep up with current trends. Obtaining the appropriate level of training to safely perform robotic surgery varies based on the technical aspects related to different specialties and operations being performed. However, fundamental knowledge of how the robot works, attaining technical experience, and knowledge of troubleshooting are of utmost importance. Over the past few decades, since the adoption of laparoscopy, the Fundamentals of Laparoscopic Surgery (FLS) has been

# US Procedure Trend

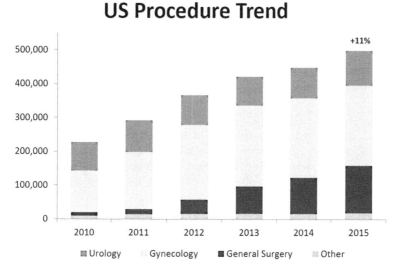

**Fig. 17.1** Estimated number of robot-assisted cases performed in the United States. (Data from Intuitive Surgical, Investor Presentation, 2016. Available at: http://investor.intuitivesurgical.com/ phoenix.zhtml%3fc%3D122359%26p%3Dirol-irhome. Accessed November 2016)

developed by the Society of American Gastrointestinal and Endoscopic Surgeons (SAGES) to ensure that all general surgery trainees have a minimum understanding and the ability to demonstrate a basic grasp of laparoscopic skills. More recently, a similar certification process for acquiring basic endoscopic skills, the Fundamentals of Endoscopic Surgery (FES), has emerged. FLS and FES certifications are now required by the American Board of Surgery (ABS) for all general surgery trainees to be eligible for board certification. No such curriculum currently exists for robotic surgery, but societies like the American Society of Colon and Rectal Surgeons (ASCRS), Society for Robotic Surgery (SRS), and SAGES are taking the lead to develop a similar, unified program.

As the da Vinci system is presently the only commercially available robotic platform with FDA approval, we will base our discussion on this system. Currently and in the past, Intuitive Surgical offers a robotic training certification course to all surgeons or trainees new to the platform. The components of the course include completing online training modules, a systems overview course, simulator exercises, and case observations, all of which could take months to complete. This is followed by a course that costs approximately $5000 USD and spans 2 days, during which time participants engage in didactic lectures, live instruction, simulation practice, and some degree of case performance on cadaveric or porcine specimens. At the end of the course, Intuitive issues a certificate stating that you have successfully completed their basic requirements for knowing how to use their platform. The certification does not make any mention (nor does it intend to) in any way that one can safely perform robotic surgery from a medicolegal standpoint. That decision is usually deferred to the surgeon's hospital credentialing committee or robotics steering committee.

As mentioned before, there are no established protocols or minimum requirements for robotic training in general surgery residency, but several academic institutions across the country have attempted to develop a protocol or curriculum to expose their trainees to basic robotic technology [5, 6]. Training of new robotic surgeons should entail both technical and nontechnical skills, including decision-making, troubleshooting, and effective communication [7]. Protocols may vary based on the specialty and should ideally be individualized based on level of training, technical proficiency, and procedures. However, we recommend that at a minimum, basic training in robotic skills should include the following:

*On Line training*—Intuitive Surgical provides free online interactive training modules that introduce learners to the various components of the robotic platform, common applications, and troubleshooting tips. Modules contain questions that assess retention of relevant information and trainees are issued a certificate of completion after all modules have been successfully completed with a minimum allotted score (https://www.davincisurgerycommunity.com/).

*Console-based simulation training*—learners should next proceed to simulation training to obtain hands-on experience with the functionality of the robotic platform. Simulation allows for progress through the learning curve and has been shown to be transferable to the clinical setting [8]. Several simulators are available (*See below section on Virtual Reality Simulation for further details*), and all have a variety of exercises dedicated to technical training for camera clutching, instrument manipulation and switching, tissue handling, and use of surgical energy.

*Bedside training*—under supervision, learners should be aware of all aspects involved with proper and optimal setup to provide safe and efficient care while being able to maximize the utility of robotic technology. Bedside training should include, but not limited to, instruction on the following:

- Operating room setup and patient position
- Choice of port placement based on case
- Effective communication with operative staff when docking the robot at bedside
- Docking robotic arms to patient ports and instrument insertion and troubleshooting
- Principles of instrument exchange/camera manipulation
- Assistant port site selection and utilization
- Bedside first assistant for at least ten cases—Total cases as a bed-side assistant may vary but trainees should be able to demonstrate a grasp of the above and be able to safely assist with bedside maneuvers.

*Operating at the console*—preferable to have a dual console system where an attending surgeon can take control at any time. Surgeons should utilize a graduated autonomy approach. A trainee should perform a minimum number of dual console cases prior to allowing independence as console surgeon.

As a sample curriculum, we have included the following requirements in place for surgical residents at the author's institution:

1. Complete all pertinent online training modules
2. Attend a hands-on workshop for introduction to docking, instrument exchange, simulator, and console training.
3. Complete designated modules on the simulator with a score of *90% or greater* (total of 14 modules)
   (a) Camera and Clutching—Camera Targeting 1 and 2
   (b) EndoWrist Manipulation—Pick and Place, Peg Board 1 and 2
   (c) Energy and Dissection—Energy switching 1 and 2 and Energy dissection 1 and 2
   (d) Needle Control—Needle targeting, Thread the rings
   (e) Needle Driving—Suture sponge 1 and 2; Tubes
4. Bedside assistant for a minimum of *10 robotic cases*, with responsibility for docking, instrument exchange, and assisting.
5. Console surgeon for a minimum of *15 cases*. An *additional 5 cases* as console surgeon must include a post case review with the attending surgeon and must be deemed as competent on the console for these cases. Cases should be performed with at least two different attendings and must be performed during the final year of residency.

If a resident or fellow successfully completes all the above, they will graduate with an equivalency certificate issued by Intuitive which is also endorsed by our general surgery program director. This eliminates the need to perform basic training in the future and graduates can apply for credentials immediately.

## Virtual Reality (VR) Simulation Training and Skills Curriculum

The surgical skills required to perform robotic surgery are unique from those needed for either open or laparoscopic procedures. As many studies have shown, basic robotic surgery skills can effectively be acquired through training on virtual reality simulators. There are currently four VR robotic surgical simulators commercially available (Table 17.1):

Mimic dVTrainer (dV-Trainer) (Fig. 17.2a)—Mimic Technologies, Inc., Seattle, WA, USA

Da Vinci Skills simulator (dVSS) (Fig. 17.2b)—Intuitive Surgical, Sunnyvale, CA, USA

Robotic Surgical Simulator (RoSS) (Fig. 17.2c)—Simulated Surgical Systems, Buffalo, NY, USA

Sim-Surgery Educational Platform (SEP)—SimSurgery, Norway

All VR simulator platforms presented here have several validation studies published in the literature. Our purpose is not to make any recommendations regarding the superiority of one over another, but instead we provide an objective yet brief description of each. *(For further information regarding in-depth comparisons and differences in functionality, see Suggested Reading's 2 and 3 provided at the end of the chapter)*

**Table 17.1** Overview of currently available VR simulators for robotic surgery training

| VR simulator platform | Year developed | Approx. cost | Basic construct | # of training exercises | Hardware/comments |
|---|---|---|---|---|---|
| Mimic dV-Trainer | 2007 | $100 K | Portable, table-top console with mobile foot pedals; 3D visualization | 65 exercises; 11 Categories: 1. EndoWrist manipulation 2. Knot tying 3. Camera control 4. Needle control 5. Clutching 6. Needle driving 7. Vessel dissection 8. Suturing 9. Energy control 10. Fourth arm control 11. System settings and controls | Measurement of hand motion less precise than RoSS and Da Vinci System |
| da Vinci surgical simulator (dVSS) | 2011 | $85 K | Single, compact hardware device that attaches directly onto the Da Vinci Surgical Console. 3D visualization | 40 exercises; 6 Categories: 1. EndoWrist Manipulation 2. Camera Clutching 3. 4th Arm Integration 4. Systems Settings 5. Needle Control and Driving 6. Energy and Dissection | Based on Mimic trainer software. Requires actual surgeon console. Simulation training cannot be performed while console being used for clinical cases |
| Robotic surgical simulator (RoSS™) | 2009 | >$100 K | Portable, All-in-one free-standing console. 3D visualization | 52 exercises; 4 categories: 1. Orientation 2. Motor Skills 3. Basic Suturing Skills 4. Intermediate Suturing Skills | Hand controls have smaller range of motion compared to da Vinci system |
| SimSurgery Educational Platform (SEP) | 2006 | $40–45 K | Stand-alone unit with portable hand controls mounted separately and external 2D monitor serving as eyepiece | 21 exercises; 3 Categories: 1. Tissue manipulation (6) 2. Basic suturing (7) 3. Advanced suturing (8) | No fourth arm component 2D visual |

| Da Vinci Skills Simulator | dV-Trainer | RoSS |
|---|---|---|

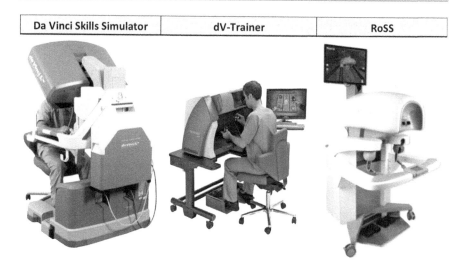

**Fig. 17.2** Photos of commercially available VR simulators. (**a**) Da Vinci Skills simulator (dVSS)—Intuitive Surgical, Sunnyvale, CA, USA). (**b**) The Mimic dv-Trainer (Mimic Technologies, Inc., Seattle, WA, USA). (**c**) The RoSS™ Robotic Surgery Simulator (Simulated Surgical Systems LLC, San Jose, CA, USA). From Smith et al. Comparative analysis of the functionality of simulators of the da Vinci surgical robot. *Surgical endoscopy.* Apr 2015;29(4):972–983. Fig. 1. Springer all rights reserved, with permission

A recent review of VR simulators showed that the dVSS, dV-Trainer, and RoSS platforms demonstrated the ability of a VR training curriculum to improve basic robotic skills, with proficiency-based training being the most effective training style [9]. In many instances, a performance score of 80% on any given task or module has been used to define proficiency. There is no formula as to why 80% was set as threshold, but rather it is based on expert consensus from high-volume robotic surgeons.

In 2014, collaborative efforts of an international multi-society consensus provided a template for developing a core curriculum in basic robotic training, *The Fundamentals of Robotic Surgery*, that focuses on competency-based training using current generation simulators needed to safely perform robotic surgery [2]. Based on their recommendations, a dedicated curriculum should include: introduction to and didactic instructions for robotic systems, cognitive skills training, psychomotor skills training, and team training/communication skills. As it relates to technical skills training, the psychomotor skills modules they recommended were:

1. FLS peg transfer
2. FLS suturing and knot tying
3. FLS pattern cutting
4. Running suture
5. Dome with four towers for ambidexterity—specifically designed device, "FRS Dome"—to allow performance of all skills on a single platform that can be easily observed

6. Vessel dissection and clipping
7. Fourth arm retraction and cutting
8. Energy and mechanical cutting
9. Docking task
10. Trocar insertion task

In 2013, Stegemann et al. developed a validated *VR-based skills curriculum* (Fundamental Skills of Robotic Surgery, FSRS) using the RoSS platform in a multi-institutional randomized control trial [10]. Their study consisted of 16 unique tasks included with four training modules (Fig. 17.3):

- Basic console orientation
- Psychomotor skills training
- Basic surgical skills
- Intermediate surgical skills

As of this writing, there are still no widely accepted standardized protocols for simulation training. The material presented here is from recent literature and societal recommendations. Every program will have different limitations in resources and although robotic training curricula may be individualized to institutional needs, the above represent a minimum recommendation of options to provide a basis for the safe training of new robotic surgeons.

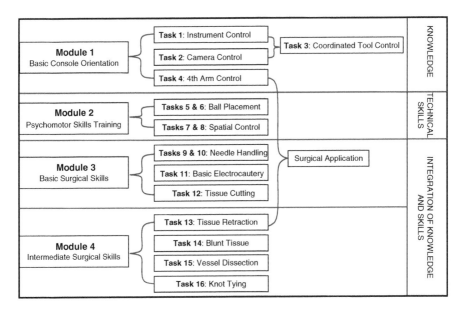

**Fig. 17.3** Four modules with included tasks for a structured Fundamental Skills of Robotic Surgery (FSRS) curriculum. From Stegemann et al. Fundamental skills of robotic surgery: a multi-institutional randomized controlled trial for validation of a simulation-based curriculum. *Urology*. Apr 2013;81(4):767–774, Fig. 1A. Elsevier all rights reserved, with permission

## Credentialing and Privileging

One of the current debates of robotic surgery centers around credentialing and privileging. Currently, there are no specific standards for approval or maintenance of privileges. In the past, guidelines were based on recommendations from Intuitive, which were loosely based on their training protocols that we described earlier. Until recently, majority of surgeons were training for robotic surgery after their residency, so no formal case logs were necessary. Competency was based on case observations by proctors, who were designated by the company. To qualify as a proctor, a surgeon had to have completed over 20 robotic cases. Individual privileges were kept if surgeons performed 1–2 cases a year. This model was based on what was accepted during the early era of the laparoscopic cholecystectomy. Surgeons at that time would train at a weekend course, perform a few cases at their home institution, and then would go teach other surgeons. As a result, new technology was being adapted quickly, but complications also increased which led to surgical groups to develop consensus statements. Even at our institution, the above remained true up till this year when new system-wide guidelines were implemented.

Several shifts have occurred recently that has provoked more thought and restructuring of credentialing across all specialties. Nowadays, many residents are exposed to robotics, especially in urology and gynecology. The number of robotic cases in general surgery is rising exponentially and is driving many of the changes, but case volumes alone cannot be predictors of competency. Privileging has shifted to evidence of competency, whether through dedicated training programs in residency vs completing the surrogate equivalency training set by Intuitive. Intuitive has responded to this by increasing the minimum number of cases required to become a proctor from 20 now to 40. In addition, a surgeon cannot be listed on their website unless they complete more than 20 cases a year. Thus, maintenance of privileges needs to align with these metrics.

Current proposals for maintaining privileges revolve around markers for competency. In most centers with robotic surgery, patient outcomes are collected and recorded. Formal steering committees are being established to monitor this data and maintain quality for the hospital. This committee also sets the parameters for maintenance of skills via the simulator. Here are the key highlights from our recently revamped program:

## Robotic Credentialing Guidelines

1. Successful completion of ACGME/AOA residency or fellowship training program
2. Physician must be board certified or eligible
3. Has privileges in similar open and laparoscopic cases
4. Proof of training
    (a) Residency or Fellowship—need letter from program director, minimum case logs as assist (10) and console surgeon (20)
    (b) No formal training—must complete successful training with Intuitive
5. Proctoring—must be proctored for first two cases by someone with active privileges

## Maintenance of Privileges

1. Completion of five core simulator skill exercises with passing score of 85% every 2 years
2. Case logs from recent 2 years must perform at least 20 procedures in the 2 years
3. Failure in above will result in case proctoring for next two cases
4. Surgeons who are inactive for more than 90 days must complete core simulator exercises with passing score above 85%
5. Surgeons performing more than 50 cases in 2 years will be exempt from the above

This was developed with input from among all specialties (gynecology, urology, thoracic, cardiac, general, otolaryngology) and from guidelines used for other invasive procedures, like central line insertions. Unfortunately, no data exists to support if this is sufficient or stringent enough to maintain quality and determine competency. Opponents may point out that no guidelines currently exist to maintain other surgical procedure privileges and this should be extended to robotic procedures. Ultimately, this discussion should occur regularly among all participating surgeons at your own institution to maintain quality and safety of the patient.

**Acknowledgement** This work is supported in part by the Foundation for Surgical Fellowships.

## References

1. Wormer BA, Dacey KT, Williams KB, et al. The first nationwide evaluation of robotic general surgery: a regionalized, small but safe start. Surg Endosc. 2014;28(3):767–76.
2. Smith R, Patel V, Satava R. Fundamentals of robotic surgery: a course of basic robotic surgery skills based upon a 14-society consensus template of outcomes measures and curriculum development. Int J Med Robot. 2014;10(3):379–84.
3. Investor presentation. Intuitive Surgical; 2016. Available at: http://phx.corporate-ir.net/phoenix.zhtml?c5122359&p5irol-irhome. Accessed 6 Nov 2016.
4. Farivar BS, Flannagan M, Leitman IM. General surgery residents' perception of robot-assisted procedures during surgical training. J Surg Educ. 2015;72(2):235–42.
5. Winder JS, Juza RM, Sasaki J, et al. Implementing a robotics curriculum at an academic general surgery training program: our initial experience. J Robot Surg. 2016;10(3):209–13.
6. Wiener S, Haddock P, Shichman S, Dorin R. Construction of a urologic robotic surgery training curriculum: how many simulator sessions are required for residents to achieve proficiency? J Endourol. 2015;29(11):1289–93.
7. Ahmed K, Khan R, Mottrie A, et al. Development of a standardised training curriculum for robotic surgery: a consensus statement from an international multidisciplinary group of experts. BJU Int. 2015;116(1):93–101.
8. Zhong W, Mancuso P. Utilization and surgical skill transferability of the simulator robot to the clinical robot for urology surgery. Urol Int. Sept 2016. (epub, ahead of print)
9. Bric JD, Lumbard DC, Frelich MJ, Gould JC. Current state of virtual reality simulation in robotic surgery training: a review. Surg Endosc. 2016;30(6):2169–78.
10. Stegemann AP, Ahmed K, Syed JR, et al. Fundamental skills of robotic surgery: a multi-institutional randomized controlled trial for validation of a simulation-based curriculum. Urology. 2013;81(4):767–74.

## Suggested Reading

Leal Ghezzi T, Campos CO. 30 years of robotic surgery. World J Surg. 2016;40(10):2550–7.
Bric JD, Lumbard DC, Frelich MJ, Gould JC. Current state of virtual reality simulation in robotic surgery training: a review. Surg Endosc. 2016;30(6):2169–78.
Smith R, Truong M, Perez M. Comparative analysis of the functionality of simulators of the da Vinci surgical robot. Surg Endosc. 2015;29(4):972–83.
Stegemann AP, Ahmed K, Syed JR, et al. Fundamental skills of robotic surgery: a multi-institutional randomized controlled trial for validation of a simulation-based curriculum. Urology. 2013;81(4):767–74.

Mihir M. Shah and Edward Lin

## Introduction

Innovations in minimally invasive surgery have led to the development of advanced robotic technology where instruments follow the commands of the surgeon situated at some distance from the actual surgery. Currently, the only commercially available robotic-assisted surgery (RAS) platforms are produced by Intuitive Surgical, Inc. (Sunnyvale, CA) and are known as the da Vinci Surgical Systems (S, Si, and Xi models) [1]. The purported benefits over standard laparoscopy include three-dimensional high-definition visualization, ergonomic control of wristed surgical instruments, minimization of surgeon hand tremor, and a sitting operating posture. While there is suggestion that basic skills can be learned more quickly using the RAS platform compared to laparoscopy, there is still a learning curve to become proficient at using the RAS platform [2, 3].

Between January 1, 2000 to August 1, 2012, 245 adverse events were reported to the FDA (Food and Drug Administration) including 71 deaths and 174 nonfatal injuries. The surgical mortalities reported were gynecologic (31%; 22/71), urologic (21.1%; 15/71), cardiothoracic (16.9%; 12/71), otolaryngologic (14.1%; 10/71), colorectal (4.2%; 3/71), and general surgical (4.2%; 3/71). The most common cause of mortality was hemorrhage (29.6%; 21/71). Reports of nonfatal injury were most common with hysterectomy (43.1%; 75/174) and prostatectomy (17.2%; 30/174). Nearly half (46.6%) of nonfatal injuries resulted in permanent damage, and 17.2% and 15.5% resulted in conversion to open and a second operation, respectively [4]. While it is difficult to understand the root cause for these adverse events, the greater our understanding of RAS and dissemination of practical insights gained from

M.M. Shah, M.D. (✉) • E. Lin, D.O., F.A.C.S.
Emory Endosurgery Unit, Division of Gastrointestinal and General Surgery, Department of Surgery, Emory University School of Medicine, Atlanta, GA, USA
e-mail: mihir253@gmail.com; ELin2@emory.edu

© Springer International Publishing AG 2018
A.D. Patel, D. Oleynikov (eds.), *The SAGES Manual of Robotic Surgery*,
The SAGES University Masters Program Series, DOI 10.1007/978-3-319-51362-1_18

experience will reduce any potential that the RAS contributes to any complications. Even if no injury occurs to the patient, the expenses related to repairing the RAS platform may prohibit its subsequent use.

## Standard Precautions

### Power Requirements

To avoid overloading electrical circuits, all three components—Surgeon Console, Patient Cart, and Vision Cart—should operate on separate, dedicated power circuits. Ancillary devices such as insufflators or energy devices should not be connected through any system component, particularly not through the Vision Cart because it has a large power requirement, and could result in overloading the circuit. Instead, ancillary devices should be connected to wall outlets on separate circuits from all system components. Use of an extension cord with any of the system components is also not recommended. Any of the above could lead to a power failure during a procedure.

### Instrument Insertion and Removal

Modification of the cannula mounts, sterile adapters, instruments, cracked wiring or housing can result in electrical hazards, performance degradation, and energy-related injuries to the patient. When inserting an instrument for the first time, the same precautions as laparoscopy should be taken to make sure the tips are visualized to prevent any unintended contact with tissue. When resistance is met during instrument insertion, it can be due to bumping up against tissue, or the cannula is dislodged out of the surgical cavity.

Prior to removing any instruments during a procedure, the assistant should communicate with the surgeon, and the surgeon must keep the instrument tip straight, release any organ, structure, or sutures, even though the instruments are designed to release the tissue as a safety feature. Along the lines of communication, the audio and microphone system should be functioning and extraneous sounds minimized.

### Energy Application

The same insulation precautions for laparoscopic instruments apply to the robotic system. The same grounding pad principles also apply. As reminders of what is commonly known, the dispersive electrode (grounding pad) is placed as close as possible to the operating field but away from any interference from the robotic system. We apply the same lowest effective energy setting as laparoscopy. The finer instruments tend to concentrate more energy at its points of contact. The surgeon should avoid energizing other robotic or endoscopic instruments directly and be cognizant that energy may also be transferred to tissue outside of the field of view. Intentional energy application is possible but make sure the instrument is away from other critical structures.

## Camera Head and Endoscope

The camera head and light cable should be handled with care, especially with the bulky camera head of the Si system, to prevent damage to the internal fiber optic cables. Furthermore, the camera head can cause injury when dropped on the patient, or if it pulls other instruments off the field due to its weight. In addition, the temperature of the distal tip of the endoscope may exceed 41 °C during full illumination, which will burn any object on brief contact; skin, tissue, clothing, and drapes. When used during a case, it is better not to clean the tip of the endoscope by rubbing it against tissue as it could cause secondary thermal damage to the tissue and leave residue on the lens. Because of the high-definition resolution of the camera and lens, it is possible to reduce the light intensity and work closer to the surgical tissue. The downside of decreasing the light output is a grainy image.

## Surgical Control

The infrared head sensors on the console perform a safety function by preventing movement of the Patient Cart arms when the surgeon's head is not in the viewer; this is often forgotten for those early on in their robot experience. Similarly, once the head is removed from the surgeon console viewer, the instruments will lock in position and cannot be moved. If the surgeon plans to step away from the console, the head should be removed first from the viewer prior to removing the hands and fingers from the masters, which takes the system out of the "following mode."

## Handling of Errors

It is inevitable that system errors will occur and most can easily be resolved. Try to resolve the problem before using the Recover button. In both the vision cart and surgeon console, the specific error will be displayed. If you are unable to resolve it, technical support can be contacted and they can usually diagnose and recover the fault if the system is connected to the internet. In the meantime, we advise removing all instruments to prevent unintended movements in case the system has to be reset. By default, the system will not move the arms if it senses instruments are being reset. If the errors cannot be managed intraoperatively, it is recommended that the surgeon proceed with laparoscopic methods since the robot trocars can easily be converted to laparoscopic ports.

## Power Outage

In the middle of the operation, if the robot shuts down, then it is safe to turn it back on, as the booting sequence will not take place while the arms are docked. If there is an electric power outage without backup, the battery life on the patient cart is automatically activated, and may last for just enough time to permit undocking and moving the patient cart away.

## Practical Pearls

While the above outlined the standard operating guidelines specific to the system, there are other safety pearls that the surgeon should be aware of.

### Docking and Arm Positioning

There are several ways to successfully position and dock the robot. The standard practice is to triangulate the arms with the surgical pathology to make sure the camera stays within the "sweet spot." The reality is you can dock the robot in many ways and achieve the same exposure, but you will have to pay more attention to the position of the robot arms. A major point is to be sure you have adequate spacing between the trocars and the elbows of the arms. Test the range of movement of the arms prior to inserting instruments and "burp" the arms to avoid collisions. Place the patient in the intended position prior to docking; otherwise, you will have to undock all of the arms if you wish to reposition the patient. The newer Xi system can be used with a synchronized bed that enables table motion in lock-step with the robot arms. However, currently you can only utilize this feature with two instruments inside the patient. If you are using all four arms, then you must remove one of the instruments to enable this feature.

The surgeon should be listening for clashes of the arms, which needs to be alleviated by bending the elbows of the robot arms, or repositioning. It is a skill, but listening to the speed and crescendos of the moving robot arms is an important indicator of the motion efficiency (i.e., wasted movements) of operating instruments in the body cavity. A fast and loud "swoosh," even though not visible inside the body cavity is transmitted to patient port site and the arms may even strike the bedside assistant unaware of the surgeon's intentions. Another sign that robot arms may be clashing is an inability or resistance to movement at the master, or instrument tremors seen in the viewer.

### Protecting Patient's Face and Extremities

As there are multiple ways to position the robot and its arms, modifications should be made to always protect the patient, especially their face and extremities. A thick sponge/foam can be used to cover the patient's face and airway. During docking, the surgeon's hand should be placed on the patient's face to ensure there is adequate distance from the patient's face to the robot arms. The same should be applied to the extremities, taking care to avoid any pinch points between the robot and table. The bedside assistant should be actively involved with positioning so they can be aware of potential issues during the case. In practice, when a stationary arm (such as one used for retraction) is ever moved, it behooves the bedside assistant to run his or her fingers between the lowest point of the robot arm with the patient's extremity or body part to prevent any body part impingement.

## Prolonged Trendelenburg Positioning

Because the patient's bed is immoveable after docking, patients were historically placed in extreme positions from the beginning of the case. Newer beds also facilitated this, especially with extreme Trendelenburg position (over 30°). This can result in increased intracranial and intraocular pressures. In addition, it has been suspected to cause postoperative airway obstruction due to facial or laryngeal edema. To avoid this, the anesthesiologist should look at the patients face several times during a prolonged case, and a surgeon should not hesitate in requesting the anesthesiologist to check the patient's face during the case. Patient slipping from the original position on the bed is another concern. In addition to routine measures to secure the patient, a gel pad below the patient can be used to avoid a slippery surface and potentially reduce slippage. Using Trendelenburg to the lowest degree that allows safe completion of the operation is another important measure that will potentially reduce complications related to this particular position. Alternatively for long cases in extreme positions, the surgeon can undock the robot and return the patient to a neutral supine position every 1–2 h for a few minutes prior to proceeding with the case.

## Operative Tips

### Control of Intraoperative Bleeding

Majority of the bleeding encountered in a case is usually related to poor tissue handling or misapplication of energy. The surgeon typically relies on visual cues to enhance tactile feedback. Also, awareness and knowledge about instruments and its grip strength will help the surgeon avoid inadvertent injury to the visceral structures. There will always be instances of bleeding during some operations. Inserting a laparotomy sponge from the assistant port, and then using the suction is very helpful. The individual at the console can use the sponge to tamponade the bleed and improve visualization of that area. This helps create more time to determine the surgeon's next maneuvers. If needed, suture can be used to repair or ligate the bleeding vessel, which is also delivered from the assistant port. The downside to a robot system is that any small amount of blood is magnified in three-dimension, which very rapidly obscures a clear view. Therefore, a capable assistant performing suction and compression with a sponge is important to keep the field clear. The use of bipolar energy, including the vessel sealer, has tremendous advantages because these instruments can serve as graspers as well as cautery simultaneously.

## Suturing Tips

Tying knots without tearing the tissue, shredding or breaking the suture is a skill in the setting of reduced tactile feedback. In knot-tying, we rely on visual cues such as the appearance of water beads on the suture and indentations created on tissues as indicators of just the right tension. While the added range of motion for suturing is a clear advantage of the robot system, these added degrees of movement exceed the anatomic limitations of the surgeon's wrist and fingers (i.e., the human wrist and fingers do not have 360° rotation). In fact, the surgeon probably has to employ more range of hand-finger motion than he or she is accustomed to from open or laparoscopic surgery. It is necessary to fully use hand-finger range of motion at the master to drive the needle and follow its entire curve with wrist rotation. Like passing a baton in a relay race, the needle needs to be passed from one instrument to another purposefully and released at the right time to avoid destroying the needle tip or creating rough glitches on the body of the needle. Remember that one of the advantages of using the robot system is tremor suppression, which means that there will be an almost imperceptible motion delay from what the surgeon's hand does to what actually occurs on the field. Any fast motions, intended or unintended, will be tempered down especially in suturing. The best advice for needle handling and suturing is to perform dry runs with the robot and understand the feel of passing the needles, where the breaking points are, and how tight (or loosely) one can hold the needle.

## Conclusions

There are several potential benefits of the RAS platform over traditional laparoscopy. There is a learning curve to become proficient at using the RAS platform. Understanding the full capabilities of the robot as well as its inflexibilities can only come with frequent use. The ability to troubleshoot problems is valuable for using the RAS platform because it will broaden the times a surgeon can use the robot (e.g., nights and weekends) and reduce dependence on costly bedside and technical support. Using the robot actually requires even greater awareness than just hand-eye coordination because it requires auditory cues as well and understanding the capabilities and limitations of the bedside assistant. It is appropriate to consider the 60–40 rule using the robot-assisted platform; 60% of the effort is occurring at the bedside, and only 40% of the case occurs at the surgeon console. It then follows that 60% or more of RAS-associated complications occurs to misadventures, recognized or not, occurring at the bedside.

**Acknowledgement** This work is supported in part by the Foundation for Surgical Fellowships.

## References

1. da Vinci Si Surgical System. User manual. Sunyvale: Intuitive Surgical; 2012.
2. Kim HJ, Choi GS, Park JS, Park SY. Comparison of surgical skills in laparoscopic and robotic tasks between experienced surgeons and novices in laparoscopic surgery: an experimental study. Ann Coloproctol. 2014;30(2):71–6.
3. Yohannes P, Rotariu P, Pinto P, Smith AD, Lee BR. Comparison of robotic versus laparoscopic skills: is there a difference in the learning curve. Urology. 2002;60(1):39–45. Discussion
4. Cooper MA, Ibrahim A, Lyu H, Makary MA. Underreporting of robotic surgery complications. J Healthc Qual. 2015;37(2):133–8.

## Suggested Reading

Park SY, Choi GS, Park JS, Kim HJ, Ryuk JP. Short-term clinical outcome of robot-assisted intersphincteric resection for low rectal cancer: a retrospective comparison with conventional laparoscopy. Surg Endosc. 2013;27(1):48–55.
Yang Y, Wang F, Zhang P, Shi C, Zou Y, Qin H, et al. Robot-assisted versus conventional laparoscopic surgery for colorectal disease, focusing on rectal cancer: a meta-analysis. Ann Surg Oncol. 2012;19(12):3727–36.

# Part III

# Common Procedures

Arturo Garcia and Aaron Carr

## Introduction

Despite the excellent results of traditional laparoscopic cholecystectomy, there have been numerous attempts to decrease the parietal trauma of the typical 4-port technique. Reducing the number of trocars used and reducing the port size have both been used to reduce the parietal peritoneal trauma. Single-incision laparoscopic cholecystectomy (SILC) has been shown to be feasible [1–7], but the technique is challenging because of reduced ability to triangulate with linear instruments, limited visualization, and internal and external collisions [8]. Despite the demonstrated safety of SILC, these limitations have decreased the wide spread adoption of SILC. Robotic single-incision instrumentation has been able to address many of these limitations.

Since its introduction over a decade ago, the popularity of robotic surgery has increased, especially in the specialties of urology and gynecology. The most robust and studied platform for single-site surgery is the da Vinci Si Surgical System (Intuitive Surgical Inc. Sunnyvale, CA). Although other platforms exist in various stages of development, none are currently approved for use in the United States. The da Vinci single-site technology for cholecystectomy overcomes many of the limitations of SILC, including triangulation, ergonomics, quality of vision, and range of motion [9]. If studies with more than 50 cases are analyzed from a PubMed search for SIRC the average docking times ranged from 5 to 15 min and average total

A. Garcia, M.D.
Department of Surgery, University of California-Davis,
2315 Stockton Blvd OP 512, Sacramento, CA 95817, USA

A. Carr, M.D. (✉)
Department of Surgery, University of California-Davis,
2221 Stockton Blvd, Sacramento, Sacramento, CA 95817, USA
e-mail: acarr@ucdavis.edu

© Springer International Publishing AG 2018                                                    243
A.D. Patel, D. Oleynikov (eds.), *The SAGES Manual of Robotic Surgery*,
The SAGES University Masters Program Series, DOI 10.1007/978-3-319-51362-1_19

**Table 19.1** Single-incision robotic cholecystectomy outcomes

| | $N$ | Robotic docking time (min) | Console time (min) | Total time (min) | Major complication (bile leak, bleeding) |
|---|---|---|---|---|---|
| Pietrabissa et al. (2012) | | | | | |
| SIRC | 100 | 15 | 31 | 71 | None |
| Gonzalez et al. (2013) | | | | | |
| SIRC | 166 | NA | NA | 63 | 1.8% |
| SILC | 166 | – | – | 37 | 1.8% |
| SILC (SPIDER) | 166 | – | – | 53 | 1.2% |
| Angus et al. (2014) | | | | | |
| SIRC | 55 | 11 | 29 | 62 | None |
| Morel et al. (2014) | | | | | |
| SIRC | 82 | 7 | 51 | 91 | 2.4% |
| Vidovszky et al. (2014) | | | | | |
| SIRC | 95 | 5 | 39 | 84 | 1.1% |
| Escobar-Dominguez et al. (2015) | | | | | |
| SIRC | 192 | NA | NA | 58–73 | None |
| Gonzalez et al. (2015) | | | | | |
| SIRC | 465 | NA | 21 | 52 | 0.8% |
| Chung et al. (2015) | | | | | |
| SIRC | 70 | 12 | 53 | 106 | None |
| LC | 70 | – | – | 112 | None |
| Svoboda et al. (2015) | | | | | |
| SIRC | 200 | NA | NA | 65 | None |
| Kubat et al. (2016) | | | | | |
| SIRC | 150 | NA | NA | 83 | 0.7% |

Data from PubMed search for SIRC studies with greater than 50 patients
*SIRC*, single-incision robotic cholecystectomy; *LC*, conventional laparoscopic cholecystectomy; *SILC*, single-incision laparoscopic cholecystectomy; *SPIDER*, single-port instrument delivery extended research (TransEnterix, Inc.); *NA*, not available

operative ranged from 63 to 106 min. The rate of bile injury, bile leak, or bleeding ranged from 0 to 1.8% (Table 19.1).

## Indications

The indications for SIRC are similar to those of traditional laparoscopic cholecystectomy. These include symptomatic cholelithiasis, cholecystitis, acalculous cholecystitis, symptomatic gallbladder polyps or polyps greater than 10 mm, porcelain gallbladder, and biliary dyskinesia [10]. Certain relative contraindications for SILC include patients with severe acute cholecystitis, BMI $\geq$ 35 kg/m$^2$, previous upper abdominal surgery, suspected bile duct stones and intrahepatic duct stones, suspected malignancy, and ASA class $\geq$ 3 [11–13]. Some of these contraindications have been alleviated by the da Vinci Si single-site cholecystectomy platform because of improved triangulation and surgeon experience with the platform. SIRC is increasingly being performed in patients with higher BMI, cholecystitis, and previous upper abdominal surgery, all with good results [14].

## Robotic Components and Operating Room Team

There are three major components to the da Vinci Surgical System. Two components are not sterile and located away from the table: Surgeon Console (SC) and Vision Cart (VC). The patient-side cart (PSC) component is covered with sterile drapes and docked at the operating room table. The SC gives the surgeon control of the instrumentation and visualization of the operative field. The VC contains supporting hardware and software such as the optical light source, electrosurgical unit, and optical integration. The PSC has four articulated mechanical arms, which control the instruments that are docked to the ports. Efficient use of the robotic system is best utilized with dedicated personnel. As previously discussed in Chapter 14, our structure consists of a robotic nurse manager, equipment specialist, circulating nurse, and scrub nurse. The nurse manager coordinates equipment and personnel several days in advance, the equipment specialist will set up the robotic subcomponents, and the circulating nurse is responsible for patient care and any additional equipment during the operation. The bedside scrub nurse must be proficient at instrument exchanges and basic bedside problem solving. This structure has been successful in achieving a mean SIRC docking time of $4.9 \pm 2.8$ min [14].

## Room Setup and Patient Positioning

The patient is positioned supine on the operating table with the right arm tucked and left arm at $90°$. The surgeon and assistant initially start on the patient's left or right side according to surgeon preference. The instrument table and scrub nurse are positioned near the feet. The PSC robotic component will always be over the patient's right shoulder, and the position of the electronics cart and surgeon console can be altered depending on room limitations. Typically the SC is to the patient's left and the VC is to the patient's left or right.

Once the single-site port has been deployed and the abdomen insufflated to $12–15$ mmHg, the PSC is driven at $45°$ and placed slightly over the patient's right shoulder. Prior to docking of the robot, the patient is placed in $10°–15°$ of reverse Trendelenburg and rotated to the left $10°–15°$. Once the docking is completed, the surgeon can transition to the console and the assistant can transition to the patient's left side with the scrub nurse remaining near the patient's feet on the left or right. The position of the patient relative to the anesthesia machine may have to be adjusted in order for the robotic patient-side cart to be positioned over the patient's right shoulder without interfering with the anesthesia machine or endotracheal tube (Fig. 19.1).

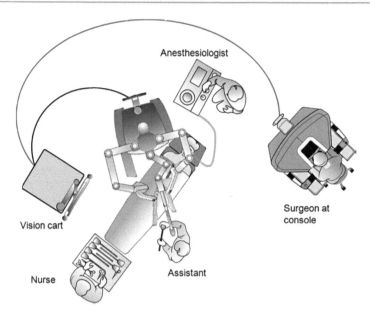

**Fig. 19.1** Single-incision robotic cholecystectomy room setup

## Technical Pearls

- Consider positioning the patient 30°–45° relative to the anesthesia machine.
- Patient positioning can be altered once the robot is docked if using the da Vinci Xi but not with the da Vinci Si robotic surgical system.

## Port Placement and Robotic Docking

A 2.5 cm skin incision is made around the umbilicus. The incision can lie vertical or horizontal depending on the surgeon's preference. Placing the incision in the most prominent skin fold at the umbilicus may provide an improved cosmetic result. Next, the underlying fascia is elevated and opened 2.5 cm horizontally, and the peritoneum is elevated and entered with sharp dissection. Retractors are used to stretch the opening large enough to allow port placement. The da Vinci single-site port (Intuitive Surgical Inc., Sunnyvale, CA) has five openings: one for the robotic 8 mm camera, one for insufflation, two for the robotic arms, and one for the assistant's standard laparoscopic grasper (Fig. 19.2). The silicon port is folded, clamped with an atraumatic clamp at its lower rim, and lubricated with water to facilitate its introduction. Care is taken to not crush the insufflation tubing during clamping. The silicone port is inserted into the abdominal cavity under direct vision by following the curve of the clamps while providing retraction at the incision with Army–Navy retractors. Once deployed, the orientation of the port is confirmed by making sure to align the arrow with the anatomical target and the carbon dioxide insufflation is begun (Fig. 19.3).

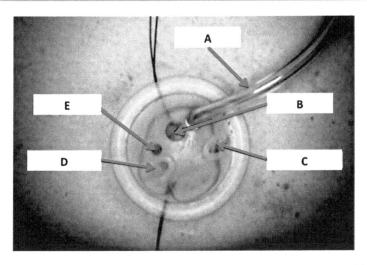

**Fig. 19.2** The da Vinci single-site port. (**a**) $CO_2$ insufflation tubing, (**b**) camera port, (**c**) curved working port—Arm 1, (**d**): curved working port—Arm 2, (**e**) assistant port

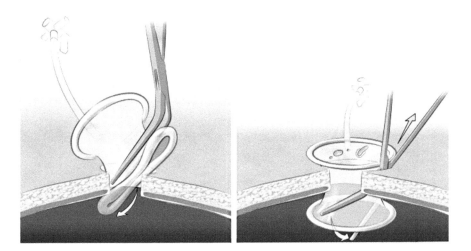

**Fig. 19.3** Insertion of single-incision port

The first 8.5 mm trocar is placed (for the camera), and the camera trocar is docked prior to placing the remaining ports. Once docked, an 8 mm 30° down facing camera is introduced and used for visualization of the remaining ports. Next, the two robotic curved trocars are placed through the port under direct vision. These cannulae cross at the fascial level to allow appropriate triangulation for the semi-rigid instruments during dissection. Because the instruments cross in the port, the intra-abdominal instrument position is reversed. The instrument that enters the abdomen from the left reaches the operative field on the right and vice versa (Fig. 19.4). The curved cannulae are docked to the robotic arms. Finally, a fourth (5 mm)

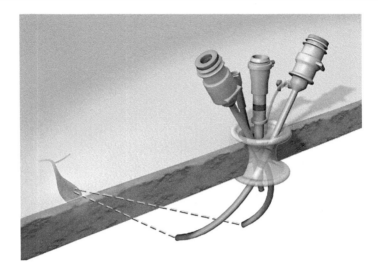

**Fig. 19.4** Single-site cannula crossing within the trocar. The end of the ports aims toward target anatomy

trocar for the bedside assistant is placed through the port, also under direct visualization. With the cannula tip in view, the Crocodile grasper is inserted in arm 1, and the monopolar cautery hook is inserted in arm 2.

## Technical Pearls

- Use clamps on each side of the silicone port to prevent slippage during trocar insertion.
- Lubricate all trocars with saline.
- For obese patients, use the long curved metal trocars, as tip deflection is less common.

## Robotic Dissection and Fluorescence Imaging

The cholecystectomy is performed in a similar manner as a routine laparoscopic cholecystectomy. The operating surgeon starts the dissection phase at the console with the assistant helping to retract the gallbladder cephalad with a grasper through the assistant port. The camera is driven under the assistant grasper, which gives the console surgeon partial control of fundal retraction. The crossing of the cannulae inside the port internally increases the distance between the instruments tips to overcome the SILC parallelism, while the curvature of the cannulae internally allows the instruments to reach the operative field in a convergent way. This restores the correct triangulation and allows exposure to Callot's triangle with the combination of

**Fig. 19.5** Intraoperative dissection of triangle of Calot (picture from the University of California, Davis, Department of Surgery Archive)

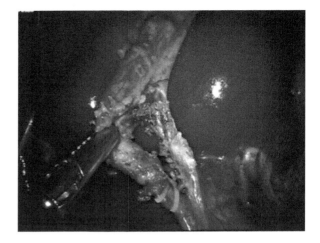

the assistant grasper and the Crocodile grasper. The da Vinci software automatically associates the surgeon's hands to the ipsilateral instrument tips to restore intuitive control of the instruments.

Although we do not routinely use indocyanine green (ICG) and near infrared fluorescence for real-time cholangiography to help identify the ductal structures, studies show that it may improve the safety of SIRC by preventing inadvertent bile duct injuries [15]. The robotic platform allows the surgeon to easily switch from white light to fluorescence imaging after the administration of IV ICG. The cystic duct and artery are dissected with monopolar hook and divided between Hem-o-lok (Weck Closure Systems, Research Triangle Park, NC) clips (Fig. 19.5). Due to the flexibility of the instruments, care must be taken with the tension applied to the monopolar hook electrocautery to prevent spring-like deflection of the tip. The gallbladder is detached from the liver bed with the hook cautery.

At this point, the patient-side cart is undocked and the curved cannula is removed. The gallbladder is subsequently removed directly out of the single-site port incision, or it can be placed into a 10-mm disposable specimen bag inserted through the assistant port. The single-site port is finally removed through the abdominal incision with the gallbladder. The size of the single incision allows for easy specimen removal, even with large gallbladders or stones. The peritoneum is closed with absorbable suture followed by careful fascial closure with interrupted absorbable or permanent sutures in a horizontal vest over pants fashion. The skin is re-approximated with subcuticular continuous suture and adhesive glue for dressing.

## Technical Pearls

- Swap the hook and grasper instruments to dissect laterally using your left hand.
- Perform extensive medial dissection prior to clipping the cystic duct or artery.

- If using ICG and near infrared fluorescence for real-time cholangiography, give 2.5 mg of ICG 45 min prior to the start of the procedure.
- If using a specimen bag, upsize the assistant port to a 10 mm port after removal of the curved cannulae, and use a specimen bag to scoop the gallbladder.

## Summary

The ideal robotic platform should have minimal setup time; a low external profile, the possibility of being deployed through a single access site, and the possibility of restoring intra-abdominal triangulation while maintaining the maximum degree of freedom for precise maneuvers and strength for reliable traction. SIRC addresses some of these requirements while maintaining similar outcomes to traditional laparoscopic cholecystectomy.

## References

1. Hong TH, You YK, Lee KH. Transumbilical single-port laparoscopic cholecystectomy: scarless cholecystectomy. Surg Endosc. 2009;23(6):1393–7.
2. Hernandez JM, Morton CA, Ross S, Albrink M, Rosemurgy AS. Laparoendoscopic single site cholecystectomy: the first 100 patients. Am Surg. 2009;75(8):681–5; discussion 685–6.
3. Tacchino R, Greco F, Matera D. Single-incision laparoscopic cholecystectomy: surgery without a visible scar. Surg Endosc. 2009;23(4):896–9.
4. Carr A, Bhavaraju A, Goza J, Wilson R. Initial experience with single-incision laparoscopic cholecystectomy. Am Surg. 2010;76(7):703–7.
5. Elsey JK, Feliciano DV. Initial experience with single-incision laparoscopic cholecystectomy. J Am Coll Surg. 2010;210(5):620–4; 624–6.
6. Erbella Jr J, Bunch GM. Single-incision laparoscopic cholecystectomy: the first 100 outpatients. Surg Endosc. 2010;24(8):1958–61.
7. Pisanu A, Reccia I, Porceddu G, Uccheddu A. Meta-analysis of prospective randomized studies comparing single-incision laparoscopic cholecystectomy (SILC) and conventional multiport laparoscopic cholecystectomy (CMLC). J Gastrointest Surg. 2012;16(9):1790–801.
8. Pietrabissa A, Sbrana F, Morelli L, Badessi F, Pugliese L, Vinci A, et al. Overcoming the challenges of single-incision cholecystectomy with robotic single-site technology. Arch Surg. 2012;147(8):709–14.
9. Gonzalez A, Murcia CH, Romero R, Escobar E, Garcia P, Walker G, et al. A multicenter study of initial experience with single-incision robotic cholecystectomies (SIRC) demonstrating a high success rate in 465 cases. Surg Endosc. 2016;30(7):2951–60.
10. Agresta F, Campanile FC, Vettoretto N, Silecchia G, Bergamini C, Maida P, et al. Laparoscopic cholecystectomy: consensus conference-based guidelines. Langenbecks Arch Surg. 2015;400(4):429–53.
11. Jung GO, Park DE, Chae KM. Clinical results between single incision laparoscopic cholecystectomy and conventional 3-port laparoscopic cholecystectomy: prospective case-matched analysis in single institution. J Kor Surg Soc. 2012;83(6):374–80.
12. Kurpiewski W, Pesta W, Kowalczyk M, Glowacki L, Juskiewicz W, Szynkarczuk R, et al. The outcomes of SILS cholecystectomy in comparison with classic four-trocar laparoscopic cholecystectomy. Videosurg Other Minim Invasive Tech. 2012;7(4):286–93.

13. Tay CW, Shen L, Hartman M, Iyer SG, Madhavan K, Chang SK. SILC for SILC: single institution learning curve for single-incision laparoscopic cholecystectomy. Minim Invasive Surg. 2013;2013:381628.
14. Vidovszky TJ, Carr AD, Farinholt GN, Ho HS, Smith WH, Ali MR. Single-site robotic cholecystectomy in a broadly inclusive patient population: a prospective study. Ann Surg. 2014;260(1):134–41.
15. Escobar-Dominguez JE, Hernandez-Murcia C, Gonzalez AM. Description of robotic single site cholecystectomy and a review of outcomes. J Surg Oncol. 2015;112(3):284–8.

# Robotic-Assisted Distal Pancreatectomy 20

Filip Bednar, Melissa E. Hogg, Herbert J. Zeh,
and Amer H. Zureikat

## Introduction

Resections of the pancreas have become more common as operative technique and perioperative care have significantly improved postoperative outcomes. The advent of minimally invasive techniques over the past three decades has revolutionized many general and oncologic surgical procedures. Laparoscopic—and now robotic-assisted—approaches to a distal pancreatic resection are a natural evolution of this trend. In this chapter, we review the indications, technique, and outcomes of robotic-assisted distal pancreatectomy (RDP).

## Indications

Robotic distal pancreatectomy is performed for both benign and malignant pancreatic pathologies. Benign etiologies include pancreatic trauma with pancreatic ductal disruption, acute and chronic pancreatitis with or without pseudocyst formation, and cystic neoplasms of the pancreas. Malignant etiologies range from pancreatic neuroendocrine tumors and pancreatic adenocarcinomas to metastatic disease to the pancreas, including renal cell carcinoma, breast carcinoma, peritoneal malignancies, and direct extension of solid GI malignancies such as colon and stomach adenocarcinomas.

F. Bednar, M.D., Ph.D.
Department of Surgery, University of Michigan,
1500 E. Medical Center Dr., 2210 Taubman Center, Ann Arbor, MI 48109, USA

M.E. Hogg, M.D., F.A.C.S. • H.J. Zeh, M.D., F.A.C.S.
Surgical Oncology, University of Pittsburgh Medical Center,
3550 Terrace St., Suite 497 Scaife Hall, Pittsburgh, PA 15261, USA

A.H. Zureikat, M.D., F.A.C.S. (✉)
UPMC Pancreatic Cancer Center, Surgical Oncology, University of Pittsburgh Medical Center, 3550 Terrace St., Suite 497 Scaife Hall, Pittsburgh, PA 15261, USA
e-mail: zureikatah@upmc.edu

© Springer International Publishing AG 2018 253
A.D. Patel, D. Oleynikov (eds.), *The SAGES Manual of Robotic Surgery*,
The SAGES University Masters Program Series, DOI 10.1007/978-3-319-51362-1_20

## Preoperative Testing

Initial evaluation of the patient consists of a thorough history and physical examination along with pertinent laboratory studies, including tumor markers, depending on the presumed pathology. Operative planning and further diagnosis are achieved with high-quality cross-sectional imaging. In our practice, all of our patients undergo a "pancreatic protocol" triple-phase high-resolution computed tomography (CT) scan prior to any surgery. This is sometimes supplemented by an endoscopic ultrasound with a fine needle aspiration for pathologic diagnosis. Further cross-sectional imaging and information can also be obtained with magnetic resonance imaging/magnetic resonance cholangiopancreatography (MRI/MRCP).

Patient preparation preoperatively consists of confirming that the patient is physiologically fit to undergo general anesthesia and laparoscopy. The key aspects of the evaluation focus particularly on cardiovascular disease and chronic obstructive pulmonary, since these may alter the operative approach or make the patient ineligible for minimally invasive surgery.

## Patient Positioning and Preparation

The patient is positioned supine on a split leg operating table. We extend the right arm out to 90° and tuck the left arm next to the body for the procedure. The lower extremities are padded and secured to allow intraoperative positioning into a steep reverse Trendelenburg position without buckling. Once well supported, the legs are abducted outward bilaterally to allow the first assistant to stand between them during the operation. Foley catheter is placed and appropriate IV access and monitoring lines are inserted. Placement of central lines is optional depending on the overall health of the patient and the judgement of the surgeon and anesthesiologist. We utilize both upper and lower body warming blankets during the operation to maintain patient normothermia. Once general anesthesia is established, we rotate the operating room table 45° to the patient's right. This allows for the unimpeded docking of the daVinci® system over the patient's head, while maintaining appropriate access (left side) for the anesthesia team to the airway and any central lines that were placed (Fig. 20.1). Standard-of-care preoperative antibiotics and DVT prophylaxis are administered.

## Operative Approach

### Peritoneal Access

We gain access to the peritoneum with a 5 mm OptiView port in the left upper quadrant under direct vision. This can also be accomplished with a Veress needle using the standard Veress insertion technique. The placement of this port is planned to allow for eventual upsizing to one of the 8 mm robot working ports (Fig. 20.2). The abdomen is insufflated to 15 mmHg of pressure, and an initial inspection of the

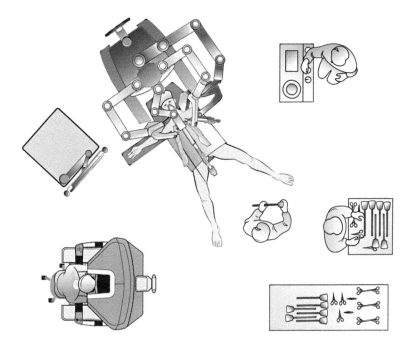

**Fig. 20.1** OR setup

**Fig. 20.2** Port placement

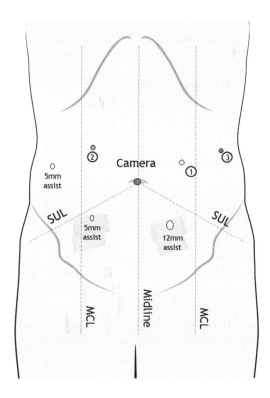

abdominal cavity is performed to determine the presence of any metastatic disease or other pathology that would alter the operative approach. If the decision is made to proceed, a periumbilical 12 mm camera port is placed. We immediately also insert a figure-of-eight 0 Polysorb/Vicryl suture using a Carter-Thomason suture passer to allow for a rapid fascial closure at the end of the case. Additional 8 mm robotic and 5 mm/12 mm assistant ports are placed as demonstrated in Fig. 20.2. A right lateral 5 mm port is used as an entry site for the liver retractor to allow for the elevation of the left lateral segment of the liver and the stomach. The left lower quadrant 12 mm port site will eventually be slightly enlarged and serve as the specimen extraction site during the operation.

## Liver Retraction and Access to the Lesser Sac

The patient is placed in a steep reverse Trendelenburg position and rotation to the left or right is utilized to optimize the visualization of the operative field. This is a key step in the operation because once the daVinci® system is docked, no further adjustments in patient or bed positioning can be made without removing all of the instruments and completely undocking the robotic arms. With all ports in place, we insert a triangular liver retractor to elevate the left lateral segment of the liver and directly visualize the anterior surface of the stomach and the spleen. We expose the anterior surface of the pancreas by dividing the greater gastrocolic omentum immediately outside of the right gastroepiploic arcade. The line of division is continued taking the short gastric vessels all the way to the left crus of the gastroesophageal hiatus. We utilize the laparoscopic LigaSure™ instrument for the omental division. The operating surgeon is typically on the right side of the patient, while the first assistant provides countertraction and exposure from a position between the patient's legs during this step. Division of the omentum provides exposure to the anterior surface of the pancreas toward the spleen.

## Isolation of the Splenic Artery

Once the stomach is mobilized, it can be placed above the triangular liver retractor to keep it out of the operative field without sacrificing an active instrument. At this point, the daVinci® system is brought into the field. Arms 1 and 3 are docked to the left of the camera; arm 2 is docked to the right. The 30° robotic camera is inserted into the 12 mm periumbilical port with a 30° downward orientation. Under direct vision, we typically place the robotic hook cautery instrument into arm 1, the fenestrated bipolar grasper into arm 2, and a second non-cautery grasper (Prograsp or Cadiere forceps) into arm 3. The assistant uses a suction irrigator device and a long 5 mm laparoscopic LigaSure™ device through the 5 and 12 mm assistant ports to keep the field clear and to assist with the hemostasis.

The first step of the dissection focuses on the isolation of the proximal splenic artery, which can typically be found above the superior border of the pancreas. For pancreatic cancers, we divide the pancreas at the neck to ensure an excellent

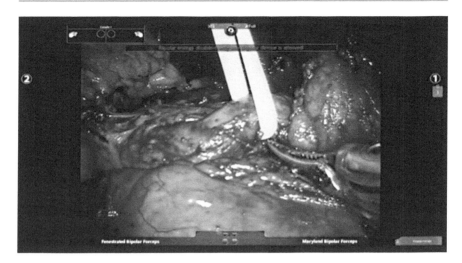

**Fig. 20.3**  Isolation of splenic artery

lymphadenectomy along the left gastric pedicle and celiac trunk. For pNETs or other non-PDA diseases, we divide the pancreas 1–2 cm to the right of the lesion. A splenectomy is performed en-bloc for all PDA cases. Careful blunt dissection and judicious use of hook cautery supplemented with the 5 mm LigaSure™ and the fenestrated bipolar device are used to circumferentially dissect the splenic artery. A vessel loop is used to provide gentle traction on the vessel (Fig. 20.3). Occasionally, a robotic Maryland forceps instrument is also used for assistance during this dissection. Once isolated, the splenic artery is divided with the 45 mm gold vascular load for the EndoGIA stapler.

## Isolation of the Pancreatic Body and Splenic Vein

The specific point of division on the pancreas will depend on the patient pathology. We often utilize an intraoperative ultrasound probe for the daVinci® system to confirm our planned point of division. The dissection of the pancreatic body begins at the inferior border of the pancreas. Specific attention is given to the location of the superior mesenteric vein (SMV), which forms the most proximal extent of the dissection. Additional vascular structures needing identification during this step are the inferior mesenteric vein (IMV) at its insertion to the splenic vein or SMV. We carry the dissection posterior to the pancreas along the avascular plane that separates it from the rest of the retroperitoneum. Along this course, we identify the splenic vein, if it has not been isolated yet. Once the superior edge of the pancreas is reached, we pass a moistened umbilical tape around the gland to provide gentle traction (Fig. 20.4). A 60 mm purple or gold (depending on thickness) EndoGIA stapler load is used for division of the gland. Alternatively, if the gland is too thick, we will transect it with electrocautery scissors and close the stump with a running 3-0 V-Loc suture with 5-0 pds suture closure of the pancreatic duct if found.

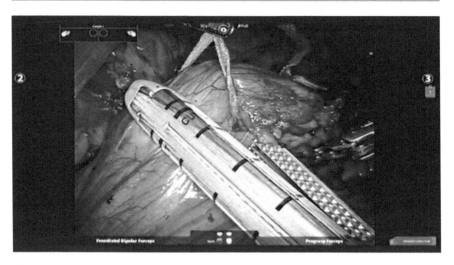

**Fig. 20.4** Isolation and division of the pancreas

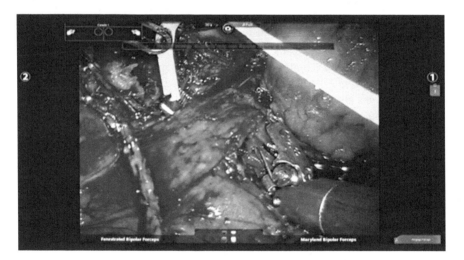

**Fig. 20.5** Isolation vein

   With the pancreas and the splenic artery divided, the only structure left to isolate is the splenic vein. At this point, the vein is typically easily visible and is again circumferentially dissected (either at its junction with the superior mesenteric vein [SMV] or to the left of the spleno-portal confluence) and then encircled with the help of a vessel loop (Fig. 20.5). Division of the splenic vein is performed with a 45 mm gold EndoGIA stapler load (Fig. 20.6). At the end of this maneuver, all of the major vascular tributaries to the spleen have been controlled, and we turn our attention to the final retroperitoneal dissection and splenic mobilization.

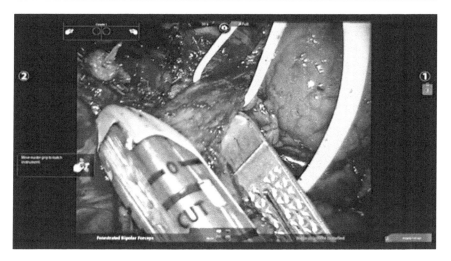

**Fig. 20.6**  Division of the of the splenic splenic vein

## Antegrade Mobilization from the Retroperitoneum, Splenic Mobilization

The extent of the retroperitoneal dissection depends on the pathology being treated. If we are performing a distal pancreatectosplenectomy for a pancreatic adenocarcinoma, we also resect the superficial retroperitoneum anterior to the adrenal gland, renal vessels, and Gerota's fascia en bloc with the pancreas. If the etiology is a benign or a malignancy other than a true pancreatic adenocarcinoma, the dissection can be simply carried along the retropancreatic avascular plane (just posterior to the splenic vein) toward the spleen. The tissue dissection is typically performed with gentle elevation of the pancreas toward the anterior abdominal wall using arm 3 grasper. The hook cautery, the 5 mm LigaSure™, and the fenestrated bipolar are all involved in hemostasis with the assistant using the suction irrigator to keep the field clear of fluid, blood, and smoke. Carrying the retroperitoneal dissection laterally eventually brings the surgeon to the posterior, superior, and inferior attachments of the spleen. These are divided with hook cautery or the 5 mm LigaSure™ to finish the mobilization of the entire specimen (Fig. 20.7).

## Specimen Extraction

The specimen is extracted in two parts. We identify the plane separating the distal pancreatic tail from the spleen at the splenic hilum and use an EndoGIA 45 mm gold or purple stapler loads to divide the splenic hilum at that point. The distal pancreas and the spleen are separately contained within two 10 or 15 mm Endocatch bag devices depending on the size of each specimen. The bags are extracted through the 12 mm left lower quadrant assistant port. This port sometimes has to be enlarged one or two centimeters to allow for the tissue extraction.

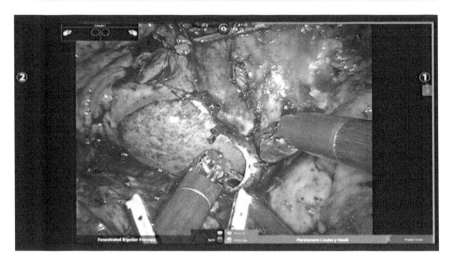

**Fig. 20.7** Retroperitoneal dissection and splenic mobilization

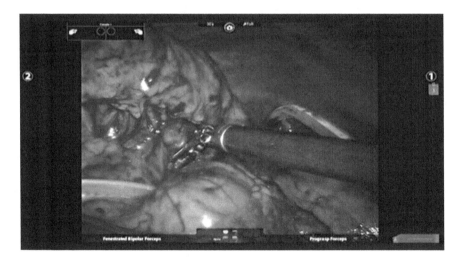

**Fig. 20.8** Drain placement

After specimen extraction, we place a round #19 channel drain into the resection bed posterior to the stomach with the tip near the transected pancreas (Fig. 20.8). This is typically placed through robotic port #3 and secured at the skin with a 2-0 nylon suture. We irrigate the resection bed and the left upper quadrant with the suction irrigator to verify hemostasis. We then undock the daVinci® system and begin the final closure.

## Closure

For the closure the patient is returned to a supine position. We close the fascia of the enlarged 12 mm port in the left lower quadrant with interrupted figure-of-eight #1 polysorb vicryl sutures. The periumbilical port site is closed with the previously placed figure-of-eight Polysorb/Vicryl suture. All skin incisions are closed using 4-0 running Monocryl/Monosorb subcuticular sutures. The drain is placed to bulb suction. We typically leave the Foley catheter in place until the following morning. Early drain removal (POD 3–4) is employed if the drain amylase level is <3 times the serum level.

## Clinical Outcomes

### Feasibility

As with any new technology, analysis of RDP outcomes initially focused on safety and feasibility of the robotic approach in comparison to the other platforms. Giulianotti and colleagues published a series of five robotic-assisted pancreatic resection cases with advanced vascular resections [1]. These included two Appleby procedures, one distal pancreatectomy with a portal vein resection, and the other Whipple pancreaticoduodenectomies with portal vein resections. The manuscript did not contain significant long-term outcomes but served to introduce the application of this technology to complex pancreatic and vascular resections.

Our group published its initial large summary of robotic pancreatic resection experience in 2013 [2]. Out of the reported 250 pancreatic resections, 83 were distal pancreatectomies. We observed no 30- or 90-day mortalities and a 13% rate of Clavien-Dindo Grade III complications [3]. Forty-three percent of our patients had a postoperative pancreatic fistula, 17% were clinically relevant Grade B/C fistulas. Our conversion rate to an open procedure was 2%. Similar to our experience, Zhan and colleagues summarized their early experience with 16 RDPs and demonstrated a pancreatic leak rate of 56% [4]. Suman and colleagues performed 49 RDPs for cancer with a postoperative morbidity of 40%, pancreatic fistula rate of 20%, and clinically relevant Grade B/C fistulas in 5% of their patients [5]. However, they converted to an open operation in 18.4% of their cases while achieving a 92% R0 resection rate. Hwang and colleagues published their experience with 22 spleen-preserving RDPs [6]. The postoperative pancreatic Grade B/C fistula rate was 9.1% and no conversions were noted. These single institution series demonstrate that a robotic-assisted approach to distal pancreatectomy can achieve results that are potentially comparable to historical controls for open distal pancreatic resections.

One key aspect in the adoption of any new technology is its associated learning curve. Our group has specifically tried to address this question by analyzing the first 100 RDPs at our institution utilizing the cumulative sum analysis (CUSUM) method for operative time. In our experience, the learning curve was approximately 40 cases [7]. Comparing the first 40 cases with the latter 60 demonstrated a significant drop in operative time from 299 to 210 min. We also lowered our rate of readmissions from 40 to 20% and the rate of Grade B/C pancreatic fistulas from 27.5 to 11.7%. For oncologic resections, we had a stable 3–5% rate of R1 resections.

In comparison to our learning curve data, Napoli and colleagues analyzed 55 RDPs from their institution [8]. Similar to our approach, they also utilized a cumulative sum analysis (CUSUM) of operative times and determined their learning curve threshold to be ten cases. They demonstrated operative time decrease from 421 to 248 min and grade B/C fistula rate of 60% and 42% for the first 10 versus the next 45 cases. It is notable that both reports analyzing the learning curves come from high-volume institutions that have also built the appropriate perioperative and operating room support system that allows for efficient progression of learning and skill acquisition under the mentorship of experienced robotic surgeons.

## Comparison with Open and Laparoscopic Distal Pancreatectomy

Robotic distal pancreatectomy represents an evolution of the minimally invasive laparoscopic paradigm. Our group compared our early robotic experience (first 30 cases) with 94 laparoscopic distal pancreatectomies (LDP) at our institution. Even though these cases represented the early part of our learning curve, we still demonstrated decreased OR times (293 vs. 372 min), lower blood loss (375 vs. 500 cc), and low conversion rate to an open resection (0 vs. 16%) when utilizing the robotic technique compared to LDP [9].

Additional single institution studies also compared various aspects of robotic, laparoscopic, and open approaches. Waters and colleagues compared 17 RDPs with 22 open distal pancreatectomy and 18 LDPs [10]. In this report, operative times were 298 min for RDP, 234 min for open distal pancreatectomy, and 224 min for LDP. Postoperative morbidity was 18% in the robotic cohort, 18% in the open cohort, and 33% in the laparoscopic cohort. Length of stay was the shortest in the robotic cohort at 4 days. Both laparoscopic and robotic procedures had a ~12% conversion rate.

Kang and colleagues analyzed 25 laparoscopic and 20 RDPs [11]. In their comparison, younger patients underwent the robotic resection more often. Operative times were 258 min for the laparoscopic resections and 349 min for the RDPs with similar associated blood loss. Rates of postoperative complications were similar in both groups at 10–16%. Duran and colleagues analyzed 16 RDPs and compared these to 13 open and 18 laparoscopic resections [12]. The robotic cohort was healthier at baseline with no ASA III patients. 12.5% underwent conversion in the RDP cohort. There were two Grade A postoperative pancreatic fistulae in the RDP cases compared with two Grade B in the laparoscopic and open cases. In the study by Lai and colleagues, 17 RDPs were compared with 18 laparoscopic resections [13]. The operative time was longer for the RDP at 221 vs. 174 min. The associated postoperative pancreatic fistula rate was 41 and 33%. Goh and colleagues compared eight RDPs with 31 laparoscopic resections [14]. There were no conversions in the RDP cohort and 42% conversion rate in the laparoscopic cohort. OR times in the RDP group were longer (452 min) than in the laparoscopic group (245 min). Postoperative pancreatic fistula rates were high at 58–63%. Percentages of 25 and 13 of the RDP or laparoscopic patients suffered a Grade III/IV complication.

The group from Memorial Sloan Kettering has recently published an analysis of their distal pancreatectomy experience [15]. They compared 637 open, 131 laparoscopic, and 37 robotic distal resections. The robotic and laparoscopic cohorts had a lower proportion of malignant histology (39% vs. 11–15%). OR time was slightly longer for the RDPs at 213 min compared with the open and laparoscopic resections (185 and 193 min). Conversion rates were similar between RDP and LDP at 38 and 31%. Grade B or higher pancreatic fistulas were present in 9% (open), 6% (laparoscopic), and 5% (robotic) of patients. Grade III/IV complications occurred in 25, 22, and 43% of patients.

Two studies attempted to compare RDP with laparoscopic distal pancreatectomies in a more controlled fashion. Butturini and colleagues performed a small nonrandomized prospective trial comparing 22 RDPs with 21 laparoscopic resections [16]. The study was again underpowered, but the observations were similar to the series presented earlier. The conversion rates were equivalent in the two cohorts at 4.5 and 4.7%. The postoperative fistula rates were 50–57% with 27–33% Grade B/C. The readmission rate and reoperative rate were higher in the robotic cohort at 18.2% vs. 4.7% and 13.6% vs. 4.6%. The significance of these differences is difficult to assess given the low numbers of patients enrolled in each cohort.

Chen and colleagues conducted a matched cohort study of 69 robotic and 50 laparoscopic distal pancreatectomies [17]. They noted a significantly higher rate of splenic preservation (65% vs. 26%), significantly lower operative time (150 vs. 200 min), and lower blood loss in the robotic cohort. They had no conversions in any of the RDPs. Postoperative morbidity was equivalent in the two groups at ~40–48%. The pancreatic fistula rate was 25–32% and Grade B fistulas were seen in 15–29%.

## Conclusion

Current clinical experience and published data suggest that the robotic approach to distal pancreatectomy is safe and feasible. The learning curve has been estimated to be between 10 and 40 cases at high volume centers. Published outcomes are limited by small numbers and selection bias; however, emerging data suggests noninferiority compared to the laparoscopic approach. Robotic approaches to pancreatic resection continue to carry significant promise of improved outcomes; however, randomized controlled trials or large-scale registries are needed to delineate the benefit of the robotic approach compared to other platforms.

## References

1. Giulianotti PC, Addeo P, Buchs NC, Ayloo SM, Bianco FM. Robotic extended pancreatectomy with vascular resection for locally advanced pancreatic tumors. Pancreas. 2011 [cited 2016 Aug 28];40(8):1264–70. Available from: http://www.ncbi.nlm.nih.gov/pubmed/21785385.

2. Zureikat AH, Moser AJ, Boone BA, Bartlett DL, Zenati M, Zeh HJ. 250 Robotic pancreatic resections: safety and feasibility. Ann Surg. 2013 [cited 2016 Aug 28];258(4):554–9; discussion 559–62. Available from: http://www.ncbi.nlm.nih.gov/pubmed/24002300.

3. Dindo D, Demartines N, Clavien P-A. Classification of surgical complications: a new proposal with evaluation in a cohort of 6336 patients and results of a survey. Ann Surg. 2004;240(2):205–13.

4. Zhan Q, Deng XX, Han B, Liu Q, Shen BY, Peng CH, et al. Robotic-assisted pancreatic resection: a report of 47 cases. Int J Med Robot Comput Assist Surg. 2013 [cited 2016 Aug 28];9(1):44–51. Available from: http://www.ncbi.nlm.nih.gov/pubmed/23225335.

5. Suman P, Rutledge J, Yiengpruksawan A. Robotic distal pancreatectomy. JSLS. 2013 [cited 2016 Aug 28];17(4):627–35. Available from: http://www.ncbi.nlm.nih.gov/pubmed/24398207

6. Hwang HK, Kang CM, Chung YE, Kim KA, Choi SH, Lee WJ. Robot-assisted spleen-preserving distal pancreatectomy: a single surgeon's experiences and proposal of clinical application. Surg Endosc Other Interv Tech. 2013 [cited 2016 Aug 28]. p. 774–81. Available from: http://www.ncbi.nlm.nih.gov/pubmed/23052527.

7. Shakir M, Boone BA, Polanco PM, Zenati MS, Hogg ME, Tsung A, et al. The learning curve for robotic distal pancreatectomy: an analysis of outcomes of the first 100 consecutive cases at a high-volume pancreatic centre. HPB (Oxford). 2015 [cited 2016 Aug 28];17(7):580–6. Available from: http://www.ncbi.nlm.nih.gov/pubmed/25906690.

8. Napoli N, Kauffmann EF, Perrone VG, Miccoli M, Brozzetti S, Boggi U. The learning curve in robotic distal pancreatectomy. Updates Surg. 2015 [cited 2016 Aug 28];67(3):257–64. Available from: http://www.ncbi.nlm.nih.gov/pubmed/25990666.

9. Daouadi M, Zureikat AH, Zenati MS, Choudry H, Tsung A, Bartlett DL, et al. Robot-assisted minimally invasive distal pancreatectomy is superior to the laparoscopic technique. Ann Surg. 2012 [cited 2016 Aug 28];257(1):1. Available from: http://www.ncbi.nlm.nih.gov/pubmed/22868357.

10. Waters JA, Canal DF, Wiebke EA, Dumas RP, Beane JD, Aguilar-Saavedra JR, et al. Robotic distal pancreatectomy: cost effective? Surgery. 2010 [cited 2016 Aug 28];148(4):814–23. Available from: http://www.ncbi.nlm.nih.gov/pubmed/20797748.

11. Kang CM, Kim DH, Lee WJ, Chi HS. Conventional laparoscopic and robot-assisted spleen-preserving pancreatectomy: does da Vinci have clinical advantages? Surg Endosc Other Interv Tech. 2011 [cited 2016 Aug 28];25(6):2004–9. Available from: http://www.ncbi.nlm.nih.gov/pubmed/21136089.

12. Duran H, Ielpo B, Caruso R, Ferri V, Quijano Y, Diaz E, et al. Does robotic distal pancreatectomy surgery offer similar results as laparoscopic and open approach? A comparative study from a single medical center. Int J Med Robot Comput Assist Surg. 2014 [cited 2016 Aug 28];10(3):280–5. Available from: http://www.ncbi.nlm.nih.gov/pubmed/24431290.

13. Lai ECH, Tang CN. Robotic distal pancreatectomy versus conventional laparoscopic distal pancreatectomy: a comparative study for short-term outcomes. Front Med. 2015 [cited 2016 Aug 28];9(3):356–60. Available from: http://www.ncbi.nlm.nih.gov/pubmed/26271291.

14. Goh BKP, Chan CY, Soh H-L, Lee SY, Cheow P-C, Chow PKH, et al. A comparison between robotic-assisted laparoscopic distal pancreatectomy versus laparoscopic distal pancreatectomy. Int J Med Robot. 2016 [cited 2016 Aug 28]. Available from: http://www.ncbi.nlm.nih.gov/pubmed/26813478.

15. Lee SY, Allen PJ, Sadot E, D'Angelica MI, Dematteo RP, Fong Y, et al. Distal pancreatectomy: a single institution's experience in open, laparoscopic, and robotic approaches. J Am Coll Surg. 2015 [cited 2016 Aug 28];220(1):18–27. Available from: http://www.ncbi.nlm.nih.gov/pubmed/25456783.

16. Butturini G, Damoli I, Crepaz L, Malleo G, Marchegiani G, Daskalaki D, et al. A prospective non-randomised single-center study comparing laparoscopic and robotic distal pancreatectomy. Surg Endosc Other Interv Tech. 2015 [cited 2016 Aug 28];29(11):3163–70. Available from: http://www.ncbi.nlm.nih.gov/pubmed/25552231.

17. Chen S, Zhan Q, Chen JZ, Jin JB, Deng XX, Chen H, et al. Robotic approach improves spleen-preserving rate and shortens postoperative hospital stay of laparoscopic distal pancreatectomy: a matched cohort study. Surg Endosc Other Interv Tech. 2015 [cited 2016 Aug 28];29(12):3507–18. Available from: http://www.ncbi.nlm.nih.gov/pubmed/25791063.

# Robotic Liver Resection and Biliary Reconstruction

Iswanto Sucandy and Allan Tsung

## Robotic Liver Resection

Until the 1980s, operative mortality after liver resections was about 20%, which was mainly related to significant intraoperative hemorrhage [1]. As liver surgery became safer because of a better understanding of liver anatomy, safer anesthesia, and more advanced perioperative care, minimally invasive techniques began to gain popularity in the mid-1990s. Application of robotic technology in the fields of hepatobiliary and complex surgical oncology is gradually gaining popularity worldwide. Robotic liver resection and biliary reconstruction are now performed in many major hepatobiliary centers for malignant and benign diseases. Published articles in modern surgical literature assessing this new approach are also rapidly expanding. This chapter provides an overview of robotic application in liver and biliary tract surgery, a contemporary summary in regards to perioperative outcomes, and a comparison against the more established conventional laparoscopic technique.

The minimally invasive approach has proven its benefits in the past two decades in almost all surgical subspecialties, including colorectal surgery, gynecology, urology, cardiothoracic surgery, bariatric surgery, and surgical oncology. Reduced postoperative pain decreased postoperative narcotic requirement, decreased length of hospital stay, lowered wound-related complications, and improved cosmesis have transformed minimally invasive surgery to become the technique of choice. The conventional laparoscopic technique, however, has several inherent limitations, such as limited range of motion, amplification of physiologic tremor, reduced ergonomics, and a steep learning curve. The need for advanced laparoscopic skills, which include suturing, knot tying, and bimanual tissue manipulations, hinders adoption of this technique for complex liver, pancreas, and biliary tract surgeries.

I. Sucandy, M.D. • A. Tsung, M.D. (✉)
Department of Surgery, University of Pittsburgh Medical Center,
Kaufmann Medical Building, 3471 Fifth Ave., Suite 300, Pittsburgh, PA 15213, USA
e-mail: sucandyi2@upmc.edu; tsunga@upmc.edu

© Springer International Publishing AG 2018
A.D. Patel, D. Oleynikov (eds.), *The SAGES Manual of Robotic Surgery*,
The SAGES University Masters Program Series, DOI 10.1007/978-3-319-51362-1_21

Operating surgeons need sufficient experience in advanced laparoscopic surgery in addition to open liver surgery in order to perform a safe laparoscopic liver resection. Robotic surgery can potentially provide a better solution for the technical limitations of conventional laparoscopic techniques. In a series reported by Choi et al., surgeons without any experience in laparoscopic major liver resections succeeded in performing robotic major hepatectomies [2]. The robotic system, therefore, may enable surgeons with insufficient experience in advanced laparoscopy to perform more complex minimally invasive procedures.

## Advantages and Disadvantages of Robotic Surgery

The robotic system provides several advantages over the traditional laparoscopic techniques, including seven degrees of freedom, enhanced suturing capability, superior visualization with a 3-D camera system, elimination of physiologic tremor, and surgeon ergonomics. These features allow for precise identification and complex dissection of inflow/outflow vessels and biliary ducts, both extra- and intrahepatically. While intrahepatic Glissonian pedicle approach is popular and effective in a non-cirrhotic liver, this technique is dangerous in cirrhotic livers. The cirrhotic liver parenchyma often resists a smooth clamp insertion or stapler passage, while a minor injury to the pedicles may cause significant bleeding in the context of portal hypertension. The extrahepatic approach appears to be ideal in this situation, as long as it can be done safely during minimally invasive liver resections. Robotic surgery provides a superior technical ease in accomplishing this key step, when compared to the conventional laparoscopic approach. Some surgeons may even advocate that portal/inflow dissection is easier and safer robotically, secondary to the enhanced 3-D visualization, better dissection angle, vision magnification, and tremor filtering by the robotic system.

Casciola et al. described that the robotic approach is most useful for lesions located high in the hepatic dome (segment 7–8) [3]. Due to the straight characteristics of most laparoscopic instruments, the convexity of the liver surface can create difficulties in reaching the hepatic dome area. Robotic endowrist features of da Vinci robotic system provide better access to this area. Additionally, the use of the robotic system seems to shorten the learning curve for most complex operations when compared to the conventional laparoscopy. The technical advantages associated with the robotic approach allow completion of a higher percentage of major hepatectomies using a purely minimally invasive approach. Tsung et al. reported that 93% of the robotic liver resections were accomplished without the need for hand-assist ports or hybrid technique, in contrast with only 49.1% of those performed using the conventional laparoscopic approach [4]. The technically challenging nature of most hepatobiliary operations provides an ideal application for robotic technology [5–8].

Higher operative costs, lack of tactile feedback, narrow operative field, and the need for a skilled bedside assistant are some of the disadvantages of robotic surgery currently. The lack of tactile feedback can generally be compensated by visual feedback, which gradually comes with practice and experience [9]. Guilianotti et al. in 2003 reported the first series of robotics in general surgery [10]. In their early report of 207 procedures, which included liver and pancreas resections, they concluded that robotic-assisted surgery is both safe and feasible. Based on the most recent international consensus in Morioka, Japan, however, major robotic liver surgery is still recommended to be done within an institutional review board-approved registry [11].

## Robot-Assisted Liver Surgery

The first report of robot-assisted liver resection was published in 2006 by Ryska et al. [12]. Fourteen major series of robotic liver resection since 2010 have then been published in the literature, with description of operative time, estimated blood loss, requirement for blood transfusion, extent of hepatic resection, perioperative morbidity, and postoperative duration of hospital stay. The 2008 International Consensus Conference on laparoscopic liver surgery held in Louisville, Kentucky led to recommendations that solitary liver lesions of 5 cm or less and peripheral tumor location are ideal for minimally invasive approach. No specific guidelines have been written to date, in regards to the use of robot-assisted liver resection [11].

Upon review of all published series on robot-assisted liver resection, approximately 72% of cases were performed for malignancies [9]. The most common pathology was hepatocellular carcinoma, followed by colorectal liver metastasis and intrahepatic cholangiocarcinoma. On the other hand, benign indications for liver resection included symptomatic hemangioma, hepatic adenoma, and fibronodular hyperplasia. Thirty-one percent of cases were classified as major resections with more than three liver segments resected. Operative time varied between 90 and 812 min. The long operative times were usually attributed to equipment unfamiliarity and longer robotic setup times. Increase in technical experience of the console surgeon, bedside assistant, and operating room team reduced the operative time [10]. Estimated blood loss ranged from 50 ml to 413 ml with transfusion rates ranged from 0 to 44%. Ji et al. in their series reported reduced blood loss using the robotic approach, in comparison with the conventional laparoscopic or classical open operation (280 ml vs. 350 ml vs. 470 ml, respectively; $p < .05$) [13]. Publication from our institution demonstrated reduced blood loss in the latter 44 robotic liver resections, when compared with the initial 13 cases (100 ml vs. 300 ml) [10]. Seven percent of open conversion rate was related to intraoperative bleeding, significant intraabdominal adhesions, technical difficulties in accomplishing resection, and concerns regarding oncologic margins [14].

Average reported rate of complications after robotic liver resections was 21%, which included liver-specific complications (bile leak, liver failure, and postoperative ascites), those related to the operation (abdominal bleeding, pleural effusion, wound infection, postoperative ileus, and bladder injury), and those related to the any surgery in general (postoperative venous thromboembolism, Clostridium difficile infection) [9]. The overall most common were bile leaks, development of bilomas, and intraabdominal abscesses. No perioperative mortality has been reported in any of the reported series. Length of hospital stay ranged from 4 to 12 days. There appeared to be variability in length of hospital stay depending on the country where the procedures were performed. The shortest hospital stay was observed in the United States. In Europe and Asia, post-hepatectomy patients were kept in the hospital longer. Experience from the University of Pittsburgh Medical Center showed a median postoperative hospital stay of 4 days [8, 10]. Ji et al. also described the duration of hospital stay to be 3 days shorter after robotic liver resection, when compared with open (7 days vs. 10 days) [13].

There have been only limited data on oncologic outcomes after robotic liver resections. Most series reported a high R0 resection with only five series reported follow-up longer than 9 months after hepatectomy (range 9.6–25 months) [2–3, 14–16]. Recurrence rates after robotic liver resection appears to be comparable with that of the laparoscopic liver resection published in the literature [17]. Given the lack of solid long-term follow-up data, more definitive conclusions on local recurrence rates and disease-free survival require further studies.

## Patient Assessment and Operative Strategy

The indications and preoperative evaluation for robotic liver resections are similar to those of open liver surgery. Imaging of the liver is best obtained with triphasic liver CT scan or MRI. Biopsy of liver mass is usually reserved only for diagnostic uncertainty, despite of high-quality imaging. Evaluation of future liver remnant and patient general health performance are similar to those of the open surgery. Decision to perform liver resection robotically is strongly influenced by the tumor location, size, vicinity to the vital structures, and experience of the robotic team. Both the console surgeon and his/her bedside assistant should be ideally proficient in open and robotic liver surgery. They should be interchangeable throughout the entire case. Central and high posterior lesions provide challenges and require significant robotic experience. The technical challenges with liver mobilization, hilar dissection, parenchymal transection, and hemostasis can be minimized by an optimal port placement, good patient positioning, and efficient operating room team. Difficult dissections that require significantly prolonged operative time, failure to progress, significant intraoperative bleeding should prompt a consideration for conversion to the open approach. The anesthesia team should also understand that a low central venous pressure should always be aimed during any liver operations, regardless of the operative approach. Temporary inflow occlusion with Pringle maneuver is sometimes necessary. In our institution, we use a flat rubber tape, which is placed around the portal pedicle via the foramen of Winslow using a blunt robotic grasper. The rubber tape is then tightened by pulling its two ends together and subsequently held in place by a laparoscopic bulldog clamp.

## Surgical Technique in Robotic Liver Resection

### Patient Positioning and Port Placement

The patient is placed supine on the operating table with 15–30 degree reverse Trendelenburg position and split legs. The bedside assistant is standing in between the patient's legs. A foot board should be routinely placed to avoid untoward patient's movements during intraoperative positional maneuvers. For lesions in right posterior sectors, the table can be slightly rotated to the left (partial left lateral decubitus) in order to increase exposure. Unlike in conventional laparoscopy where the operating table adjustments can be readily made at any time during the operation, in robotic surgery, the arms must be undocked before any positional changes.

A total of six ports are used (two 12 mm ports, three 8 mm robotic ports, and one 5 mm port) in standard robotic major liver resection. Trocar positioning for both right and left liver resections is shown (Figs. 21.1 and 21.2). Access into the abdominal cavity can be safely established using either the standard Hasson or the Optiview technique. After 15 mmHg pneumoperitoneum is achieved, a 30-degree robotic camera is inserted. The camera port should be placed approximately 15–20 cm from the target anatomy. The additional five ports are placed under direct visualization with the robotic ports should be placed at least 8 cm apart from each other to minimize external collisions. The da Vinci robotic system is docked from the cranial aspect of the patient, making sure an adequate clearance from anesthesia apparatus. A properly docked robotic system should in line with the working axis (Fig. 21.3). In right liver resection, the 12 mm camera port is usually introduced in the right periumbilical position in order to place the camera in the middle of the target anatomy. The main working arms (arm 1 and 2 are placed to the left and right of the camera port). The third robotic arm is placed to the left of the arm 2, approximately 10 cm away. This arm is used for field exposure and tissue retraction. The two assistant ports (12 mm port to allow insertion of linear stapling device and 5 mm for laparoscopic suction/hemostatic instruments) are placed caudolateral to the camera port facing the target anatomy. For left hepatectomies, the camera port is placed in supraumbilical position because the operative frame is slightly shifted toward the left abdomen. The assistant's instruments must be able to reach the working area for suctioning, clipping, compression, stapling, or ultrasonographic mapping without difficulty.

### Right Hepatic Lobectomy

The operation begins with division of the round and falciform ligaments. Attachments between the liver and the hepatic flexure, right kidney, duodenum, or omentum are taken down using a hook electrocautery. The third robotic arm is positioned to provide upward and medial retraction to the right liver in order to explore the right triangular ligament laterally and short hepatic veins medially (Fig. 21.4). Appropriate

**Fig. 21.1** Trocar
positioning for right liver
resection

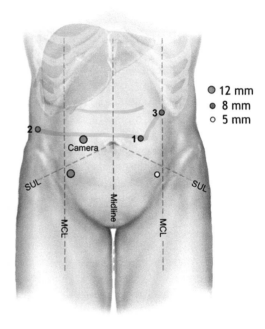

**Fig. 21.2** Trocar
positioning for left liver
resection

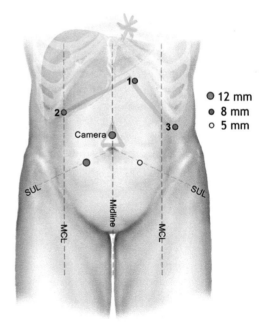

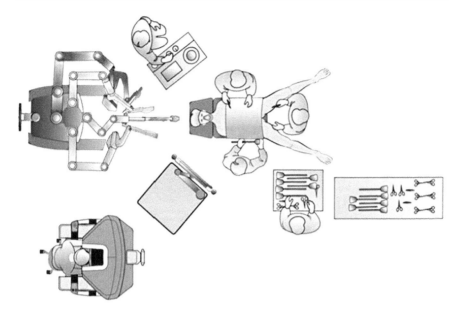

**Fig. 21.3**   Operating room setup and robotic system docking position

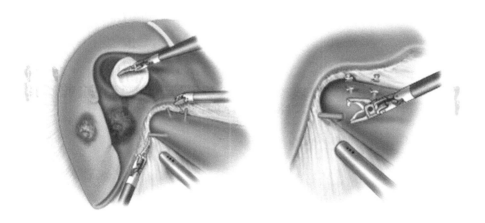

**Fig. 21.4**   Exposure and mobilization of the right lobe of the liver

adjustment is made by the third arm as the dissection proceeds cranially toward the hepatic hilum. The right side of the inferior vena cava (IVC) is dissected carefully off the inferior aspect of the liver. The short hepatic veins are individually isolated and divided between clips and silk ties.

Portal dissection is started by appropriately lifting the inferior aspect of the liver cranially using the third robotic arm. The gallbladder when still present can be used

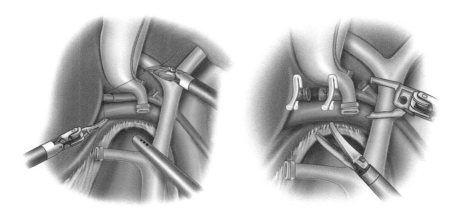

**Fig. 21.5** Portal dissection and division of the right hepatic artery

as a natural grasping handle by the third arm. The proper hepatic artery, which leads to the right hepatic artery, is identified. The right hepatic artery branch is isolated using a Maryland dissector and encircled with a vessel loop. A clamping test must be performed to ensure an intact arterial flow in the left hepatic artery prior to division. Silk tie with placement of metal clips or Hemolock clips are commonly used for this step (Fig. 21.5). A close attention must be exercised to avoid injury to the replaced or accessory right hepatic artery that is present in up to 25% of patients. The right portal vein is then carefully dissected and isolated prior to division using a linear vascular stapler (Fig. 21.6). Small branches to the caudate lobe often need to be divided in order to provide an adequate space for division. Finally the right hepatic duct is isolated, ligated, and divided after an intraoperative cholangiogram confirming presence of an intact contralateral biliary system (Fig. 21.7). Other authors have described the extra-Glissonian approach, where the right hepatic duct is divided using a linear stapler, without having to do a portal dissection with individual structure identification/ligation [2].

The right hepatic vein is then isolated and encircled with a vessel loop. A linear vascular stapler is used to divide the right hepatic vein by the bedside assistant, which safely accomplishes the outflow control. The line of parenchymal transection is then marked with the hook electrocautery, which follows a demarcation line on the liver surface. Placement of figure of eight silk sutures on both sides of the transection plane can be helpful for retraction (Fig. 21.8). Intraoperative ultrasonography is performed to confirm adequate tumor margins and to anticipate any large underlying crossing vessels. The Tilepro® feature of da Vinci system is helpful in transferring the ultrasonographic images to the console. The liver parenchymal transection is started using a combination of a Maryland bipolar forceps, application of silk ties and metal clips, and the robotic vessel sealer device. Use of rubber bands for lateral traction of the liver in minimally invasive hepatectomy has been introduced by Choi et al. [18,

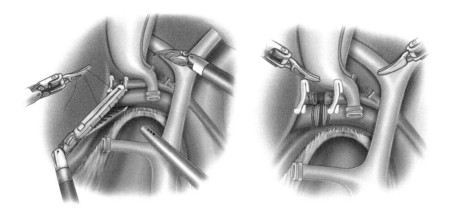

**Fig. 21.6** Isolation of the right portal vein and division using linear vascular stapler

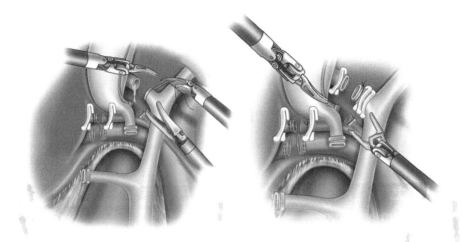

**Fig. 21.7** Isolation and division of the right hepatic duct

19]. As the parenchymal transection progresses, the traction of each rubber band was adjusted to optimize the exposure. The bedside assistant should help with tissue hemostasis and dynamic exposure of the transection plane. Medium- and large-sized crossing vessels/branches found intrahepatically are individually secured using ties and clips before division. Alternatively, they can also be handled using linear vascular stapler, fired by the bedside assistant. Thorough hemostasis and meticulous search for bile leak are performed along the cut surface prior to placing an abdominal drain. The resected specimen is placed in a large endo bag retrieval system and removed via either the enlarged camera port at the umbilical location or via a Pfannenstiel incision.

**Fig. 21.8** Placement of two stay stitches on both sides of transection plane

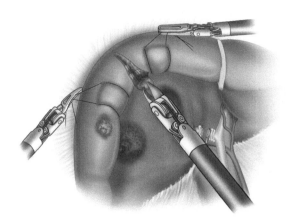

## Left Hepatic Lobectomy

The round and falciform ligaments are taken using similar technique as the right liver resection. A complete stomach decompression via a naso/oro-gastric tube is important at the beginning of the case. The left triangular ligament is divided using the hook electrocautery. It is important to not injury the branch of the phrenic veins often located nearby. Access into the lesser sac is obtained by dividing the gastrohepatic ligament. An accessory or replaced left hepatic artery is ligated and clipped prior to division when present in about 10–15% of patients. The lesser sac is opened all the way cephalad, toward the origin of the left hepatic vein. The goal is to obtain a complete mobilization of the left hemiliver. The portal dissection and parenchymal transection are performed using similar techniques as the right liver resection. The transverse portion of the left portal inflow allows a technically safer dissection. The right posterior sectoral bile duct empties into the left hepatic duct in approximately 13–19% of the population [20, 21]. Therefore, it is safer to divide the left bile duct close to the junction of the transverse and umbilical portion of the portal pedicles. Outflow dissection is subsequently performed after division of Arentius' ligament. With the left lobe reflected toward the right, the origin of the left and middle hepatic veins is carefully dissected. In majority of patients, the left and middle hepatic veins create a common trunk before entering the inferior vena cava. A linear vascular stapler is used to divide the hepatic vein after encirclement using a vessel loop (Fig. 21.9). If a safe outflow dissection cannot be achieved extrahepatically, the hepatic veins can also be divided intra-hepatically as the parenchymal transection proceeds cephalad (Fig. 21.10). Hemostasis and bilestasis are meticulously ensured prior to completion.

## Left Lateral Sectionectomy and Nonanatomic Liver Resection

In a left lateral sectionectomy, the transection line is located just to the left of the falciform ligament after left hemiliver mobilization. The divided round ligament

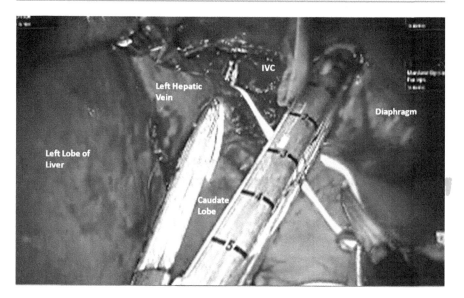

**Fig. 21.9** Isolation of the left hepatic vein outflow before parenchymal division

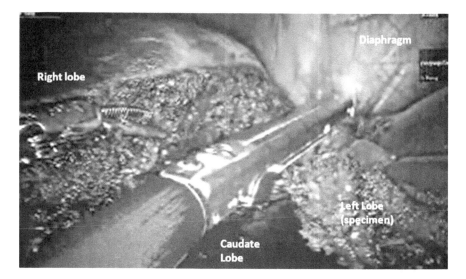

**Fig. 21.10** Parenchymal transection with division of hepatic vein common trunk

can be used as a handle toward the right anterior direction, which opens up the transection plane. Segment 2 and 3 pedicles were taken (either together or individually) with vascular load linear staplers, following the extra-Glissonian technique. The parenchymal transection is performed using similar steps, similar to those in formal left or right hepatectomies. Crossing vessels to segment 4A and 4B usually are usually encountered, but they can be easily managed with clips, vessel sealing devices, or linear staplers. The left hepatic vein is divided intrahepatically toward the end of the parenchymal transection. For nonanatomic liver resection, intraoperative ultrasonography is frequently used to ensure adequate margins and to detect underlying major vessels to and from the segments of pathology. Adequate planning for vascular control of medium/large vessel branches shown by the ultrasound should be in place prior to transection. Complete hemostasis and detection of bile leak must be ensured after parenchymal division. When a bile leak is identified from a biliary branch, careful placement of silk or vicryl sutures are effective. For hemostasis, we prefer to use saline-cooled radiofrequency device, which gives excellent results. Thermal energy, however, must be carefully applied in areas near the hepatic hilum and vessel staple lines. It is a good practice to lower the pneumoperitoneum while observing the liver cut surface for occult bleeding prior to closure [22].

It is critical to have a skilled bedside assistant surgeon with this type of advanced operations in liver surgery. Intraoperative bleeding during parenchymal transection is the primary reason for conversion to open surgery during major laparoscopic liver resection. Similar situation applies for major robotic liver resections. Conversion rates in laparoscopic major hepatectomy range from 33% in the early experience by Dulucq et al. [23] to a lower rate of 14% reported more recently by Gayet et al. [24]. In the totally robotic right hepatectomy of 24 patients reported by Giulianotti et al. [25], open conversion only occurred in 1/24 patients, which was related to oncologic concerns (inability to carefully evaluate the resection margins).

## Robotic Biliary Reconstruction

Robotic application in hepatobiliary surgery has included complex biliary tract reconstructive operations for benign and malignant biliary pathology. In 1995, the first report of minimally invasive choledochal cyst excision with Roux-en-Y hepaticoenterostomy was published by Farello et al. [22]. Unfortunately, adoption of this technique is slow, because of its technical complexity. In the past 5 years, however, several studies have emerged due to the availability of robotic system in many developed countries, which clearly facilitates performance of complex minimally invasive biliary tract operations [26, 27]. Alizai et al. reported 27 total cases of robot-assisted resection of choledochal cysts with hepaticojejunostomy in children, with five cases converted to open because of technical difficulties [28]. Reported average operative time was 5 h. Positive outcomes after 2.7 years of mean follow-up were reported with one child developed anastomotic stricture and subsequent bile leak after an open redo hepaticojejunostomy. Median hospital stay was 6 days and cosmetic results were excellent. Another report of robot-assisted complete excision of type 1 choledochal cyst with significantly shorter operative time (180 min) was published by Akaraviputh et al. [29]. A postoperative complication, which required percutaneous drainage of fluid collection and administration of systemic antibiotic, was noted, with otherwise excellent 1 year follow-up outcomes.

Inflammation of the porta hepatis, variable biliary anatomy, inadequate exposure and visualization, overly aggressive attempts at dissection/hemostasis, and surgeon inexperience are the commonly cited risk factors for biliary injury during cholecystectomy.

Roux-en-Y hepaticojejunostomy is the standard treatment for common hepatic duct injury type E2 according to the Strasberg classification. Most biliary injuries occur high in the biliary tree, close to the porta hepatis, thus not allowing a tension-free anastomosis with the duodenum for a choledochoduodenostomy. Prasad et al. reported the first case of robotic hepaticojejunostomy reconstruction for common bile duct injury after a cholecystectomy [30].

In a palliative setting of advanced malignant biliary obstruction, biliary drainage procedure can also provide durable restoration of life. The minimally invasive method may provide an optimum palliation with minimal trauma, low morbidity, and rapid recovery. Robot-assisted Roux-en-Y hepaticojejunostomy provides a better solution for the obstacles related to the technically challenging laparoscopic hepaticojejunostomy. Lai et al. in 2015 reported nine patients who were successfully treated using the robotic-assisted technique [31]. Roux-en-Y hepaticojejunostomy with gastrojejunostomy (double bypass) was performed in four patients, and the other five underwent hepaticojejunostomy only. The mean operative time was 213 min with blood loss of <40 ml. Bile leak was seen in 1/9 patient with no mortality. They concluded that robot-assisted hepaticojejunostomy for malignant biliary obstruction is a viable alternative to the percutaneous or endoscopic approach with low complication rates and improved quality of life.

## Surgical Technique in Biliary Tract Reconstruction

### Excision of Choledocal Cyst with Roux-en-Y Hepaticojejunostomy

The patient is positioned in reverse Trendelenburg prior to docking to allow the intestines and right colon to fall caudally. Ports are placed in similar configuration as that for right hepatectomy (Fig. 21.1). Using the third robotic arm, the liver is retracted cephalad, which results in exposure of the porta hepatis. The portal dissection is started by carefully identifying and dissecting the choledochal cyst off the hepatic artery medially and portal vein posteriorly. Once the hepatic artery and portal vein are separated from the cyst, the common bile duct dissection is continued distally toward the pancreas. The distal common bile duct is then ligated and clipped prior to division. The divided common bile duct with cyst attached to it is retracted cephalad. Careful dissection is carried out toward the biliary bifurcation until normal caliber common hepatic duct is identified. The gallbladder (if present) is then dissected and removed. The common hepatic duct is transected with scissors. The resected specimen is placed in an endo bag specimen retrieval system for later removal. A Roux-en-Y jejunal limb is then brought up in an antecolic fashion and prepared for an end-to-side hepaticojejunostomy. Tension and torsion of the jejunal limb must be avoided at all cost. anastomosis. can be done using either running or interrupted technique depending on diameter of the bile duct. Robotic system greatly facilitates precise suturing of the bile duct to the jejunal limb. A Jackson–Pratt drain is placed next to the anastomosis, prior to specimen removal.

## Robotic Roux-en-Y Hepaticojejunostomy for Bile Duct Injury After Cholecystectomy

After Anastomosis establishing a pneumoperitoneum up to 15 mmHg, the operating table is placed in a reverse Trendelenburg position and slightly rotated to the left if possible. The robotic system is then docked and the usual three working arms are installed. The porta hepatis is freed up from the duodenum and transverse colon if they are found to be adhered. The anatomy of the biliary duct must be sorted out and the site of bile duct injury/transection is identified. The source of bile leakage must be ensured and thorough exploration for additional injuries to the bile duct or surrounding structures must be performed. The cut edge of the common hepatic duct is freshened with scissors. Devitalized tissue caused by excessive thermal injury from hemostasis attempts must be resected until a healthy segment is seen. Doppler examination of the hepatic artery must also be performed to ensure the presence of intact right and left hepatic artery branches. A Roux-en-Y jejunal limb is then brought up using similar technique described previously. The hepaticojejunostomy can be done using either running or interrupted fashion, similar to that in choledochal cyst resection. A Jackson–Pratt drain is placed next to the anastomosis for an early detection and drainage of bile leak if it were to develop postoperatively.

## Robot-Assisted Hepaticojejunostomy for Advanced Malignant Biliary Obstruction

The patient and the trocars were positioned in a similar fashion as previously described. It is preferable to place the bedside assistant between the patient's legs. After establishing pneumoperitoneum, staging laparoscopy and laparoscopic ultrasonographic assessment of the tumor were performed. Only after these steps and decision to proceed is made by the operating surgeon, then robotic system is docked. Approximately 40–60 cm Roux limb is prepared in a standard fashion and brought up toward the hilum in an antecolic tension-free configuration. In a case of malignant distal biliary obstruction with significantly dilated common bile duct, a side-to-side choledochoduodenostomy can be performed. For more proximal biliary obstruction, an end-to-side hepaticojejunostomy is performed after transection of the common bile duct. If a double bypass is planned, then the hepaticojejunal anastomosis is completed before the gastrojejunal anastomosis. For a thin bile duct, monofilament sutures are preferred, while for a thickened bile duct, continuous 3–0 V-Loc™ sutures (Covidien, Dublin, Ireland) are preferred.

Robotics is one of the most recent developments in the field of minimally invasive surgery and many surgeons have started to see its advantages over the conventional laparoscopic approach. Robotic-assisted approach in complex hepatobiliary surgery can potentially overcome many limitations of the laparoscopic technique. Publications are emerging and promising outcomes are being reported from major centers worldwide. Further, large multi-institutional randomized trials are needed to establish robotic liver and biliary tract operations as new standards in modern minimally invasive hepatobiliary surgery.

# References

1. Fortner JG, Blumgart LH. A historic perspective of liver surgery for tumors at the end of the millennium. J Am Coll Surg. 2001;193(2):210–22.
2. Choi GH, Choi SH, Kim SH, et al. Robotic liver resection: technique and results of 30 consecutive procedures. Surg Endosc. 2012;26(8):2247–58.
3. Casciola L, Patriti A, Ceccarelli G, et al. Robot-assisted parenchymal-sparing liver surgery including lesions located in the posterosuperior segments. Surg Endosc. 2011;25(12):3815–24.
4. Tsung A, Geller DA. Reply to Letter: "Does the robot provide an advantage over laparoscopic liver resection?". Ann Surg. 2015;262(2):e70–1.
5. Giulianotti PC, Coratti A, Angelini M, et al. Robotics in general surgery: personal experience in a large community hospital. Arch Surg. 2003;138(7):777–84.
6. Zureikat AH, Moser AJ, Boone BA, et al. 250 robotic pancreatic resections: safety and feasibility. Ann Surg. 2013;258(4):554–9.
7. Daouadi M, Zureikat AH, Zenati MS, et al. Robot-assisted minimally invasive distal pancreatectomy is superior to the laparoscopic technique. Ann Surg. 2013;257(1):128–32.
8. Packiam V, Bartlett DL. Tohme, et al. Minimally invasive liver resection: robotic versus laparoscopic left lateral sectionectomy. J Gastrointest Surg. 2012;16(12):2233–8.
9. Ocuin LM, Tsung A. Robotic liver resection for malignancy: current status, oncologic outcomes, comparison to laparoscopy, and future applications. J Surg Oncol. 2015;112(3):295–301.
10. Tsung A, Geller DA, Sukato DC, et al. Robotic versus laparoscopic hepatectomy: a matched comparison. Ann Surg. 2014;259(3):549–55.
11. Wakabayashi G, Cherqui D, Geller DA, et al. Recommendations for laparoscopic liver resection: a report from the second international consensus conference held in Morioka. Ann Surg. 2015;261(4):619–29.
12. Ryska M, Fronek J, Rudis J, et al. Manual and robotic laparoscopic liver resection. Two case-reviews. Rozhl Chir. 2006;85(10):511–6.
13. Ji WB, Wang HG, Zhao ZM, et al. Robotic-assisted laparoscopic anatomic hepatectomy in China: initial experience. Ann Surg. 2011;253(2):342–8.
14. Troisi RI, Patriti A, Montalti R, Casciola L. Robot assistance in liver surgery: a real advantage over a fully laparoscopic approach? Results of a comparative bi-institutional analysis. Int J Med Robot. 2013;9(2):160–6.
15. Berber E, Akyildiz HY, Aucejo F, et al. Robotic versus laparoscopic resection of liver tumours. HPB (Oxford). 2010;12(8):583–6.
16. Lai EC, Yang GP, Tang CN. Robot-assisted laparoscopic liver resection for hepatocellular carcinoma: short-term outcome. Am J Surg. 2013;205(6):697–702.
17. Nguyen KT, Gamblin TC, Geller DA. World review of laparoscopic liver resection-2,804 patients. Ann Surg. 2009;250(5):831–41.
18. Choi SH, Choi GH, Han DH, et al. Laparoscopic liver resection using a rubber band retraction technique: usefulness and perioperative outcome in 100 consecutive cases. Surg Endosc. 2015;29(2):387–97.
19. Lee JH, Han DH, Jang DS, et al. Robotic extrahepatic Glissonean pedicle approach for anatomic liver resection in the right liver: techniques and perioperative outcomes. Surg Endosc. 2015;30(9):3882–8.
20. Gazelle GS, Lee MJ, Mueller PR. Cholangiographic segmental anatomy of the liver. Radiographics. 1994;14(5):1005–13.
21. Puente SG, Bannura GC. Radiological anatomy of the biliary tract: variations and congenital abnormalities. World J Surg. 1983;7(2):271–6.
22. Farello GA, Cerofolini A, Rebonato M, et al. Congenital choledochal cyst: video-guided laparoscopic treatment. Surg Laparosc Endosc. 1995;5(5):354–8.
23. Dulucq JL, Wintringer P, Stabilini C, et al. Laparoscopic liver resections: a single center experience. Surg Endosc. 2005;19(7):886–91.

24. Bryant R, Laurent A, Tayar C, et al. Laparoscopic liver resection-understanding its role in current practice: the Henri Mondor Hospital experience. Ann Surg. 2009;250(1):103–11.
25. Giulianotti PC, Sbrana F, Coratti A, et al. Totally robotic right hepatectomy: surgical technique and outcomes. Arch Surg. 2011;146(7):844–50.
26. Diao M, Li L, Cheng W. Laparoscopic versus open Roux-en-Y hepatojejunostomy for children with choledochal cysts: intermediate-term follow-up results. Surg Endosc. 2011;25:1567–73.
27. Liem NT, Pham HD, Dung LA, Son TN, Vu HM. Early and intermediate outcomes of laparoscopic surgery for choledochal cysts with 400 patients. J Laparoendosc Adv Surg Tech A. 2012;22:599–603.
28. Alizai NK, Dawrant MJ, Najmaldin AS. Robot-assisted resection of choledochal cysts and hepaticojejunostomy in children. Pediatr Surg Int. 2014;30(3):291–4.
29. Akaraviputh T, Trakarnsanga A, Suksamanapun N. Robot-assisted complete excision of choledochal cyst type I, hepaticojejunostomy and extracorporeal Roux-en-Y anastomosis: a case report and review literature. World J Surg Oncol. 2010;8:87.
30. Prasad A, De S, Mishra P, et al. Robotic assisted Roux-en-Y hepaticojejunostomy in a post-cholecystectomy type E2 bile duct injury. World J Gastroenterol. 2015;21(6):1703–6.
31. Lai EC, Tang CN. Robot-assisted laparoscopic hepaticojejunostomy for advanced malignant biliary obstruction. Asian J Surg. 2015;38(4):210–3.

# Robotic-Assisted Pancreaticoduodenectomy (Whipple)

**22**

Jonathan C. King, Melissa E. Hogg, Herbert J. Zeh, and Amer H. Zureikat

Pancreaticoduodenectomy (PD) has long been considered the *sine qua non* of surgical mastery among abdominal operations. The procedure has challenged some of the greatest surgeons in the modern era due to the need for meticulous dissection and flawless reconstructive techniques. With the advent of laparoscopic techniques, interest in the application of laparoscopy to PD has grown [1]; however, the technical complexity of the operation has prevented its widespread adoption and dissemination [2]. Robotic-assisted laparoscopic surgery offers some advantages over traditional laparoscopic surgery by providing improved degrees of freedom of motion, greater precision through computer assistance, and improved visualization, allowing a greater number of practitioners to incorporate minimally invasive techniques in the management of pancreatic diseases. Multiple single institutional high-volume center reports of robotic-assisted PD (RAPD) have confirmed its safety and efficacy (with outcomes comparable to the open operation [3]) though there remains a significant learning curve that must be negotiated, ideally in the setting of dedicated fellowship training or in a mentored or proctored setting [4].

J.C. King, M.D.
Department of Surgery, David Geffen School of Medicine at UCLA,
304 15th St., Suite 102, Santa Monica, CA 90404, USA

M.E. Hogg, M.D., F.A.C.S. • H.J. Zeh, M.D., F.A.C.S.
Surgical Oncology, University of Pittsburgh Medical Center,
3550 Terrace St., Suite 497 Scaife Hall, Pittsburgh, PA 15261, USA

A.H. Zureikat, M.D., F.A.C.S. (✉)
UPMC Pancreatic Cancer Center, Surgical Oncology, University of Pittsburgh Medical Center, 3550 Terrace St., Suite 497 Scaife Hall, Pittsburgh, PA 15261, USA
e-mail: zureikatah@upmc.edu

© Springer International Publishing AG 2018
A.D. Patel, D. Oleynikov (eds.), *The SAGES Manual of Robotic Surgery*,
The SAGES University Masters Program Series, DOI 10.1007/978-3-319-51362-1_22

## Patient Selection and Preparation

Successful outcomes following RAPD are intimately linked to appropriate and judicious patient selection, particularly early in the learning curve. The selection process begins with a thorough assessment of the patient's medical and surgical history along with cardiopulmonary risk stratification. Predictors of mortality following open PD include age, male sex, preoperative albumin, tumor size, sepsis, and comorbidities, particularly renal insufficiency [5]. Among these factors, preoperative nutrition is the only modifiable risk factor. Therefore, particular attention to concomitant weight loss, biliary obstruction, steatorrhea, new-onset or worsening diabetes mellitus, and poor alimentation are important. Long-standing biliary obstruction with or without malnutrition is best managed with temporary biliary stenting and nutritional supplementation [6]. However, if an operation is planned within 7–10 days and biliary obstruction has been sub-acute, biliary stenting is best avoided [7].

Cross-sectional imaging with intravenous contrast should be performed for all potential candidates. Computed tomography (CT) or magnetic resonance (MR) imaging depending on institutional availability, patient factors, and preference may be used. CT and MR accurately assess the primary pathology and are highly predictive of resectability [8]. Involvement of major vascular structures (superior mesenteric vein [SMV], portal vein [PV], hepatic artery [HA], and superior mesenteric artery [SMA]) is generally a contraindication to RAPD though some expert surgeons have reported on the feasibility of vascular resection and reconstruction with minimally invasive techniques [9]. Endoscopic ultrasound (EUS) may also be utilized, particularly if tissue diagnosis is required. While assessment of large-vessel vascular invasion by EUS is very sensitive and specific for some practitioners, it is also highly operator dependent [10]. For this reason the authors rely on triphasic cross-sectional imaging interpreted by an expert pancreatic-biliary radiologist to evaluate resectability in the preoperative setting.

Prior abdominal operations and anatomic abnormalities must be noted, and while these are not absolute contraindications to RAPD, ulcer operations, large hiatal hernias, severe scoliosis, and roux en-Y gastric bypass surgery may add undue complexity to a robotic-assisted approach. The indication for operation should be considered as well. It is the opinion of the authors that early in the practitioner's RAPD experience, benign lesions or those with low malignant potential (i.e. low-grade pancreatic neuorendocrine tumors [PNET], cystic neoplasms, ampullary adenoma, etc.) are ideal due to lack of vascular involvement. Unfortunately, these 'non-PDA' cases may be associated with higher pancreatic leak rates due to a soft pancreatic gland and the presence of a non-dilated pancreatic duct. In summary, a thoughtful and exclusionary approach to patient selection maximizes the opportunity to perform RAPD safely.

## Instrumentation

Our practice has led to a standardized approach to instrumentation: the dissection is carried out with a monopolar cautery hook dissector, a fenestrated bipolar cautery grasper, and a utility grasper forceps. Suturing is performed with large needle drivers

**Table 22.1** Equipment for robotic-assisted pancreaticoduodenectomy (RAPD)

| Robotic instruments | Laparoscopic instruments | Disposable equipment | Durable equipment | Sutures/supplies |
|---|---|---|---|---|
| 12 mm, 30° down scope | 5 mm 0° and 30° scope | GIA staplers (3.5 mm, 2.5 mm staple height) | Split-leg OR table | 2-0 silk, 3-0 silk; 8″ length |
| Hook monopolar cautery | Graspers | 5- and 7-French ERCP Stent | Carter-Thomason | 3-0 V-Loc 180; 6″ length × 2 |
| Fenestrated bipolar forceps | Scissors | Laparoscopic specimen bag (10 cm, 15 cm) | Self-retaining liver retractor | 4-0 V-Loc 180; 6″ length × 2 |
| Prograsp™ forceps | Maryland dissector | 19-French Blake drain | Ultrasound | 5-0 polyglactin or polydiaxonone 5″ length |
| Maryland dissector | 5 mm trocar × 2 | 10 mm clip applier | | ¼″ Umbilical tape |
| Scissors (monopolar) | 12 mm trocar × 2 | GelPoint® Mini™ | | |
| Large needle driver × 2 | | Vessel sealer | | $\frac{1}{8}''$ Vessel loops |
| 8 mm trocar × 3 | | | | |
| Ultrasound probe | | | | |

*GIA* gastrointestinal anastomosis

with and without integrated cutting blades and additional tools such as scissors and Maryland dissectors are used as needed. The bedside assistant's tools consist of standard laparoscopic instruments: graspers, scissors, suction–irrigator, and a vessel sealing device such as Ligasure (Covidien-Medtronic; Minneapolis, MN). We employ a self-retaining liver retractor (Mediflex; Islandia, NY) routinely to retract segment 4B of the liver. Instruments and supplies are listed in Table 22.1. Additionally, retractors and instrument trays for an open PD, including vascular instruments, should be immediately available in case of the need to convert to laparotomy.

## Operating Room Configuration

The patient is positioned with the right arm padded and tucked and the left arm extended at the shoulder on a split-leg table that allows the bedside assistant to stand between the legs of the patient. The patient is secured to the table with straps, and foot supports are utilized to allow reverse Trendelenburg positioning. Extreme care must be taken to pad all pressure points. The robotic (da Vinci Si) patient cart is positioned over the patient's head and the robotic arms are aligned as shown in Fig. 22.1. The laparoscopic monitors are positioned to allow the bedside assistant an unobstructed view in an ergonomically neutral posture. The robotic console should be placed to allow unimpeded communication between the console surgeon and bedside assistant.

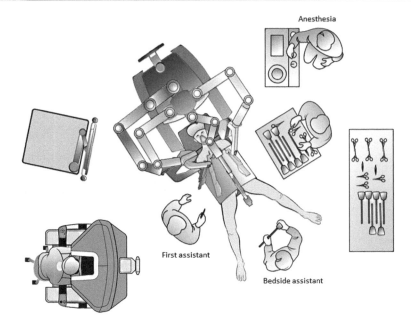

**Fig. 22.1** Operating room setup

## Operative Steps

The operative steps outlined in the following text represent a general flow of the operation, though specific parts may be re-arranged or modified as clinically indicated. Experienced pancreatic surgeons will quickly realize that the steps are very familiar to its open counterpart and, in fact, RAPD is essentially identical to open PD as performed by the authors with few exceptions.

## Port Placement/Laparoscopy

The operation starts with the patient bed in neutral position, and a 5 mm optical trocar is placed to the left of the midline through the rectus sheath 2–3 cm above the level of the umbilicus. Upon entry into the abdomen the peritoneum is explored for evidence of metastatic disease. Barring any contraindications to resection additional laparoscopic/robotic ports are placed as shown in Fig. 22.2. Approximately 10 cm (roughly one hand-breadth) is required between robotic ports to minimize collisions between the robotic arms. The right lateral trocar is placed with the patient in reverse Trendelenburg and the right side rotated upwards to allow it to be positioned as far laterally as possible. The initial entry 5 mm trocar is changed to an 8 mm trocar for robotic instruments.

The initial dissection and exploration are performed laparoscopically. Any adhesions between the liver and stomach are divided to allow placement of the liver

**Fig. 22.2** Laparoscopic/
robotic trocar positioning

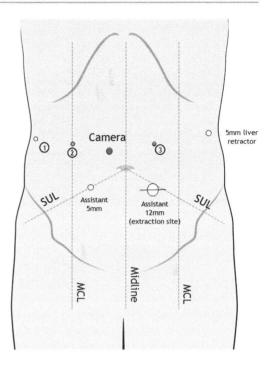

retractor. The lesser sac is entered through the gastrocolic ligament below the level of the gastroepiploic arcade and opened widely. The right colon is mobilized completely to the cecum. Next, a marking stitch is placed in the jejunum 80 cm distal to the ligament of Treitz (LOT). Proximal to the marking stitch the jejunum is tacked to the greater curve of the stomach with another stitch. This maneuver facilitates identification and orientation of the jejunal loop for creation of the gastrojejunostomy (GJ).

## Docking/Bedside Assisting

The robot is docked and robotic instruments are inserted: monopolar cautery hook dissector in arm 1, fenestrated bipolar cautery grasper in arm 2, and Prograsp™ forceps in arm 3. A 30°, down-angled stereoscopic laparoscope is used. The bedside assistant, standing between the legs of the patient, operates the vessel sealer and suction–irrigator or laparoscopic graspers through the right lower quadrant 5 mm trocar and the left lower quadrant 12 mm trocar. The bedside assistant is responsible for clearing the surgical field of blood/fluids, providing dynamic retraction, dividing blood vessels and achieving hemostasis with the vessel sealer, operating staplers, exchanging robotic instruments, passing sutures, and extracting the specimens. Bedside assistant requires sound surgical instinct, a thorough knowledge of surgical anatomy and the steps of the operation, as well as maneuvers to stem blood loss or manage emergencies. It is not an appropriate role for most surgical scrub technicians, physician assistant, or junior surgical residents.

## Kocher Maneuver

Once the robot arms are positioned, hook cautery is used to dissect the duodenum and the head of the pancreas off of the retroperitoneum until the left renal vein is visible and the LOT is reached. The proximal jejunum is delivered into the dissection field whereupon a point 10 cm distal to the LOT can be chosen to create a mesenteric window and divide the bowel with a stapler (2.5 mm staple height). The vessel sealer is used to divide the mesentery. This linearizes the distal duodenum and facilitates the lateral SMV dissection later.

## Transect Stomach/Hepatic Artery/GDA

The lesser omentum is opened in the *pars flaccida* taking care not to divide a replaced/accessory left hepatic artery (HA), if present. A stapler with 3.5 mm staples is used to divide the stomach 2–3 cm proximal to the pylorus. The antrum is retracted to expose the underlying neck of the pancreas. The hepatic artery lymph node (level VIIIa) is identified and the peritoneum is opened along its inferior border. The entire lymph node is excised exposing the [common] HA beneath it. Once the HA is identified, it is traced distally to the takeoff of the gastroduodenal artery (GDA) which is skeletonized. The HA [proper] is also traced further distally where the right gastric artery may be found and divided with a vessel sealer. The importance of using Doppler flow ultrasound to confirm flow in the HA while occluding the GDA cannot be understated. It is also the author's practice to rotate the specimen medially (to the left) and dissect the lateral border of the hepatoduodenal ligament to confirm the presence or absence of an accessory/replaced right HA *before* the GDA has been ligated. Once these steps have confirmed the arterial anatomy, a stapler with 2.5 mm staples can be used to transect the GDA. The bedside assistant applies a 10 mm vascular clip to the GDA stump.

## Hepatoduodenal Ligament/Bile Duct/Superior Neck

With the GDA transected the portal vein (PV) is easily identified immediately deep to the previous dissection. The hook cautery is used to dissect in the peri-adventitial plane of the vein, and soft tissue at the superior neck of the pancreas is divided. This is a convenient time to create the superior aspect of the superior mesenteric vein (SMV) tunnel as well. Next, the lateral border of the PV is dissected, freeing it from the bile duct anterio-laterally. This dissection may be difficult in patients with bile duct tumors; care must be taken not to injure the PV where it may be adherent to the common bile duct (CBD). At this point the lymph node posterior to the PV and CBD (level XI) may be dissected and retracted caudally to be taken with the specimen. Again, identification and protection of a replaced right HA are necessary and may be aided by placing vessel loop around it. If no CBD stent has been placed the bile duct is divided with a stapler with 2.5 mm staples. If a stent is present the bile duct may be transected with a stapler above the stent or with cautery. Cholecystectomy can then be performed in a standard fashion.

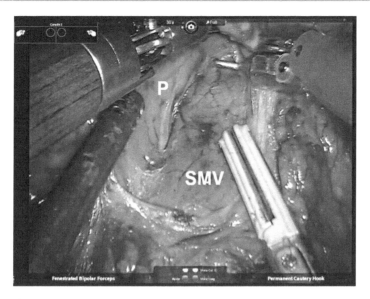

**Fig. 22.3** Creating the tunnel behind the neck of the pancreas. The bedside assistant applies gentle traction downwards and uses the opposite hand to elevate the neck of the pancreas to expose the tunnel. *SMV* superior mesenteric vein, *P* neck of pancreas

## Inferior Neck/Tunnel

Next, with the third arm retracting the specimen cephalad the inferior neck of the pancreas is exposed. The peritoneum at the inferior border of the pancreas is opened until the SMV is identified, allowing creation of the pancreatic neck tunnel. This is accomplished by using a grasper to gently lift the pancreas while the hook cautery bluntly develops the avascular plane anterior to the SMV using gentle downward movements progressively more proximal on the vein wall (Fig. 22.3). Several maneuvers assist in making the tunnel dissection safer and easier: create a wide window in the peritoneum at the inferior border of the pancreas— this will open the dissection to allow greater access to the tunnel and effectively make the tunnel shorter. Also, use the vessel sealer or bipolar cautery to divide the soft tissue at the inferior neck of the pancreas medial to tunnel. There are typically several small vessels here which bleed profusely if divided with monopolar cautery. Finally, pan outwards with the camera to identify the PV at the superior neck of the gland, as this will establish the trajectory of the SMV and help to avoid creating a tunnel that does not connect to the superior dissection. The superior and inferior tunnels are joined and the bedside assistant places a laparoscopic grasper through the tunnel so an umbilical tape may be passed through.

## Transection of Pancreas/PV: SMV Dissection

The neck of the pancreas is transected with the robotic scissors using monopolar cautery. The umbilical tape suspends the pancreas to avoid injuring the SMV/

PV. When approaching the main pancreatic duct (MPD) the scissors are used without energy to avoid cauterizing the duct itself. Once transection of the pancreas is complete, an *en face* margin from the specimen side may be obtained for frozen section analysis, if indicated.

Retracting the specimen laterally, the robotic scissors are used with the tips opened 3–5 mm to bluntly 'roll' the vein off of the pancreas. The bedside assistant applies gentle retraction on the vein medially allowing progressive dissection towards the uncinate process. Inferiorly, this dissection will expose the middle colic and gastroepiploic veins as they drain into the SMV. Next, the entire specimen is rotated medially and the lateral wall of the SMV is identified and skeletonized. This maneuver is important to avoid mistaking the first jejunal vein for the SMV which can set the stage for ligating the true SMV under the assumption that it is an expendable mesocolic tributary. Once the SMV is positively identified the specimen is rotated laterally again and the middle colic and gastroepiploic veins may be ligated.

Cephalad, if a replaced right (or common) HA is present, it will be encountered as it passes lateral to the PV and continues posteriorly towards the SMA. Arterial branches in this location should not be ligated unless involved by tumor *and* alternate arterial inflow to the liver is confirmed.

## Uncinate Dissection/SMA

The uncinate process is typically the most challenging portion of the dissection. The bedside assistant plays an active role in retracting the SMV/PV medially and maintaining a bloodless field, while the third robotic arm retracts the specimen laterally 'up and out' (analogous to the surgeons left hand during open PD). The console surgeon applies liberal use of bipolar cautery both for obtaining hemostasis and to 'pre-coagulate' visible uncinate vessels prior to dividing them. Fortunately, the visualization of the SMA is unparalleled in comparison to the traditional open technique where these steps are performed with a combination of 'feel' and blind dissection. This enhanced visualization allows the dissection to follow a plane immediately adjacent to the artery, which enables maximize the retroperitoneal surgical margin. While most bleeding can be avoided with careful use of cautery, there is usually some level of 'oozing' that may persist until the specimen is completely freed. As a result, overzealous attempts to achieve a bloodless field may unnecessarily prolong this step and paradoxically result in more blood loss.

## Removal of Specimen

Completion of the uncinate dissection marks the end of what is typically the most challenging portion of the operation. Most major blood loss, physiologic perturbation, and operative risk are incurred up to this point. The continued strain of operating on the robotic console may contribute to some level of 'robot fatigue'. This phenomenon is quite reproducible though not measured formally and is based on our own observations after cooperating on many cases. Typical signs are missed cues and 'unforced errors' that are uncharacteristic for the skill of the operating surgeon. In our experience, the best strategy to mitigate the effects of robot fatigue is to switch the roles of the bedside assistant and console surgeon at this point in the operation.

The specimens are placed in retrieval bags, and the incision around the left lower quadrant 12 mm trocar is enlarged transversely to allow removal. A gel port with an airtight lid (GelPoint™ Applied Medical; Rancho Santa Margarita, CA) may be used to seal the incision and allow re-insufflation of the abdomen. The 12 mm assistant trocar is placed through the gel port.

## Pancreaticojejunostomy

Many methods of pancreatic-enteric anastomosis have been described and there remain numerous variations. We have standardized our approach using a modified Blumgart two-layer PJ technique.

The jejunal limb is oriented so the antimesenteric border lies next to the pancreatic duct and loops gradually and without kinking past the bile duct. Two to four centimeters of the pancreatic stump is dissected from surrounding tissues. Interrupted horizontal mattress sutures of 3-0 silk are placed using trans-pancreatic bites of pancreas and seromuscular bites of jejunum. A 5-French Hobbs ERCP stent (Hobbs Medical; Stafford Springs, CT) is placed in the main pancreatic duct (MPD) to help prevent inadvertent occlusion. The sutures are tied so that the bowel wall is directly opposed to the posterior pancreas without any dead space. The best way to ensure this is to lift both tails of the sutures prior to securing the first knot (Fig. 22.4). The needles are left

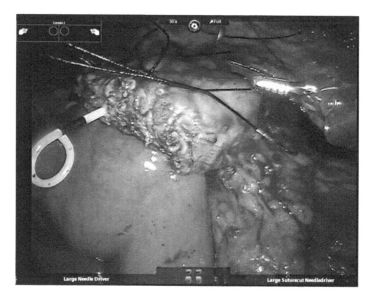

**Fig. 22.4** Placement of buttressing sutures of 3-0 silk. Note how the surgeon lifts the ends of the suture prior to tying the first knot to close any dead space between the serosa of the jejunum and pancreas posteriorly. The pancreatic duct stent prevents occlusion of the main pancreatic duct

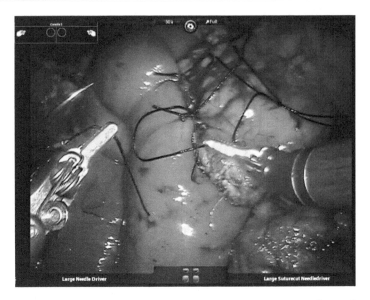

**Fig. 22.5** Seromuscular bites of jejunum are used to imbricate the bowel wall over the anterior surface of the pancreas

on these sutures and used for the anterior seromuscular layer later. Three sutures are placed in the posterior row with the middle stitch straddling the MPD.

Next, a 2–3 mm enterotomy is made in the jejunum using monopolar cautery. The inner suture line is constructed with interrupted 5-0 polydiaxonone or polyglactin sutures incorporating the pancreatic duct and full-thickness jejunum. The choice of suture material is based on surgeon preference with each offering some minor advantages and disadvantages. Both have been used extensively in our experience with good results. It is usually possible to place three to five sutures in the posterior row. After the posterior suture line is complete the Hobbs stent is inserted with the curved end in the jejunum. Another three or four 5-0 sutures anteriorly complete the inner layer. These are placed without tying until all sutures have been placed. Then, the sutures at the superior and inferior aspect of the duct are tied followed by the middle sutures, which are tied last. It may be helpful for the bedside assistant to gently push the bowel medially to remove any tension while the sutures are being tied. Finally, the anterior row mattress sutures are created using the previously placed posterior row needles (Fig. 22.5).

## Hepaticojejunostomy

The biliary anastomosis is constructed in one layer and may be interrupted or continuous depending on the diameter of the bile duct. For large ducts, we perform a running hepaticojejunostomy (HJ). We prefer using absorbable 4-0 V-Loc 180 sutures (Covidien-Medtronic; Minneapolis, MN) as the barbed monofilament

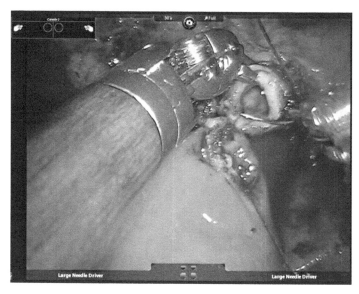

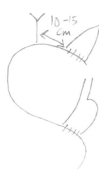

**Fig. 22.6** Single-layer continuous hepaticojejunostomy anastomosis

obviates the need for maintaining continuous traction on the suture as it is sewn (Fig. 22.6). Smaller ducts should be reconstructed with interrupted 5-0 polydiaxonone. Our practice has been to place the biliary anastomosis at least 10–15 cm downstream of the PJ anastomosis. Although not classically described in the literature, in the opinion of the authors, this space between the two anastomoses helps to prevent reflux of biliary fluid into the pancreatic anastomosis. Little clinical evidence exists to support this practice, but it is an important anecdotal observation that may decrease the incidence of massive pancreatic anastomotic disruption.

## Gastrojejunostomy

The jejunum that had been tacked to the greater curve of the stomach is freed, and the marking stitch position is noted to identify the efferent end of the jejunal loop, so it may be placed downstream of the planned gastrojejunostomy. A posterior row of 3-0 silk seromuscular sutures are placed along the length of the planned anastomosis (Fig. 22.7). Once the posterior row is complete (typically five sutures) the gastric staple line is removed with monopolar cautery. A corresponding longitudinal enterotomy is created on the jejunum.

Two 3-0 V-Loc 180 sutures are placed to complete the corner of the anastomosis using full-thickness jejunum and stomach. These stitches are placed close together, and the suture is pulled taught after each throw to eliminate any gaps. The posterior row stitch is sewn continuously to the opposite corner and around to the anterior part of the anastomosis. At this point the suture is set aside and the anterior row

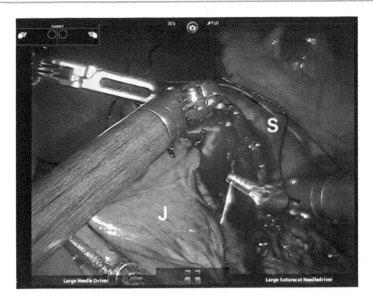

**Fig. 22.7** Gastrojejunostomy posterior-row sutures of 3-0 silk. Note this row of sutures is placed near the mesenteric border of the jejunum to avoid narrowing the anastomosis. *J* jejunum, *S* stomach

suture is used to perform a Connell stitch to complete the inner layer of the anastomosis. Finally, 3-0 silk Lembert sutures are used to complete the anterior row taking care not to narrow the anastomosis.

## Falciform Flap/Drain Placement/Closure

We routinely create a vascularized tissue flap from the falciform ligament to exclude the GDA stump from potential PJ anastomotic leakage. Several 3-0 silk sutures may be used to secure the flap to the retroperitoneum as needed. Given routine drain placement has been associated with a decrease in severe complications following PD [11], we place a 19-French Blake channel drain (Ethicon; Sommerville, NJ) through the right flank robotic port directed under the right lobe of the liver, anteriorly past the HJ and anterior to the PJ. The end of the drain is tucked behind the gastrojejunostomy to hold it in place. A Carter-Thomason device is used to re-approximate the fascia of the 12 mm camera incision, and the left lower quadrant extraction incision is closed with appropriate fascial sutures in an open fashion.

## Post-operative Care

Post-operative care is similar to that of open PD patients. Routine intensive care unit admission is generally unnecessary, and we find post-operative regional analgesia to be useful (paravertebral catheters placed preoperatively). As much of the post-operative care is standardized as this has been shown to improve care and facilitate timely discharge [12]. Prophylactic low molecular–weight heparin is routinely administered.

Surgical drain management is standardized as well: a serum and drain fluid amylase activity are assayed on the morning of post-operative day 3, and if the drain fluid amylase activity is ≤3 times the serum value and the patient is improving clinically, the drain is removed on post-operative day 4, regardless of the volume of its output. This protocol has been adapted and modified from a protocol published by Bassi et al. [13, 14].

## Learning Curve

Numerous studies have investigated and defined the number of cases that are needed to be performed before proficiency may be attained for complex procedures. Open PD has been reported to require between 30 and 60 procedures [15–18] and RAPD may add as many as 80 more cases to a surgeon's cumulative experience before mastery is attained [3, 4]. However, cautious interpretation of these numbers is warranted given evidence showing that much of the improvement in perioperative outcomes seen with increased experience has to do with the overall volume of the hospital and the quality of its ancillary services (advanced endoscopy, interventional radiology, critical care medicine, etc.) [19, 20]. Furthermore, our experience with RAPD was reported in the absence of formal training and curricula, and without the aid of mentorship in robotic-assisted surgery. In the current era, surgical trainees have the advantage of greater exposure to the robotic platform as well as the opportunity for apprenticeship with experienced surgeons. As a result the number of cases needed to graduate from the learning curve is expected to fall significantly. Nonetheless, it is important for surgeons who intend to start practicing robotic-assisted pancreatic surgery to seek and attain appropriate mentorship from experienced pancreatic and minimally invasive surgeons.

## Drawbacks/Limitations

The most frequently cited limitation of RAPD (and robotic-assisted surgery, in general) is the significant cost associated with purchase of the console ($1.2 million) and maintenance/equipment costs ($100,000–150,000 per year) above and beyond expenditures for operating room time and other supplies and equipment. These costs are magnified in the early phase of the adoption of RAPD given the longer operative times. However, robotic-assisted surgery has been shown to be profitable, particularly when operative efficiency has been optimized [21], and the institutional investment required for starting an RAPD program can be balanced by cost savings associated with shorter length of stay [22].

The complexity of RAPD represents another hurdle in the widespread adoption of robotic-assisted approaches. As with laparoscopic PD, there are currently only selected centers performing RAPD regularly. As residency training programs implement standardized robotics training curricula and trainee exposure to robotic-assisted techniques grows, we expect there will be an increased comfort with the robotic interface that will allow greater dissemination of RAPD in the future. Evidence to support the role of resident/fellow training as well as institutional implementation of robotics in the growth of robotic-assisted surgery is accumulating [23, 24].

## Outcomes

The primary goal in developing RAPD is to improve patient outcomes. To date the largest series reporting outcomes following RAPD have shown that open and robotic-assisted techniques are largely equivalent [3, 25]. However, it is important to note that endpoints such as operative times and blood loss as well as perioperative complications such as pancreatic fistula and even mortality as reported in these series represent the learning curve phase of their experience. This is illustrated by operative times that averaged $529 \pm 103$ min for the entire cohort of 132 RAPD but decreased to about 400 min after the learning curve of 80 cases was surpassed at the University of Pittsburgh [3]. Mature data to compare RAPD and open PD is still forthcoming and no direct comparisons of open PD and RAPD have been completed. A recently published systematic review of robotic and laparoscopic approaches to pancreatic surgery shows RAPD is associated with longer operative time with no associated increase in perioperative morbidity or mortality. Hospital length of stay has been observed to be decreased in some, but not all series [26]. Oncologic outcomes such as margin positivity and lymph node harvest also appear to be similar among RAPD and open PD series, though direct comparative data are lacking.

Long-term survival following PD is the most important outcome to measure, particularly for cancer patients. The receipt of adjuvant chemotherapy has implications on cancer-specific survival, and the morbidity associated with PD delays or prevents the administration of chemotherapy in a significant proportion of patients. There is evidence that laparoscopic PD is associated with fewer delays in the initiation of adjuvant therapy, and this may prove to be true for RAPD as well, though data is lacking at this time [27].

## Conclusions

Though technically challenging, RAPD represents a step forward in the management of pancreatic disease. In appropriately selected patients, RAPD may be performed safely and cost-effectively. We predict greater cumulative clinical experience will be required to realize the full potential of RAPD as the techniques and technology are still in their relative infancy. With continued dissemination of RAPD, there will be an opportunity for direct comparison of outcomes to open and laparoscopic approaches, which will help to define the role of robotic-assisted approaches to PD.

# References

1. Kendrick ML, Cusati D. Total laparoscopic pancreaticoduodenectomy: feasibility and outcome in an early experience. Arch Surg. 2010;145:19–23.
2. Zureikat AH, Breaux JA, Steel JL, Hughes SJ. Can laparoscopic pancreaticoduodenectomy be safely implemented? J Gastrointest Surg. 2011;15:1151–7.
3. Zureikat AH, Moser AJ, Boone BA, et al. 250 robotic pancreatic resections: safety and feasibility. Ann Surg. 2013;258:554–9.
4. Boone BA, Zenati M, Hogg ME, et al. Assessment of quality outcomes for robotic pancreaticoduodenectomy: identification of the learning curve. JAMA Surg. 2015. doi:10.1001/jamasurg.2015.17.
5. Venkat R, Puham MA, Schulick RD, et al. Predicting the risk of perioperative mortality in patients undergoing pancreaticoduodenectomy. Arch Surg. 2011;146(11):1277–84.
6. Moss AC, Morris E, MacMathuna P. Palliative biliary stents for obstructing pancreatic carcinoma. Cochrane Upper Gastrointestinal and Pancreatic Diseases Group. Chocrane Database Syst Rev. 2006;(2):CD004200.
7. van der Gaag NA, Rauws EA, van Eijck CH, et al. Preoperative biliary drainage for cancer of the head of the pancreas. N Engl J Med. 2010;362(2):129–37.
8. Zhao WY, Luo M, Sun YW, et al. Computed tomography in diagnosing vascular invasion in pancreatic and periampullary cancers: a systematic review and meta-analysis. Hepatobiliary Pancreat Dis Int. 2009;8:457–64.
9. Croome KP, Farnell MB, Que FG, et al. Pancreaticoduodenectomy with major vascular resection: a comparison of laparoscopic versus open approaches. J Gastrointest Surg. 2015;19(1):189–94. discussion 194
10. Li JH, He R, Li YM, et al. Endoscopic ultrasonography for tumor node staging and vascular invasion in pancreatic cancer: a meta-analysis. Dig Surg. 2014;31(4–5):297–305.
11. Van Buren G, Bloomston M, Hughes SJ, et al. A randomized prospective multicenter trial of pancreaticoduodenectomy with and without routine intraperitoneal drainage. Ann Surg. 2014;259(4):605–12.
12. Kennedy EP, Rosato EL, Sauter PK, et al. Initiation of a critical pathway for pancreaticoduodenectomy at an academic institution—the first step in multidisciplinary team building. J Am Coll Surg. 2007;204(5):917–23. discussion 923–4
13. Molinari E, Bassi C, Salvia R, et al. Amylase value in drains after pancreatic resection as predictive factor of postoperative pancreatic fistula: results of a prospective study in 137 patients. Ann Surg. 2007;246(2):281–7.
14. Bassi C, Molinari E, Malleo G, et al. Early versus late drain removal after standard pancreatic resections: results of a prospective randomized trial. Ann Surg. 2010;252(2):207–14.
15. Hardacre JM. Is there a learning curve for pancreaticoduodenectomy after fellowship training? HPB Surg. 2010;2010:230287.
16. Fisher WE, Hodges SE, Wu MF, Hilsenbeck SG, Brunicardi FC. Assessment of the learning curve for pancreaticoduodenectomy. Am J Surg. 2012;203(6):684–90.
17. Tseng JF, Pisters PW, Lee JE, et al. The learning curve in pancreatic surgery. Surgery. 2007;141(4):456–63.
18. Cameron JL, Riall TS, Coleman J, Belcher KA. One thousand consecutive pancreaticoduodenectomies. Ann Surg. 2006;244(1):10–5.
19. Ho V, Heslin MJ. Effect of hospital volume and experience on in hospital mortality for pancreaticoduodenectomy. Ann Surg. 2003;237(4):509–14.
20. Coe TM, Fong ZV, Wilson SE, et al. Outcomes improvement is not continuous along the learning curve for pancreaticoduodenectomy at the hospital level. J Gastrointest Surg. 2015;19:2132–7.
21. Geller EJ, Matthews CA. Impact of robotic operative efficiency on profitability. Am J Obstet Gynecol. 2013;209:20.e1–5.

22. Waters JA, Canal DF, Wiebke EA, et al. Robotic distal pancreatectomy: cost effective? Surgery. 2010;148:814–23.
23. Hogg ME, Zenati M, Novak SM, et al. Mastery-based virtual reality robotic simulation curriculum: the first step toward operative robotic proficiency. J Surg Educ. 2016 Nov 21. pii: S1931-7204(16)30265-3.
24. King JC, Zeh HJ III, Zureikat AH, et al. Safety in numbers: Progressive implementation of a robotics program in an academic surgical oncology practice. Surg Innov. 2016;23(4):407–14.
25. Giulianotti PC, Sbrana F, Bianco FM, et al. Robot-assisted laparoscopic pancreatic surgery: Single-surgeon experience. Surg Endosc. 2010;24:1646–57.
26. Wright GP, Zureikat AH. Development of minimally invasive pancreatic surgery: laparoscopic vs. robotic—an evidence-based systematic review. J Gastrointest Surg. 2016;20(9):1658–65.
27. Croome KP, Farnell MB, Que FG, et al. Total laparoscopic pancreaticoduodenectmoy for pancreatic ductal adenocarcinoma: oncologic advantages over open approaches? Ann Surg. 2014;260:633–40.

Julietta Chang and Matthew Kroh

## Introduction

Laparoscopic gastric surgery was first described in the resection of early gastric cancer in 1994 in a distal gastrectomy with Billroth I reconstruction [1]. While laparoscopic resections for various intra-abdominal procedures such as colectomy have gained widespread adoption, minimally invasive gastrectomy remains less so, likely as it is a technically challenging laparoscopic procedure with a steep learning curve. Additionally, fewer patients present with pathology related to gastric disease than colonic pathologies. Regardless, laparoscopic gastric resection has been shown to have reduced morbidity, improved recovery with decreased hospital stay and, in the case of gastric cancer, equivalent oncologic outcomes compared to open gastrectomy [2].

The da Vinci® Surgical System robotic platform was introduced in the early 2000s (Intuitive Surgical, Inc) and it is the most commonly used system currently. This device allows for stereoscopic three-dimensional visualization, tremor-filtration, enhanced instrument movement with 7° of instrument articulation, among other advantages. The first robotic gastrectomy was shortly thereafter described in 2003 for early gastric cancer [3]. This chapter will aim to discuss the indications for

---

**Electronic supplementary material:** The online version of this chapter (doi: 10.1007/978-3-319-51362-1_23) contains supplementary material, which is available to authorized users. Videos can also be accessed at http://link.springer.com/chapter/10.1007/978-3-319-51362-1_23.

J. Chang, M.D.
Section of Surgical Endoscopy, Department of General Surgery, Digestive Disease Institute, Cleveland Clinic, Cleveland, OH, USA

M. Kroh, M.D. (✉)
Section of Surgical Endoscopy, Department of General Surgery, Digestive Disease Institute, Cleveland Clinic, Cleveland, OH, USA

Digestive Disease Institute, Cleveland Clinic, Abu Dhabi, UAE
e-mail: KROHM@ccf.org

© Springer International Publishing AG 2018
A.D. Patel, D. Oleynikov (eds.), *The SAGES Manual of Robotic Surgery*,
The SAGES University Masters Program Series, DOI 10.1007/978-3-319-51362-1_23

the application of robotic gastrectomy in both malignant and benign disease, the technical aspects in the use of the robot in these surgeries, the potential advantages of the use of the robot in these cases, and future directions.

## Indications in Malignancy

The Japanese Gastric Cancer Guideline from 2010 regards minimally invasive gastrectomy for gastric cancer as an investigational treatment, although up to 20% of gastrectomies in Japan are now performed with minimally invasive techniques. Laparoscopic resection is recommended for T1 tumors or smaller. The incidence of early gastric cancer, defined as cancer limited to the mucosa or submucosa regardless of nodal involvement, is increasing in Japan and Korea due to earlier detection secondary to aggressive national screening protocols, such that up to 50% of newly diagnosed gastric cancers are T1 lesions [2] and thus potentially suitable for a minimally invasive resection. However, in Western countries, the proportion of early gastric cancer remains relatively fixed at 15–21% [4]. A D1 lymphadenectomy encompassing lymph node stations 1 through 7 is the standard of care for T1 lesions [2, 5] (Fig. 23.1). However, due to understaging, some authors recommend routine D2 lymphadenectomy involving resection of D1 lymph nodes as well as stations 8 through 12 [6]. However, a Dutch randomized controlled trial examining D1 versus D2 lymphadenectomy for gastric cancer found increased perioperative morbidity and mortality following D2 lymphadenectomy without survival benefit [7].

**Fig. 23.1** Lymph node stations in gastric cancer

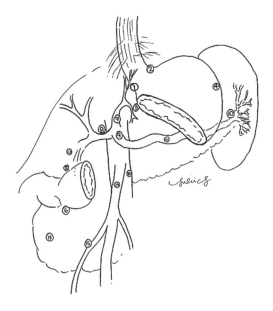

## Oncologic Outcome

As robotic gastrectomy is a relatively new approach, long-term oncologic outcome is lacking for robotic gastrectomy specifically. However, meta-analyses demonstrate no significant difference in histopathologic margins or lymph nodes retrieved between laparoscopic and robotic gastrectomy, nor are there significant differences in 3- or 5-year disease-free and overall survival [8, 9]. One meta-analysis demonstrated that robotic gastrectomy was associated with a significantly larger distal resection margin compared to laparoscopic resection [10].

One of the main advantages of robotic surgery is enhanced three-dimensional visualization allowing for precise dissection around the splenic vessels and successful removal of D2 lymph nodes. This was recently demonstrated in a prospective trial by Kim et al., who showed that a D2 lymphadenectomy was able to be completed successfully in a higher percentage of robotic-assisted gastrectomy resections compared to laparoscopic cases [11]. Another group reported greater number of retrieved lymph nodes in a D2 spleen-preserving dissection compared to laparoscopy alone [12]. One meta-analysis demonstrated a trend towards greater number of retrieved lymph nodes with an open approach versus robotic, but this did not reach statistical significance [9]. Laparoscopic gastrectomy for early gastric cancer has been found to have equivalent long-term survival compared to open gastrectomy as well [13], while a recent Cochrane review found laparoscopic versus open gastrectomy for gastric cancer to have no difference in short-term or long-term outcomes [14].

## Description of Technique

### Extent of Resection

Curative resection for gastric cancer involves resection of at least two thirds of the stomach with adequate lymphadenectomy. Depending on the location of the tumor, this may range from a total gastrectomy, distal gastrectomy, pylorus-preserving distal gastrectomy, or proximal gastrectomy. According to the Japanese Gastric Cancer Guideline, a proximal margin of at least 3 cm is recommended for T2 or greater lesions. For T1 tumors, a gross resection margin of at least 2 cm is required. Any local invasion into surrounding structures such as pancreas or colon mandates a total gastrectomy regardless of tumor location with en bloc resection of the involved organ [5].

### Distal Gastrectomy

A distal gastrectomy involves resection of the distal two thirds of the stomach. Ports are placed as shown in Fig. 23.2, with robotic and laparoscopic trocars identified as such. Initial diagnostic laparoscopy is performed to rule out metastatic disease. The robot is typically docked directly over the patient or over the left shoulder. The assistant grasps the greater curve of the stomach, while the surgeon using an advanced energy source

**Fig. 23.2** Robot trocar placement: (**a**) laparoscopic 12 mm trocar for stapler and free-needle suture; (**b**) robotic trocar; (**c**) nathanson liver retractor; (**d**) robotic camera; (**e**) robotic trocar; (**f**) laparoscopic 5 mm trocar (for distal gastrectomy) or 15 mm trocar (for total gastrectomy in anticipation of using EEA stapler for Roux-en-Y reconstruction)

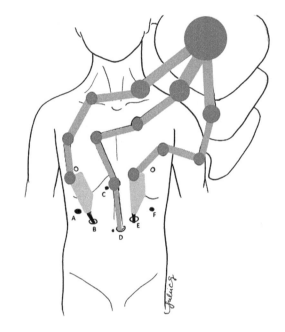

**Fig. 23.3** Intraoperative creation of the retroduodenal tunnel during robotic gastrectomy

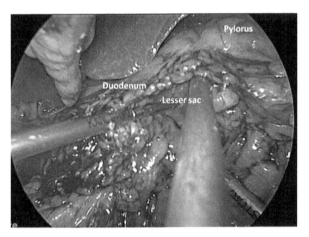

divides the gastrocolic ligament under the omentum. Dissection is carried towards the pylorus, where the right gastroepiploic artery is identified, ligated, and divided. Associated lymph nodes are kept with the specimen. Using a dissector, a retroduodenal tunnel is created from inferior to superior in the avascular plane at the point of transaction (Fig. 23.3). Attention is then taken to the superior border of the duodenum, including lymph nodes along the porta hepatis. The right gastric artery is identified, ligated, and divided between ties or clips. The advanced energy source then completes the retroduodenal tunnel. A 60 mm stapler is introduced and the duodenum is divided. The stomach is then retracted cephalad, and any attachments between the stomach and the

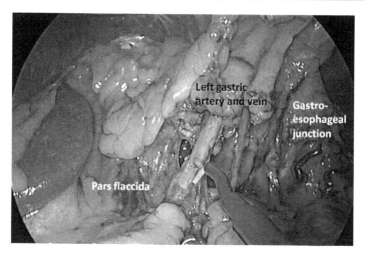

**Fig. 23.4** Dissection of the left gastric artery and vein during robotic gastrectomy

pancreas are divided. The lesser omentum is dissected close to the liver to include associated lymph nodes along the hepatic artery and the left gastric artery in the resected specimen. Either hook electrocautery or ultrasonic shears can be used for this dissection. The necessity to take the left gastric vasculature and associated lymph nodes is typically dictated by location of the lesion, with more distal lesions allowing for preservation of the vessels, and body and proximal lesions requiring inclusion. A linear stapler is introduced through the left lower port and the stomach is transected with appropriate height staple loads. The specimen is removed through the left lower port. Reconstruction is left to the discretion of the operating surgeon and may include gastro-jejunostomy, gastro-duodenostomy, or Roux en-Y. Intraoperative pathology of frozen margins should be obtained to ensure that the submucosa is free of residual tumor, after which reconstruction is carried out as detailed below.

## Total Gastrectomy

The initial steps of a total gastrectomy are described above. After omentectomy and division of the right gastroepiploic artery and duodenum, the lesser omentum is divided close to the liver to the esophagogastric junction. The left gastric artery is ligated and divided close to its origin at the celiac trunk (Fig. 23.4). Attention is turned to the greater curvature, and the short gastric arteries are taken close to spleen with an advanced energy source. After the fundus is fully mobilized, nodal tissue along the splenic artery (station 11) and adjacent to the splenic hilum (station 10) are dissected and removed with the specimen. Once the stomach is fully mobilized, the intra-abdominal esophagus is divided with a linear stapler, with associated lymph nodes in

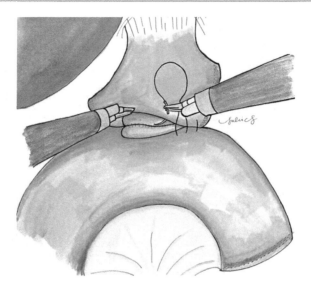

**Fig. 23.5** Robotic Roux-en-Y reconstruction

the phreno-esophageal ligaments included in the specimen. Intraoperative pathology analysis of specimen margins should be performed prior to reconstruction.

## Reconstruction

Reestablishment of gastrointestinal continuity after resection depends on the extent of gastric resection, patient anatomy, and surgeon preference. Following distal gastrectomy, reconstructive options include a Billroth I gastro-duodenostomy, Billroth II gastro-jejunostomy, or Roux-en-Y gastro-jejunostomy (most common option). Reconstruction may be done wholly intracorporeally, extracorporeally, or a combination of both. One advantage of robotic surgery with its increased dexterity and visualization is the ability to complete wholly intracorporeal anastomoses during reconstruction (Fig. 23.5), which is technically much more demanding when performed laparoscopically.

## Potential Benefits

Two randomized-controlled trials (RCTs) comparing long-term survival after minimally invasive surgery for advanced gastric cancer are currently underway in Japan and Korea. Short-term outcomes from the Korean trial demonstrate decreased morbidity with similar mortality between laparoscopic and open distal gastrectomy groups in patients with stage 1 gastric cancer [15].

Meta-analyses, prospective, and retrospective studies all consistently demonstrate a significantly decreased intraoperative blood loss in the robotic gastrectomy compared with laparoscopic or open approaches (Table 23.1). Bleeding during

**Table 23.1** Review of open versus laparoscopic versus robotic gastrectomy

| Authors | Year | Study type | Operations (n) | Op time (min) | EBL | Retrieved LN | Prox margin | Distal margin | Morbidity | LOS (days) | ROBF (days) |
|---|---|---|---|---|---|---|---|---|---|---|---|
| Xiong et al. [8] | 2012 | Meta-analysis | RAG (268) vs LAG (650) | RAG > LAG (WMD = 68.77[a]) | LAG > RAG (WMD = −41.88[a]) | RAG = LAG | NR | NR | RAG = LAG | RAG = LAG | NR |
| Xiong et al. [17] | 2013 | Meta-analysis | RAG (736) vs LAG (1759) | RAG > LAG (WMD = 48.64[a]) | RAG < LAG (WMD = −33.56[a]) | RAG = LAG | RAG = LAG | RAG < LAG (WMD = 1.13[a]) | RAG = LAG | RAG = LAG | RAG = LAG |
| Hyun et al. [18] | 2013 | Meta-analysis | RAG vs LAG vs open | RAG > LAG (WMD = 61.99[a]), RAG > open (WMD = 65.73[a]) | RAG = LAG, open > RAG (WMD = −154.18[a]) | RAG = LAG, RAG = open | RAG = LAG, RAG = open | RAG > LAG (WMD = −1.14[a]), RAG = open | RAG = LAG, RAG > open (WMD = 1.82[a]) | RAG = LAG, open > RAG (WMD = −2.18[a]) | NR |
| Shen et al. [10] | 2014 | Meta-analysis | RAG vs LAG | RAG > LAG (WMD = 48.46[a]) | RAG < LAG (WMD = −38.4[a]) | RAG = LAG | RAG = LAG | RAG > LAG (WMD = 1.04[a]) | NR | RAG = LAG | NR |
| Marano et al. | 2013 | Meta-analysis | RAG vs LAG vs open | RAG > LAG (WMD = 63.7[a]), RAG > open (WMD = 95.83[a]) | LAG > RAG (WMD = −35.53[a]), RAG = Open | RAG = LAG, RAG = Open | NR | NR | RAG = LAG, RAG = open | RAG = LAG, Open > RAG (WMD = −2.92[a]) | NR |
| Zong et al. [19] | 2014 | Meta-analysis | RAG vs LAG vs OG | RAG > OG (WMD = 68.47[a]), RAG > LAG (WMD = 57.15[a]) | OG > RAG (WMD = 68.47[a]), RAG = LAG | RAG = OG, RAG = LAG | NR | NR | RAG = OG, RAG = LAG | RAG < OG (WMD = −106.63[a]), RAG = LAG | NR |
| Junfeng et al. [20] | 2014 | Retrospective | RAG (120) vs LAG (394) | RAG (234.8) > LAG (221.3)[a] | LAG (137.6) > RAG (118.3)[a] | RAG (34.6) > LAG (32.7)[a] | RAG = LAG | RAG = LAG | RAG = LAG | RAG = LAG | RAG = LAG |
| Kim et al. [11] | 2016 | Prospective | RAG (223) vs LAG (211) | RAG 226 > LAG 180[a] | LAG 60 > RAG 50 | 49.3% D2 in RAG > 39.3% D2 in LAG[a] | Not involved in 0.5% LAG > 0% RAG | Not involved in LAG or RAG | LAG 14.2% > RAG 13.5% | RAG (6) = LAG (6) | RAG (6) = LAG (6) |
| Shen et al. [21] | 2016 | Retrospective | RAG (93) vs LAG (330) | RAG (257.1) > LAG (226.2)[a] | LAG (212.5) > RAG (176.6)[a] | RAG (33) > LAG (31.3)[a] | RAG = LAG | RAG = LAG | RAG = LAG | RAG = LAG | RAG = LAG |

*RAG* robotic-assisted gastrectomy, *LAG* laparoscopic-assisted gastrectomy, *NR* not reported, *WMD* weighted mean difference

[a]Statistically significant difference

laparoscopic gastrectomy is commonly described from injury to branches of the left gastric artery, coronary vein, or short gastric arteries [2]. Decreased blood loss in robotic gastrectomy is likely due to enhanced stereoscopic visualization and tremor filtration allowing for precise dissection of vascular structures, as well as improved dexterity to control bleeding should it occur. This potentially may lead to a decreased need for transfusions and associated transfusion-related complications, which is an advantage in the treatment of any malignancy.

Robotic surgery may also allow the surgeon to complete anastomoses intracorporeally due to enhanced ergonomics and visualization [10] rather than performing an extracorporeal anastomosis. In addition, robotic anastomoses may be less technically challenging compared to the laparoscopic approach.

Robotic gastrectomy has been shown to have longer operative times compared to laparoscopic and open approach. This is likely due to increased time during robot docking and patient positioning. However, as surgeon's experience with robotic procedures accrues, operative times have decreased approaching those of laparoscopic techniques [16].

The learning curve in robotic surgery is less steep compared to laparoscopy [15], which may allow centers to offer minimally invasive gastrectomy where previously only open approaches were performed.

## Indications for Benign Disease

### Peptic Ulcer Disease

The treatment of peptic ulcer disease (PUD) has evolved, starting from the development of histamine blockers in the 1970s, to the development of proton-pump inhibitors in the 1980s, and finally to the discovery of *H pylori* [22]. Once routinely a surgical disease, PUD is now successfully treated with medical therapy in the majority of cases. Today, two-thirds of surgical interventions for peptic ulcer disease are due to perforation, while one-third is due to uncontrolled bleeding. Laparoscopic intervention for perforated peptic ulcer disease has been shown to have equivalent outcomes with shorter hospital stays and decreased postoperative pain compared to open repair [23]. However, there is only one case series detailing a single institution experience with general surgery robotic cases. The authors report a robotic partial gastrectomy for perforation from peptic ulcer disease; however, this was unable to be completed robotically and required conversion to laparoscopy [24]. The concepts and techniques regarding robotic washout and repair are comparable to laparoscopic approaches, but the relative rarity of surgical PUD has made description of robotic management rare in the literature as well.

## Gastric Gastrointestinal Stromal Tumor

Gastrointestinal stromal tumors (GIST) arise from the interstitial cells of Cajal and most commonly occur in the stomach [25, 26]. Due to hematogenous spread, lymphadenectomy is not indicated, and these require resection to grossly negative margins as the status of microscopically positive margins has not been shown to affect long-term survival [25]. These are usually discovered incidentally on abdominal imaging or endoscopy. Symptomatic GIST may present with bleeding due to ulceration or obstruction depending on size and location. The preoperative workup of a GIST tumor should include both computed tomography imaging and endoscopy. Endoscopic ultrasound (EUS) can be useful in differentiating between GIST and other tumors. GISTs appear as smooth submucosal lesions on EUS in the muscularis propria layer. An EUS-guided fine-needle aspiration of the lesion can provide tissue diagnosis as well as information about the malignant potential of the tumor itself [25].

Laparoscopic gastric GIST resection is well-described in the literature [24]. Two series describe a series of patients who successfully undergo robotic-assisted GIST resection, in which the tumor was excised with 1–2 cm margins using a Harmonic scalpel with the defect closed with a single-layer running suture [26, 27]. Another case report describes a posterior-wall GIST excised using electrocautery and the defect was closed with absorbable suture [28], demonstrating the advantage of using the robot which facilitates intracorporeal suturing. Another describes five patients who undergo robotic gastric GIST resection with on-table endoscopy used to help facilitate localization of the tumor [29].

Applications for robotic surgery are particularly compelling in treating lesions at the esophago-gastric junction or antrum. Due to the narrowed luminal space and possibility of creating obstruction at either location, precise definition of tumor boundaries is important. Combined endoscopic and laparoscopic or robotic GIST removal has also been described in which balloon-tipped trocars are placed directly through the anterior wall of the stomach. The lesion is then either enucleated or excised laparoscopically or robotically [25]. Within the narrowed space of these challenging anatomic locations, the dexterity of the robotic platform may facilitate accurate closure. Combined laparoscopic-endoscopic GIST resection, with intragastric laparoscopic resection of the tumor and repair of the resultant defect, has been described in a series of 13 patients [30], with good long-term results and no evidence of disease recurrence [31] (Video 23.1).

## Future Directions and Conclusions

Robotic gastrectomy for gastric adenocarcinoma has been shown to have equivalent oncologic outcomes compared to laparoscopic resection, with some studies showing better lymph node retrieval. In addition, it is associated with a lower intraoperative blood loss compared to open and, in some centers, laparoscopic approaches to treatment of gastric cancer. It has been described in a variety of benign disease processes as well. Robotic techniques are mainly limited by longer operating times as well as the common need to re-dock during the course of the procedure. However, the latter may be mitigated in the new Xi robot which allows greater flexibility and access to all quadrants of the abdomen with minimal repositioning of the robot. This adaptability may increase adoption of robotic-assisted procedures in more general surgical cases, including gastric surgery.

Minimally invasive gastrectomy for gastric cancer has been slower to adopt in the United States, where the incidence of early gastric cancer is lower than in Japan and Korea. Laparoscopic gastrectomy is offered for early stage cancer. Robotic gastrectomy may allow centers to perform minimally invasive gastrectomy as it has been shown to be associated with a shorter learning curve compared to laparoscopic gastrectomy.

In conclusion, robotic gastrectomy is feasible in both malignant and benign diseases, with the potential benefits of shorter learning curves compared to laparoscopic technique as well as improved optics and instrument articulation. Reported benefits include decreased intraoperative blood loss and, in cancer, potentially better lymph node retrieval. Further prospective trials are warranted, but as robotic technology continues to improve, we would expect advantages of robotic gastrectomy to become more evident.

## References

1. Kitano S, Iso Y, Moriyama M, Sugimachi K. Laparoscopy-assisted Billroth I gastrectomy. Surg Laparosc Endosc. 1994;4:146–8.
2. Kitano S, Shiraishi N, Uyama I, Sugihara K, Tanigawa N. A multicenter study on oncologic outcome of laparoscopic gastrectomy for early cancer in Japan. Ann Surg. 2007;245:68–72. doi:10.1097/01.sla.0000225364.03133.f8.
3. Hashizume M, Sugimachi K. Robot-assisted gastric surgery. Surg Clin North Am. 2003;83:1429–44. doi:10.1016/S0039-6109(03)00158-0.
4. Noguchi Y, Yoshikawa T, Tsuburaya A, Motohashi H, Karpeh MS, Brennan MF. Is gastric carcinoma different between Japan and the United States? Cancer. 2000;89:2237–46.
5. Japanese Gastric Cancer Association. Japanese gastric cancer treatment guidelines 2010 (ver. 3). Gastric Cancer. 2011;14:113–23. doi:10.1007/s10120-011-0042-4.
6. Douglass HO, Hundahl SA, Macdonald JS, Khatri VP. Gastric cancer: D2 dissection or low Maruyama Index-based surgery—a debate. Surg Oncol Clin N Am. 2007;16:133–55. doi:10.1016/j.soc.2006.10.005.
7. Hartgrink HH, van de Velde CJH, Putter H, Bonenkamp JJ, Klein Kranenbarg E, Songun I, et al. Extended lymph node dissection for gastric cancer: who may benefit? Final results of the randomized Dutch gastric cancer group trial. J Clin Oncol. 2004;22:2069–77. doi:10.1200/JCO.2004.08.026.
8. Xiong B, Ma L, Zhang C. Robotic versus laparoscopic gastrectomy for gastric cancer: a meta-analysis of short outcomes. Surg Oncol. 2012;21:274–80. doi:10.1016/j.suronc.2012.05.004.
9. Marano A, Choi YY, Hyung WJ, Kim YM, Kim J, Noh SH. Robotic versus laparoscopic versus open gastrectomy: a meta-analysis. J Gastric Cancer. 2013;13:136–48. doi:10.5230/jgc.2013.13.3.136.
10. Shen W-S, Xi H-Q, Chen L, Wei B. A meta-analysis of robotic versus laparoscopic gastrectomy for gastric cancer. Surg Endosc. 2014;28:2795–802. doi:10.1007/s00464-014-3547-1.

11. Kim H-I, Han S-U, Yang H-K, Kim Y-W, Lee H-J, Ryu KW, et al. Multicenter prospective comparative study of robotic versus laparoscopic gastrectomy for gastric adenocarcinoma. Ann Surg. 2016;263:103–9. doi:10.1097/SLA.0000000000001249.
12. Son T, Lee JH, Kim YM, Kim H-I, Noh SH, Hyung WJ. Robotic spleen-preserving total gastrectomy for gastric cancer: comparison with conventional laparoscopic procedure. Surg Endosc. 2014;28:2606–15. doi:10.1007/s00464-014-3511-0.
13. Lee J-H, Yom C-K, Han H-S. Comparison of long-term outcomes of laparoscopy-assisted and open distal gastrectomy for early gastric cancer. Surg Endosc. 2009;23:1759–63. doi:10.1007/s00464-008-0198-0.
14. Best LM, Mughal M, Gurusamy KS. Laparoscopic versus open gastrectomy for gastric cancer. Cochrane Database Syst Rev. 2016;3:CD011389. doi:10.1002/14651858.CD011389.pub2.
15. Kim W, Kim H-H, Han S-U, Kim M-C, Hyung WJ, Ryu SW, et al. Decreased morbidity of laparoscopic distal gastrectomy compared with open distal gastrectomy for stage I gastric cancer: short-term outcomes from a multicenter randomized controlled trial (KLASS-01). Ann Surg. 2016;263:28–35. doi:10.1097/SLA.0000000000001346.
16. Hyun M-H, Lee C-H, Kwon Y-J, Cho S-I, Jang Y-J, Kim D-H, et al. Robot versus laparoscopic gastrectomy for cancer by an experienced surgeon: comparisons of surgery, complications, and surgical stress. Ann Surg Oncol. 2013;20:1258–65. doi:10.1245/s10434-012-2679-6.
17. Xiong J, Nunes QM, Tan C, Ke N, Chen Y, Hu W, et al. Comparison of short-term clinical outcomes between robotic and laparoscopic gastrectomy for gastric cancer: a meta-analysis of 2495 patients. J Laparoendosc Adv Surg Tech A. 2013;23:965–76. doi:10.1089/lap.2013.0279.
18. Hyun MH, Lee CH, Kim HJ, Tong Y, Park SS. Systematic review and meta-analysis of robotic surgery compared with conventional laparoscopic and open resections for gastric carcinoma. Br J Surg. 2013;100:1566–78. doi:10.1002/bjs.9242.
19. Zong L, Seto Y, Aikou S, Takahashi T. Efficacy evaluation of subtotal and total gastrectomies in robotic surgery for gastric cancer compared with that in open and laparoscopic resections: a meta-analysis. PLoS One. 2014;9:e103312. doi:10.1371/journal.pone.0103312.
20. Junfeng Z, Yan S, Bo T, Yingxue H, Dongzhu Z, Yongliang Z, et al. Robotic gastrectomy versus laparoscopic gastrectomy for gastric cancer: comparison of surgical performance and short-term outcomes. Surg Endosc. 2014;28:1779–87. doi:10.1007/s00464-013-3385-6.
21. Shen W, Xi H, Wei B, Cui J, Bian S, Zhang K, et al. Robotic versus laparoscopic gastrectomy for gastric cancer: comparison of short-term surgical outcomes. Surg Endosc. 2016;30:574–80. doi:10.1007/s00464-015-4241-7.
22. Zittel TT, Jehle EC, Becker HD. Surgical management of peptic ulcer disease today—indication, technique and outcome. Langenbeck's Arch Surg. 2000;385:84–96.
23. Siu WT, Leong HT, Law BKB, Chau CH, Li ACN, Fung KH, et al. Laparoscopic repair for perforated peptic ulcer: a randomized controlled trial. Ann Surg. 2002;235:313–9.
24. Braumann C, Jacobi CA, Menenakos C, Ismail M, Rueckert JC, Mueller JM. Robotic-assisted laparoscopic and thoracoscopic surgery with the da Vinci system: a 4-year experience in a single institution. Surg Laparosc Endosc Percutan Tech. 2008;18:260–6. doi:10.1097/SLE.0b013e31816f85e5.
25. Dholakia C, Gould J. Minimally invasive resection of gastrointestinal stromal tumors. Surg Clin North Am. 2008;88:1009–18, vi. doi:10.1016/j.suc.2008.05.006.
26. Huh WJ, Coffey RJ, Washington MK. Ménétrier's disease: its mimickers and pathogenesis. J Pathol Transl Med. 2016;50:10–6. doi:10.4132/jptm.2015.09.15.
27. Al-Thani H, El-Menyar A, Mekkodathil A, Elgohary H, Tabeb AH. Robotic management of gastric stromal tumors (GIST): a single Middle Eastern center experience. Int J Med Robot. 2016; doi:10.1002/rcs.1729.
28. Moriyama H, Ishikawa N, Kawaguchi M, Hirose K, Watanabe G. Robot-assisted laparoscopic resection for gastric gastrointestinal stromal tumor. Surg Laparosc Endosc Percutan Tech. 2012;22:e155–6. doi:10.1097/SLE.0b013e3182491ff6.

29. Desiderio J, Trastulli S, Cirocchi R, Boselli C, Noya G, Parisi A, et al. Robotic gastric resection of large gastrointestinal stromal tumors. Int J Surg. 2013;11:191–6. doi:10.1016/j.ijsu.2013.01.002.
30. Walsh RM, Ponsky J, Brody F, Matthews BD, Heniford BT. Combined endoscopic/laparoscopic intragastric resection of gastric stromal tumors. J Gastrointest Surg. n.d.;7:386–92.
31. Mino JS, Guerron AD, Monteiro R, El-Hayek K, Ponsky JL, Patil DT, et al. Long-term outcomes of combined endoscopic/laparoscopic intragastric enucleation of presumed gastric stromal tumors. Surg Endosc. 2016;30:1747–53. doi:10.1007/s00464-015-4416-2.

# Robotic Approach to Transhiatal Esophagectomy

Jeffrey R. Watkins and D. Rohan Jeyarajah

## Introduction

The first transhiatal esophagectomy (THE) was performed in 1933 by Turner, but quickly replaced by the thoracic approach [1]. Orringer and Sloan re-popularized the transhiatal technique in their 1978 series, bringing about a change in the approach to treating esophageal disorders [2]. The transabdominal route requires no thoracic incisions and thus avoids the drawbacks associated with trans-thoracic esophagectomy: mainly postoperative pulmonary complications and mediastinitis from intrathoracic leak. Failure of the cervical anastomosis in transhiatal esophagectomy results in a fistula easily managed with open drainage. Consider this in contrast to the devastating sequelae of a thoracic anastomotic leak resulting in mediastinitis with a mortality rate up to 42% [3].

The oncologic appropriateness of the transhiatal approach has previously been questioned and remains a point of contention. Critics argue that a complete thoracic lymphadenectomy cannot be performed adequately with the transhiatal approach [4, 5]. Orringer and others argue, however, that long-term survival is based upon the status of the disease at the time of resection with 46% of patients with Stage III or IV disease at the time of operation and 35% of patients with occult lymph node metastasis [6]. There are no randomized control studies which show a superior survival benefit of either approach. A recent meta-analysis looking at over 200 papers with five randomized trials concluded that overall mortality was equivalent in both operative techniques except for a possible survival benefit with the transthoracic

J.R. Watkins, M.D.
Methodist Dallas Medical Center,
221 W. Colorado Blvd., Pavilion II, Suite 933, Dallas, TX 75208, USA

D.R. Jeyarajah, M.D. (✉)
Surgical Oncology, Methodist Dallas Medical Center,
1441 N. Beckley Ave, Dallas, TX 75208, USA
e-mail: rohanjeyarajah@gmail.com

© Springer International Publishing AG 2018
A.D. Patel, D. Oleynikov (eds.), *The SAGES Manual of Robotic Surgery*,
The SAGES University Masters Program Series, DOI 10.1007/978-3-319-51362-1_24

309

approach in a subgroup of limited node-positive patients [7]. The analysis also concludes that, short-term, the transhiatal approach is associated with reduced perioperative morbidity as evidenced by a shorter hospital stay and decreased in-hospital mortality rates. For gastroesophageal junction tumors, there may even be a survival advantage for Type III tumors [8].

The first series of laparoscopic transhiatal esophagectomy was described by DePaula in 1995 and, since that time, the literature has showed improvement in length of stay, postoperative morbidity and mortality of minimally invasive techniques over open esophagectomy [9, 10]. Recently, the advances in robotic technology have allowed surgeons to approach the hiatus with this new technology. Since first being described in 2002, robotic transhiatal esophagectomy has found its place among minimally invasive techniques [11]. Advanced robotic techniques such as recurrent laryngeal nodal dissection and extensive transhiatal thoracic nodal dissections including those as described by Mori et al. are pushing the boundaries of robotic surgery [12, 13]. The robot offers several advantages over traditional laparoscopy for hiatal work including stereoscopic vision, improved camera and operator stabilization, wristed instruments resulting in greater mobility, and improved surgeon ergonomics. On the other hand, diminished haptic feedback, increased cost of individual operations, and a steep learning curve have all been criticisms aimed at the platform. Regardless, the robot has been proven a powerful tool for esophageal surgery.

## Indications/Patient Selection

All patients with benign and malignant disease should be considered candidates for robotic transhiatal esophagectomy. Patients with benign disease including caustic injuries, chronic strictures from previous anti-reflux surgeries, complications relating to achalasia, and sigmoid esophagus should all be considered for resection. The debate regarding the transhiatal approach in advanced stage carcinoma has been previously addressed, but there is no clear evidence that there is a survival benefit from one technique over another. Absolute contraindications to robot surgery parallel those of laparoscopic surgery, including the inability to tolerate abdominal insufflation and advanced stage/metastatic disease. Relative contraindications include extensive previous surgery or a hostile abdomen.

Preoperative staging is a necessity for all esophageal neoplasms. It is the authors' practice to obtain preoperative computed tomography of the chest, abdomen, and pelvis along with positron emission tomography scans. Endoscopic evaluation with tissue biopsy is necessary for determination of tumor location and biology. Endoscopic ultrasound (EUS) allows for improved tumor staging including presence of local invasion and nodal status. The authors' use of EUS is mostly for early stage lesions. The use of neoadjuvant chemotherapy and radiation in any lesions greater than T2 or node-positive lesions decreases the importance of EUS. Locally advanced tumors and invasion into the trachea-bronchial tree or surrounding tissues represent a contraindication to THE. Patients with neoplastic disease routinely receive neoadjuvant chemoradiation. While it would seem that morbidity would increase with surgery after neoadjuvant therapy, this has not been shown in the literature.

# Room Setup

## Patient Positioning

The patient is placed on the operating table in a supine position with arms tucked. There are some groups that place the patient in "French" position with the legs split. This is especially useful when there is a bedside assistant with an additional port. This is not the authors' preference as a bedside surgeon is not utilized. A foam padding is placed around the upper extremities and under the patient to assist in patient comfort as well as providing a non-skid surface to keep the patient in position when placed in severe reverse Trendelenburg. These pads are specifically used to both provide cushioning and prevent sliding of the patient. If the patient's body habitus is too large, plastic sleds may assist in keeping the arms at the patient's side. When using the Si system, it is important to keep patient as close to the head of the bed as possible, otherwise there may not be enough reach with the camera arm. Foam padding and goggles are placed over the patient's face to avoid undue pressure from the robot on the eyes or other facial structures. A shoulder roll can be used to improve neck extension for the cervical portion of the dissection and anastomosis. A foot board is placed at the feet with padding under the heels and soles in order to provide support when positioned steeply.

One of the most important factors in the authors' experience with robotic foregut surgery was the acquisition of a properly adjustable sliding operating table. The table should be able to slide in both cephalad and caudal directions and achieve extreme reverse Trendelenburg with the patient nearly "standing up" (Fig. 24.1). Positioning should be checked in conjunction with anesthesia in order to assure proper patient security. Once the patient is positioned satisfactorily, waist straps are applied and the rails on the patient's right side are cleared of any obstruction, as the liver retractor will be placed here.

## Robot Positioning

When using the Si system, the table will likely need to be positioned at an oblique angle to the anesthesiologist to allow the robot to dock in a linear fashion over the patient's head (Fig. 24.2). The surgeon should ensure that the Si robot, which will dock from above the head, will leave enough room for the anesthesiologist to access the airway and face. In addition, there must be enough space for the cervical anastomotic portion of the case. When using the Xi system, the robot can approach from a lateral position with the arms turned 90° to facilitate easier docking (Fig. 24.3). The table is placed in maximal reverse Trendelenburg, then lowered as far down to the ground as possible. Sometimes it is necessary to adjust the sliding position of the table up or down. This is especially important because, unlike the Xi system, the Si boom cannot be raised or lowered. Once the positioning is confirmed, the patient may be prepped and draped.

### Key Points
See Table 24.1.

**Fig. 24.1** Positioning
patient in steep reverse
Trendelenburg on sliding
operating table

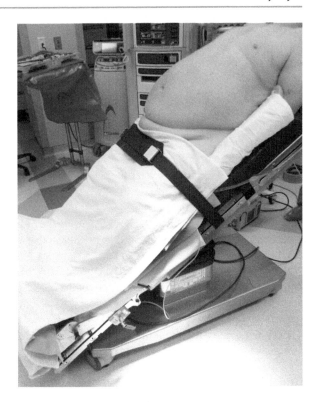

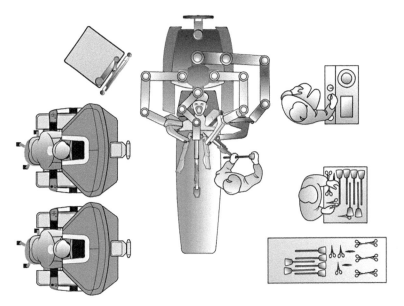

**Fig. 24.2** Room setup for Si system. The robot approaches and docks from above the patient's
head

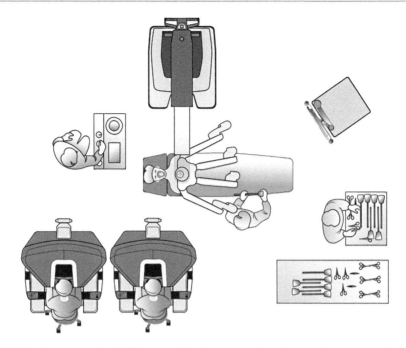

**Fig. 24.3** Room setup for the Xi system. The robot approaches and docks from the patient's side

**Table 24.1** Docking key differences

| Si | Xi |
| --- | --- |
| Dock from above patient's head | Dock from patient's left |
| Turn table | Table position unchanged |
| Patient in steep reverse Trendelenburg | Patient in steep reverse Trendelenburg |

## Console Setup/Third Arm Approach

At the authors' training institution, the use of a dual-console system is advocated in order to facilitate the involvement of trainees. The dual-console setup allows several advantages over a single-console setup. Once the trainee has fulfilled the requisite number of docking and instrument exchanges at the bedside, it is imperative that they participate in the surgery. Taking their place at the console allows involvement and graduated responsibility. Traditionally, using the "3rd arm" has referred to the utilization of the unused arm on the Si system by the assistant on the second console. The arm numbering has been changed on the Xi system and thus the term "assistant arm" will be used in place of the term third arm on the Si and fourth arm on Xi.

The use of the assistant arm allows seamless swapping of instruments between surgeon and assistant. The trainee is able to start with a single arm in order to become more familiar with the mechanics of the robot controls and gradually move to the primary arms with the acquisition of more experience. Placing a trainee bedside with an additional assistant port places emphasis on laparoscopy rather than robotics and does nothing to increase the robotic skillset. The dynamic interchange between robot arms allows the surgeon to take over the main arms during more difficult portions of the case. This technique enhances interplay between surgeon and trainee while facilitating education. It also overcomes the "loneliness" of the robot which can occur when the surgeon is isolated in the console without any other human contact. There may be some surgeons that gravitate towards robotics as a means to be alone and escape human interaction. The authors are not in this group and would encourage the more "social" surgeon to use the assistant arm as a technique of training. It is more convenient to position the two consoles near each other for ease of communication, but is not a requirement and operating room space limitations may preclude this arrangement. The voice communications system within the console may be inadequate for some, and the use of a separate hands-free wireless communication system for improved voice communication has been suggested.

It is important to customize the console settings for the individual surgeon. On both the Si and the Xi, surgeons are able to log in using unique profiles and adjust ergonomics and other settings as needed. In our experience, it is convenient to switch off the Firefly quick switching option to avoid inadvertent camera switching when finger clutching. We also use normal (1:1) motion scaling.

**Key Points**
- Use dual-console setup
- Trainee should use assistant arm until proficiency shown
- Trainee should then advance to using primary arms (1 and 2 for Si, 1 and 3 for Xi)

## Operative Technique

### Port Placement

The abdomen can be entered by any manner in which the surgeon is comfortable. The authors prefer to use a 5 mm direct entry optical entry through a supraumbilical stab incision. The abdominal wall is grasped laterally by the surgeon and the assistant and elevated as the trocar and camera are slowly advanced through the layers of the abdominal wall under direct visualization. Once the abdomen is entered, pneumoperitoneum of 15 mmHg is achieved. The underlying bowel and omentum is visualized to rule out inadvertent injury. In the authors' practice, no documented complications or injuries over hundreds of procedures using this technique have occurred. A thorough exploration of the abdomen with the laparoscope should be undertaken in the patient with malignancy. It is very easy to proceed mechanically without this step and overlook metastatic disease.

A 12 mm robotic trocar is placed in the left upper abdomen which will be used for the energy device and stapler (Fig. 24.4). The location will vary depending on the energy device used. A more cephalad position along the mid-clavicular line (MCL) towards the costal margin is required for the ultrasonic dissector in order to

**Fig. 24.4** Port placement for the Si and Xi system. If using the Harmonic device, the 12 mm port will be placed more cephalad than if using the Vessel Sealer. The camera port will be a bariatric length 11 mm trocar for the Si, or an 8 mm robotic trocar if using the Xi

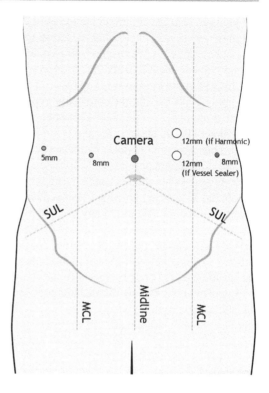

maximize the extent of its reach. It is the authors' preference to use the Harmonic ACE™ ultrasonic dissector device in this position. If using the robotic vessel sealer, the port can be placed in a more caudal position just superior to the horizontal level of the midline camera port. The ultrasonic dissector is shorter than the vessel sealer and so the left mid-clavicular port must be placed more cephalad if the former device is being used. An 8 mm robotic port will be used to "piggyback" through the 12 mm port. The 8 mm robotic port is placed inside the 12 mm port and the arm is docked to the robotic port in the normal fashion. In order to gain more reach when using the ultrasonic shears, the 12 mm port may be "burped" by the assistant which involves retracting the shears and clutching the arm and advancing the port in order to gain more distance for the instrument. Regardless of the robotic system used, this trocar should be spaced at least 10 cm away from the camera port.

An 8 mm trocar is then placed in the far left abdomen, below the costal margin at least 10 cm from the energy device port. This port should be placed far laterally while safely avoiding bowel. If the trocar is placed too far laterally, however, docking of this port can be challenging and there can be external collisions with the patient's left arm. A ProGrasp™ instrument will be used through this port and will be controlled by the assistant if using a dual-console setup. This port will be placed at the same location on the abdomen regardless of whether the Si or Xi system is used.

An 8 mm port is placed in the right abdomen on the right MCL at the level of the camera port. This will be the surgeon's right hand and a fenestrated bipolar grasper will be used. In order to maximize the effectiveness of the bipolar instrument, the tips must be slightly open when coagulating tissue; otherwise the electrocautery will not be as effective. This port will be placed in a more caudal position resulting in a more linear angle if using the Xi system.

A liver retractor system is set up by securing the clamp to the rails of the table in cooperation with the anesthesiologist to avoid clamping any of the patient lines. A flexible triangular liver retractor (Snowden-Pencer®) is placed in the abdomen and, under direct visualization, is positioned under the left lobe of the liver to expose the hiatus. This is secured in place by the assistant using the Fast Clamp system.

The 5 mm camera port is then upsized to a robotic port under direct visualization. In the Si system, a bariatric length 12 mm trocar is placed and a 12 mm camera is used. In the Xi system, an 8 mm trocar is placed and an 8 mm scope is used with the advantage of being able to use any of the 8 mm ports as the camera port. A disposable 5 mm port is placed in the far right abdomen in a subcostal position. A 5 mm AirSeal® port can be placed for improved insufflation and evacuation. If using the AirSeal® system, the surgeon should place this port last. Once AirSeal® is initiated, placement of ports becomes very difficult as the system will maintain the pressure of 15 mmHg and not allow for elevated pressures associated with trocar placement. The authors prefer this system as this is very efficient at steam evacuation without affecting pneumoperitoneum.

## Docking

Once the liver retractor is placed, the patient is placed in reverse Trendelenburg. It may be necessary for the table to be lowered and slid down towards the floor in order to achieve the correct height to accommodate the robot.

### Si System

For the Si system, the patient is approached in a linear manner from the head of the bed, i.e., dock from above the head. The robot should be advanced with the bed in the flat position. Once the camera arm appears to be in good position, the table is then placed in steep reverse Trendelenburg position and, with the surgeon watching carefully, ensures that the camera arm is still dockable. The robot will likely need to be advanced once the table position is achieved. The robot should be centered in line with the center camera port. Once the robot is positioned, the brake is applied and the camera arm is docked to the midline port, with the arm indicator in the blue "sweet spot". With a very tall patient, the surgeon may have to dock with the camera arm in the straight position. This is not a major concern, but the robot must be advanced as close to the head of the bed as possible. Use of a bariatric 12 mm trocar at the midline position helps achieve greater mobility and decreases the likelihood of port slippage. Once the camera arm is docked, the remaining arms are docked. Arm three should be positioned to the patient's left side. If there are external collisions, the arms may need to be adjusted. A 12 mm camera is placed through the camera port and the remaining instruments are placed under direct visualization. All four arms are used.

## Xi System

For the Xi system, the patient is approached from either the right or left side (see Fig. 24.3), depending on the room setup. The driver will input the location of the surgery (upper abdomen) and the direction of the approach (right or left). The green laser guides are then aligned with the midline camera port and arm 2 is docked to the 8 mm robotic port. The 8 mm camera is inserted and the targeting sequence is initiated by aiming the camera towards the hiatus and pressing the target button on the camera while holding the trocar firmly in place. The remaining free arms will move as the boom rotates. Once the targeting sequence is completed, the remaining arms are docked. Arm 3 will be docked to a free 8 mm port and "piggybacked" into a 12 mm left mid-clavicular line port.

## Key Points

See Table 24.2.

## Instrumentation

For the purpose of this section, the authors will use the arm terminology for the Si robot. Arm 1 is the right MCL port; arm 2 is the left MCL port; arm 3 is the left abdominal port.

The surgeon will use arms 1 and 2, while the assistant will use arm 3. The fenestrated bipolar instrument is used in arm 1 in the right abdomen. It is less traumatic than the ProGrasp™ and has the ability to apply bipolar energy. In order to maximize the effectiveness of the bipolar instrument, the tips must be slightly open when coagulating tissue, otherwise the electrocautery will not be effective. The surgeon uses the energy device in arm 2, which can either be an ultrasonic dissector or a bipolar vessel sealer. The Vessel Sealer is a wristed instrument which can effectively seal vessel up to 7 mm in diameter. It exhibits minimal thermal spread without any active blades. It is possible to perform blunt dissection and has a longer reach and more mobility than the harmonic dissector. The activating sequence is more complex and requires three pedal presses for each complete cycle. The ultrasonic dissector has no "wrist" ability and less overall mobility. In addition, it has an exposed active blade, so care must be taken not to cause any inadvertent thermal tissue damage. The activating mechanism requires a single pedal press and tissue dissection and vessel coagulation proceed at a much more accelerated rate. If additional length is needed for the ultrasonic dissector, the 12 mm trocar may be "burped" in farther for a longer reach.

**Table 24.2** Port placement key differences

| Si | Xi |
|---|---|
| Midline 12 mm bariatric port | Midline 8 mm robot port |
| Bring robot in then position patient | Position patient first |
| Arm 3 swings to the left | No need to rearrange arms |

The assistant arm 3 will use the ProGrasp™ instrument. It exhibits the most gripping power of the graspers, but in turn is the most traumatic to tissues. Care must be taken to limit tissue trauma by avoiding direct manipulation of hollow-viscous organs. The flexible triangular liver retractor is used in the far-right abdominal 5 mm port and held in place using the Fast Clamp system on the right-sided bed rails. A 12 mm linear-lipped vascular load-powered stapler is used through the left upper abdominal 12 mm port when transecting the right gastric vessels. Finally, if the pyloroplasty is performed intracorporeally, large cutting needle drivers can be placed through the 12 mm port along with suture.

## Operative Details

After docking the robot and placing the instruments, the right gastroepiploic vessels are identified. It is important not to manipulate or place excessive retraction around this area as it will serve as the vascular pedicle for the gastric conduit. In our practice, we prefer a left-sided approach wherein the short gastric vessels are divided and the crus is approached from the greater curvature before moving on to the right crus via the pars flacida.

Once the right gastroepiploic vessels are identified, the greater curvature is grasped and elevated by the surgeon, while the assistant retracts the gastrocolic ligament using arm 3 in the Si system (4 for Xi). The lesser sac is entered using the energy device and the short gastric vessels are divided, continuing the dissection towards the lefts crus. It is helpful for the surgeon to grasp the posterior wall of the stomach and retract medially and towards the abdominal wall. This will allow dissection and division of the posterior gastric attachments. Short gastric vessels up to 5 mm can be divided using the ultrasonic dissector or up to 7 mm using the bipolar Vessel Sealer. The authors propose an unusual approach to the left crus: they start along the greater curvature and then work more medially. Effectively, the assistant lifts the stomach up towards the ceiling in line with the left edge of the aorta (Fig. 24.5). The energy device is used to take the vessels to the left of this area. The maneuver allows for lengthening of the short gastric vessels at the spleen by taking the posterior short gastric vessels that emanate off the splenic artery first. This allows for little chance of injury to spleen itself. Once the left crus is identified, the phrenoesophageal ligament is incised. The right crus is then approached from the lesser curvature of the stomach. The gastrohepatic ligament is divided using an energy device, being careful to identify the presence of an accessory or replaced left hepatic artery. Once the right crus is identified, the phrenoesophageal ligament is divided (Fig. 24.6). Care must be taken in patients who have a hiatal defect as the left gastric vascular bundle can be elongated and enter the chest via the defect. It is possible to injure these vessels in this case.

The left gastric artery is then identified and a window is made by dissecting caudad to this vascular bundle in order to place the stapler. The cephalad dissection of the left gastric vascular bundle is created by developing the plane in the pars flaccida. A lipped vascular-load linear stapler is placed through the left upper abdominal 12 mm

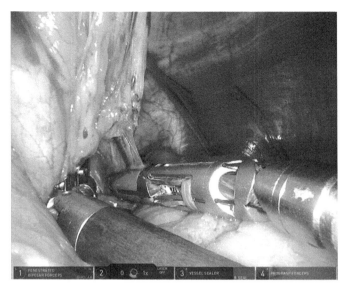

**Fig. 24.5** The initial left-side first approach is demonstrated. The stomach is retracted towards the ceiling, lengthening the posterior short gastric vessels and minimizing injury to the spleen

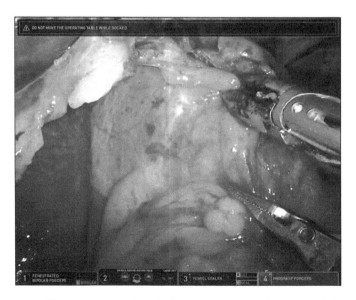

**Fig. 24.6** Approaching the right crus from the lesser curvature. The right crus and phrenoesophageal ligament are shown

port by the bedside assistant and the left gastric vessels are taken near their origin, including the celiac and common hepatic nodal basins (Fig. 24.7). Some surgeons perform an extensive celiac nodal dissection; it is the authors' preference to place the stapler as flush with the hepatic artery to capture these nodes.

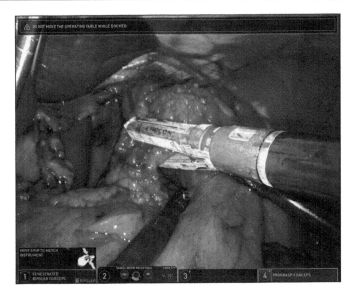

**Fig. 24.7** The left gastric vessels are isolated by the assistant and divided using a linear vascular load stapler

The esophageal hiatal mobilization and dissection begins, maintaining en bloc lymphatics. The assistant (arm 3 on the Si) will retract caudad using the esophageal fat pad, while the operating surgeon retracts the hiatus to the left and right (Fig. 24.8). In this manner, each can provide counter-traction and allow for use of the energy to divide the esophageal attachments. One of the advantages of the robotic system is the ability to gain improved hiatal visualization by placing the scope in the mediastinum and continuing the dissection. It is helpful for the assistant to retract the gastroesophageal fat pad caudally, while the surgeon retracts the crus and dissects with the energy device. Care must be taken to avoid entering the pleural spaces on each side, as the pleura are very intimately associated with the esophageal tissues. Magnification with the robotic camera allows for visualization of a thin white line that is the pleural edge. Entering the pleura does not mandate placement of a chest tube; it is rare that a post-operative clinically relevant pneumothorax will need intervention.

Specific circumstances that may cause difficulty with hiatal dissection are:

1. Preoperative Chemoradiotherapy

    In this circumstance, the esophagus can be quite thick and there can be dense adhesions to adjacent structures. Indeed, the majority of cases in the authors' experience are post-chemoradiation; as such, this has become commonplace in the esophagectomy procedure. It is important to note that the surgery should occur in the 6–12 week time frame post-radiation. After the 12 week mark, there is dense scarring that can make the surgery more challenging. The authors use the analogy of a lasagna: when fresh, all the layers can be seen. However, when

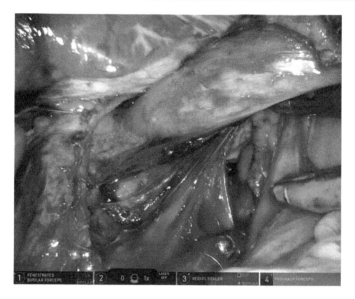

**Fig. 24.8**  The decussation of the crural fibers is identified and hiatal dissection is performed. The assistant elevates the esophagus, while the surgeon uses a combination of energy and blunt dissection

frozen (akin to long interval from radiation), there are no visible planes. Similarly, the anatomy becomes very tough the further one operates from the end of radiation therapy.

2. Presence of a Stent

   While this is becoming more commonplace, a bulky stent can lead to substantial issues when manipulating the esophagus. The stent can be rather rigid and make the traction/counter-traction more challenging than necessary. Presence of a stent should not preclude robotic surgery, but the surgeon should be prepared for a more challenging surgery.

Once the proximal extent of the hiatal dissection is completed, a pyloroplasty can be performed. The gastric antrum is identified and followed distally towards the pylorus and duodenum. Kocherization of the duodenum is achieved by dividing the peritoneum laterally using blunt and sharp dissection. The precise location of the pylorus is confirmed by the presence of the vein of Mayo. Stay sutures (the authors' preference is 2-0 silk on an SH needle) are placed and a longitudinal gastrotomy is made either using electrocautery or ultrasonic shears. This is extended through the pylorus and onto the duodenum, creating a generous 4–5 cm incision. This is then closed in the manner of Heineke-Mikulicz using interrupted 2-0 braided permanent sutures. A suture-cut needle driver is convenient in order to avoid frequently switching instruments in and out of the port. Once completed, the stay sutures are removed and the instruments withdrawn from the abdomen and the robot undocked. If an intracorporeal pyloroplasty proves unfeasible, an open approach can be performed or endoscopic botulinum toxin can be injected.

The authors have experience with a fully robotic approach, but have found that the use of a mini-laparaotomy saves time and has no consequences on postoperative recovery or pain. Therefore, the authors have evolved to the following technique that some may call "hybrid" as there is a small laparotomy scar. In fact, the authors would argue that this incision is needed to extract the specimen and there are no retractors placed. As such, there has been no difference noted in postoperative recovery.

An upper midline mini-laparotomy is made that is enough to permit a hand into the abdomen and chest. This is generally just 10 cm with a fascial undercut. Anterograde blunt hiatal dissection is then performed. The hand in placed into the abdomen and the hiatus is manually dilated. The entire hand must be placed into the mediastinum and the esophagus should be grasped from within the palm of the hand. The dissection proceeds from posterior to lateral and finally anteriorly. Much like in the pelvis, the key structures are anterior and therefore this should be left for last. The left mainstem bronchus should be palpable anterior to the esophagus. Care is taken not to enter the pleura or disrupt the bronchus.

At the same time, the neck dissection can be performed and mobilization of the cervical esophagus is achieved. A limited anterior sternocleidomastoid incision is made. The carotid is retracted laterally and the thyroid medially. Care should be taken in using energy in the tracheoesophageal groove as the recurrent laryngeal nerve is in this location. Despite careful dissection, there is a risk of palsy of this nerve of at least 10% in the authors' experience. The esophagus is mobilized from above into the thoracic inlet again working posteriorly first. The hand from above can then meet the hand from below and complete the dissection.

The nasogastric tube is pulled back and the esophagus is divided in the neck using a linear thoracic anastomosis 30 mm stapler with a blue load. The esophagus is transected leaving the staple line in the distal (specimen) side of the esophagus. A sterile nasogastric tube is sewn to the distal esophagus and the specimen is retrieved from the abdomen and laid on the abdominal wall. It is necessary to complete the antral dissection by dissecting the right gastroepiploic vessels to their origin from the gastroduodenal artery in order to gain maximal mobilization. The surgeon should not skeletonize this origin too much as it can tear when the conduit is pulled up into the neck. The conduit is then created by dissecting and stapling the lesser curvature of the stomach. The authors do not tubularize the stomach, but rather resect the proximal stomach. The staple line is oversewn using 2-0 silk in the manner of Cushing. The sterile nasogastric tube which is lying in the posterior mediastinum is then sewn to the greater curvature of the stomach and the conduit is guided into the hiatus and pulled up into the neck. Stay sutures of 3-0 silk are used to tack the stomach to the posterior wall of the esophagus. A gastrotomy is made and the anastomosis is created using a blue intestinal load linear stapler. The enterotomy is then closed using interrupted absorbable braided suture (3-0 Vicryl). A flat drain placed to bulb suction is left in the cervical wound until patient tolerating soft diet. A feeding jejunostomy tube is then placed using a jejunal loop 30 cm distal to the ligament of Trietz. A nasal gastric tube is placed at the level of the pyloroplasty and bridled into place at the nares. The fascia is closed using a running absorbable barbed fascial closure suture with one full-thickness external retention sutures.

## Postoperative Care

Postoperatively, all patients are sent to the Intensive Care Unit for close monitoring. A nasogastric tube (NGT) is left bridled in place, and special care is given to ensure proper fluid management and avoidance of hypotension. One of the most feared early postoperative complications is conduit necrosis. This presents as early tachycardia, hypotension, leukocytosis, and respiratory failure. Adjunct pain medications are maximized including parenteral formulations of acetaminophen and ibuprofen to minimize opiates. Patients with an uncomplicated post-op course are transferred to a surgical bed on the floor after the first postoperative day. Continuous trickle tube-feeding is started early and advanced to full tube feeds as tolerated.

The authors regularly obtain a water-soluble upper gastrointestinal series on the fifth postoperative day to assess the esophagogastric anastomosis as well as the pyloroplasty. Once cleared, the NGT is discontinued and a clear liquid diet is started with advancement to soft mechanical as tolerated. The cervical incision staples are removed and the drain is discontinued. Continuous tube feeds are changed to nocturnal feeds and if the patient is tolerating per os diet, the patient can be discharged on a soft diet without home tube feeding. A multi-disciplinary approach to postoperative care is recommended and members from physical therapy, nutrition, speech therapy, and social work are included.

## Complications to Avoid

With the use of the robot come additional complications one must be aware of in order to avoid. The docking process can be complicated to the uninitiated and care must be taken to avoid external arm collisions with each other as well as with the patient. When using the Si, the camera arm lies directly over the patient's head and can inadvertently cause injury if not positioned correctly. When initially placing instruments in the abdomen and with each subsequent replacement, extreme care must be taken to visualize the instrument in order to avoid blunt injury to the intraperitoneal organs. When using energy, especially electrocautery, care must be taken not to arc with other instruments. The lack of haptics (force feedback) can be challenging for the beginner robotic surgeon who is used to laparoscopy. Care must be taken to avoid undue traction on the tissues as it is much easier to damage soft tissue without the "feel" of the instruments.

## Current Data/Outcomes

Perioperative outcomes of robotic transhiatal esophagectomy in the literature have been favorable. The first series of robotic THE was presented by Galvani et al. in 2008 with 18 patients [14]. The mean operative time was 267 min, no early mortality, and minimal postoperative complications. The average ICU stay and total hospital length of stay was 1.8 and 10 days, respectively. Another series was presented by Dunn et al. in 2013 with 40 patients undergoing robotic THE [15]. The indication for the majority of the patients was esophageal carcinoma. Mean operative time was 311 min and length of stay was similar to the Galvani series. Complication rates were higher than average with a postoperative stricture rate at 68% and leak rate of 25%. Early postoperative mortality was only 2.5%.

A new robotic technique described by Mori et al. as the Non transthoracic esophagectomy (NTTE) shows promise [13]. This technique first described in 2013 with a follow-up series combines a "video-assisted cervical approach for the upper mediastinum and a robot-assisted transhiatal approach for the middle and lower mediastinum". The technique claims the benefit of an improved transhiatal nodal dissection without the disadvantages of a thoracic approach.

In the authors' own experience, outcomes from a single institution's experience with laparoscopic versus robotic THE are currently in publication. Eighteen consecutive patients who underwent robotic esophagectomy were included in the study. All procedures were performed for malignancy and mean operative time was 168 min. There was one anastomotic leak which required no further invasive intervention and no early mortalities. Mean hospital and ICU length of stay was 10 and 1.7 days, respectively. An average of 14.2 lymph nodes were harvested with no gross positive margins and 94.4% disease-free microscopic margins.

## References

1. Turner GG. Excision of thoracic esophagus for carcinoma with construction of extrathoracic gullet. Lancet. 1933;2:1315.
2. Orringer MB, Sloan H. Esophagectomy without thoracotomy. J Thorac Cardiovasc Surg. 1978;76:643–54.
3. Macrí P, Jiménez MF, Novoa N, Varela G. [A descriptive analysis of a series of patients diagnosed with acute mediastinitis]. Arch Bronconeumol. 2003;39(9):428–430.
4. Hagen JA, Peters JH, DeMeester TR. Superiority of extended en bloc esophagogastrectomy for carcinoma of the lower esophagus and cardia. J Thorac Cardiovasc Surg. 1993;106(5):850–8; discussion 858–9.
5. Altorki NK, Girardi L, Skinner DB. En bloc esophagectomy improves survival for stage III esophageal cancer. J Thorac Cardiovasc Surg. 1997;114(6):948–55. discussion 955–6
6. Orringer MB, Marshall B, Iannettoni MD. Transhiatal esophagectomy: clinical experience and refinements. Ann Surg. 1999;230(3):392–400; discussion 400–3.
7. Colvin H, Dunning J, Khan OA. Transthoracic versus transhiatal esophagectomy for distal esophageal cancer: which is superior? Interact Cardiovasc Thorac Surg. 2011;12(2):265–9.
8. Wei MT, Zhang YC, Deng XB, Yang TH, He YZ, Wang ZQ. Transthoracic vs transhiatal surgery for cancer of the esophagogastric junction: a meta-analysis. World J Gastroenterol. 2014;20(29):10183–92.
9. DePaula AL, Hashiba K, Ferreira EA, de Paula RA, Grecco E. Laparoscopic transhiatal esophagectomy with esophagogastroplasty. Surg Laparosc Endosc. 1995;5(1):1–5.
10. Gurusamy KS, Pallari E, Midya S, Mughal M. Laparoscopic versus open transhiatal oesophagectomy for oesophageal cancer. Cochrane Database Syst Rev. 2016;(3):CD011390.
11. Melvin WS, Needleman BJ, Krause KR, Schneider C, Wolf RK, Michler RE, Ellison EC. Computer-enhanced robotic telesurgery. Initial experience in foregut surgery. Surg Endosc. 2002;16(12):1790–2.

12. Mori K, Yamagata Y, Aikou S, Nishida M, Kiyokawa T, Yagi K, Yamashita H, Nomura S, Seto Y. Short-term outcomes of robotic radical esophagectomy for esophageal cancer by a non-transthoracic approach compared with conventional transthoracic surgery. Dis Esophagus. 2016;29(5):429–34.
13. Mori K, Yamagata Y, Wada I, Shimizu N, Nomura S, Seto Y. Robotic-assisted totally transhiatal lymphadenectomy in the middle mediastinum for esophageal cancer. J Robot Surg. 2013;7:385–7.
14. Galvani CA, Gorodner MV, Moser F, Jacobsen G, Chretien C, Espat NJ, Donahue P, Horgan S. Robotically assisted laparoscopic transhiatal esophagectomy. Surg Endosc. 2008;22(1):188–95.
15. Dunn DH, Johnson EM, Morphew JA, Dilworth HP, Krueger JL, Banerji N. Robot-assisted transhiatal esophagectomy: a 3-year single-center experience. Dis Esophagus. 2013;26(2):159–66.

# Robotic Adrenalectomy

25

Neil D. Saunders

## Introduction

Since its initial description by Gagner in 1992, the laparoscopic adrenalectomy has gained wide acceptance and is currently established as the preferred approach for benign adrenal tumors. Like the cholecystectomy, adrenalectomy is an operation that was revolutionized by laparoscopy. A minimally invasive approach offers the benefits of improved visualization, decreased post-operative pain, shorter length of stay, and decreased overall morbidity [1]. With the advent of the da Vinci Robotic technology (Intuitive Surgical, Sunnyvale, CA), additional benefits are now available including improved ergonomics for the operating surgeon, 3D visualization, and enhanced dexterity with endowrist manipulation. This often proves particularly useful in dissecting more difficult adrenal veins where the improved visualization and accuracy leads to greater confidence. The first robotic adrenalectomy was performed in 1999 [2] and is currently performed in many centers worldwide. It has been shown to be a safe alternative to laparoscopic adrenalectomy, with some data demonstrating improvements in blood loss and length of stay with no difference in morbidity [3, 4].

## Indications

Conditions and tumors for which one would approach an adrenalectomy robotically are similar to those for laparoscopic surgery. Small- to moderate-sized, benign adrenal masses and functional adrenal tumors including aldosteronomas, cortisol secreting cortical adenomas, pheochromocytomas, and other hormone producing tumors

N.D. Saunders, M.D. (✉)
Department of Surgery, Emory University School of Medicine,
1365 Clifton Road NE, Clinic Building A, 4th Floor, Atlanta, GA 30322, USA
e-mail: neil.saunders@emory.edu

© Springer International Publishing AG 2018                                    327
A.D. Patel, D. Oleynikov (eds.), *The SAGES Manual of Robotic Surgery*,
The SAGES University Masters Program Series, DOI 10.1007/978-3-319-51362-1_25

can be approached with a minimally invasive technique. Adrenocortical cancer continues to be a pathology for which open exposure is generally the preferred operation and for which we would not recommend a robotic approach.

## Robotic Left Adrenalectomy, Transabdominal Approach

Approaching the left adrenal tends to be less anxiety provoking for the surgeon due to the configuration of the left adrenal vein and its drainage into the left renal vein. The operative technique is similar to the laparoscopic approach.

### Positioning the Patient

The patient is placed on the bed in a position such that the gap between the iliac crest and costal margin is positioned over the break in the bed and kidney rest. An orogastric tube is placed. The patient is then rolled into a right lateral decubitus position on a beanbag or other appropriate padding system to hold them in place. The left arm is supported either on an armboard or with pillows. Before connecting the bean bag to suction, the kidney rest is raised and the operating table flexed such that the iliac to costal margin space expands, allowing for increased working space. The beanbag is then connected to suction and hardened to provide support to the patient while still allowing access to the midline of the abdomen. To secure the patient to the table, multiple straps are used: one at the level of the upper thorax, at the hips, and on the lower leg. These are appropriately padded to decrease risk of pressure necrosis or neuropathy. We then test the security of the patient by rotating the patient to the left slightly to ensure they do not move.

The bed is angled so that the robot can be positioned over the field in a configuration to provide optimum position of the camera arm. This is achieved by aligning the approach path of the robot with the adrenal gland and the camera port in a straight line as shown in Fig. 25.1. The patient is then prepped and draped in the normal sterile fashion.

### Port Placement

Entry to the abdomen is done in the manner most familiar for the surgeon. Optical trocar entry, Veress needle, or open Hasson technique are all safe ways to enter the abdomen and chosen per surgeon preference [5]. For entry into the abdomen, we rotate the patient to the left slightly and enter the abdomen using the optical trocar technique with a 10/12 mm port near the midclavicular line approximately two to three fingerbreadths below the costal margin as shown in Fig. 25.2. Once we have established pneumoperitoneum, a 10 mm 30° laparoscope is inserted to survey the abdomen. We then place our two 8 mm robotic trocars. One is placed medially and one laterally to the camera port at a similar distance from the costal margin as shown in Fig. 25.2. The splenic flexure and proximal left colon may need to be

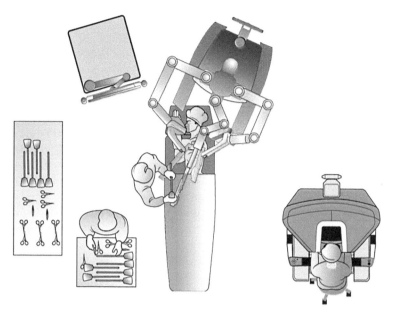

**Fig. 25.1** Operating room layout and angle of robot approach for left adrenalectomy

**Fig. 25.2** Patient positioning and port placement for transabdominal robotic left adrenalectomy

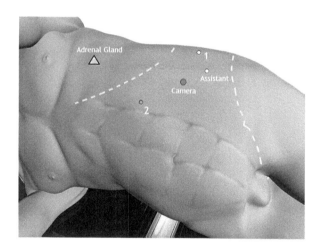

mobilized or adhesions taken down before the lateral trocar can be placed safely. To minimize collisions of the robot arms, at least 8–10 cm of space should be placed between the camera port and the working trocars. An optional fourth port is sometimes necessary for retraction or suction. This can be a standard laparoscopic 5 or 10 mm assistant port through which suction or other instruments can be introduced to the abdomen. The assistant port can also be useful for holding the colon mesentery and pancreas out of the way as one approaches the renal vein and adrenal vein. The best place for this port is typically halfway between the camera port and the lateral robot port.

## Docking the Robot

After placement of the ports, mobilization of the splenic flexure and left colon to gain exposure to the retroperitoneum can be done quickly and easily with laparoscopic instruments. Once this is accomplished, the robot is docked. If the patient was rotated slightly to the left for entry into the abdomen, the operating table is positioned back to upright in the right lateral decubitus position. The entire bed is then placed in reverse Trendelenburg position to allow the bowel to fall out of the field with the aid of gravity. The robot is then guided into place along an imagined straight line connecting the camera port to the adrenal to the base of the robot. This allows for the camera arm to be positioned into an optimum configuration and allows the greatest camera freedom of movement. A 30-degree robot scope is then docked to the camera port in a downward facing orientation. The other two robot arms are similarly docked. Robot instruments are then introduced into the abdomen being sure to keep them under direct vision during the initial placement.

## Robotic Instrument Selection

Through the medial robot port, a double fenestrated grasper is good to start the operation with. An endowrist cautery hook or scissor cautery can be used through the lateral robot port. Throughout the operation one may need a second double fenestrated grasper available as well as a Maryland bipolar or a curved bipolar forcep. The bipolar forceps can be used to stop most bleeding in this area. A robotic vessel sealer may be used but is often not necessary. As robotic instruments improve and vessel sealing energy devices advance, the bipolar forcep can be replaced. A medium or large locking polymer clips and clip applier will be used for adrenal vein ligation and robotic shears are used to cut the vein once sealed.

## Operative Technique

The left robotic adrenalectomy is approached using the previously described "open book" technique of laparoscopy [6]. After mobilization of the colon caudad, the spleen is then mobilized lateral to medial. This can be done by providing gentle medial retraction of the spleen with the medial robotic arm and dividing the avascular attachments of the spleen to the lateral abdomen with hook or scissor cautery (Fig. 25.3). Caution should be used when retracting the spleen due to the lack of haptic feedback with the robot. One should be diligent to not put too much pressure on the spleen while retracting as splenic capsular tears can easily occur. Staying in the avascular, filmy plane will allow mobilization of the spleen with minimal blood loss. This is continued up to the diaphragm cranially and at this point the superolateral aspect stomach will come into view. Continue mobilization of the spleen

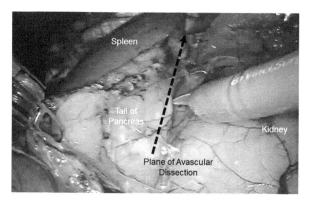

**Fig. 25.3** Mobilization of the spleen and tail of the pancreas medially to expose the retroperitoneum. Image courtesy of Yusef Kudsi, MD

medially until the spleen will lie medially under its own weight without retraction. Often, when progressing through this avascular plane, the tail of the pancreas and splenic artery are encountered. These structures may need to be gently dissected free and mobilized in continuity with the spleen to allow adequate exposure to the adrenal gland. Great care should be taken not injure the tail of the pancreas in this maneuver. This entire mobilization can usually be done with the endowrist cautery hook or scissor cautery. If small vessels are encountered, they may be sealed with bipolar cautery.

Once the mobilization of the spleen is completed, exposing and identifying the adrenal vein is the next step. As the tail of the pancreas is swept medially, the adrenal gland should come into view as well as the left kidney. The left adrenal vein is typically found at the inferomedial aspect of the adrenal gland. Dissection along the medial plane in the groove between the adrenal and the pancreas as well as dissection along the lateral aspect of the adrenal gland near the kidney can help to isolate the area of the adrenal vein (Fig. 25.4). Careful dissection, both blunt and with cautery, will allow identification of the adrenal vein as it empties into the left renal vein. Once identified and dissected circumferentially as shown in Fig. 25.5, the locking polymer clips are loading on the robotic clip applier and used to doubly ligate the vein on the stay side and once on the adrenal side (Fig. 25.6). The vein is then divided with the robotic shears. After division of vein, the tissue overlying the adrenal gland is grasped and used to elevate the adrenal gland. Bipolar cautery can be used to divide the attachments posterior to the retroperitoneal fat. The lateral aspect of the adrenal gland is similarly dissected free from the kidney. This is continued up toward the diaphragm. One may encounter a branch of the phrenic vein through this dissection, and if necessary, can be sealed and taken with bipolar cautery. Once the specimen is free, it is placed in an endocatch bag and removed through the camera port. Depending on the size of the specimen, the camera port may need to be enlarged for removal.

**Fig. 25.4** Separating the lateral aspect of the left adrenal gland from the left kidney. Image courtesy of Yusef Kudsi, MD

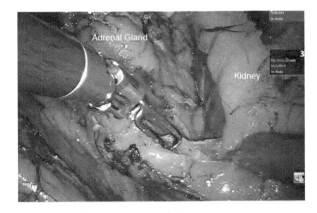

**Fig. 25.5** Left adrenal vein exposed. Image courtesy of Yusef Kudsi, MD

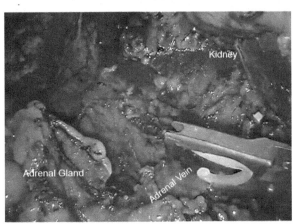

**Fig. 25.6** Dividing the left adrenal vein after placement of locking robotic clips. Image courtesy of Yusef Kudsi, MD

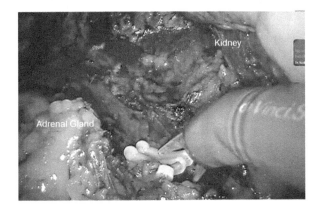

## Robotic Right Adrenalectomy, Transabdominal Approach

Similar to the transabdominal robotic left adrenalectomy, the right-sided operation is conducted in a manner analogous to its laparoscopic counterpart.

## Positioning the Patient

After intubation and orogastric tube placement, the patient is placed in the left lateral decubitus position on a beanbag or similar method to hold the patient in position. The gap between the patient's iliac crest and costal margin is placed at the level of the kidney rest on the operative table or at the break in the bed. This allows flexing of the patient to widen the iliac crest-to-costal margin space to create more working room. The right arm is placed on an arm sling or board and the patient is secured to the bed at the level of the chest, hips, and lower extremities such that the patient can be rotated to the left or right and be secure on the operating table.

## Port Placement

The right-sided adrenalectomy generally requires four ports due to the need for the liver retractor. Ports required are a 10/12 mm port for the robot camera, two 8 mm working ports for the robotic instruments, and a 5 mm assistant port for liver retraction and/or suction as shown in Fig. 25.7. The lateral working port is placed in between the anterior axillary line and mid axillary line approximately two fingerbreadths below the costal margin. The 10/12 mm camera port is placed medial to this just lateral to the mid-clavicular line. The medial robot port is positioned near the midline in the epigastric area. A 5 mm port for the liver retractor can be placed between the camera port and the medial robotic port. An optional additional assistant port is placed between the camera port and the lateral robotic port, this can be a 5 or 10 mm port.

## Docking the Robot

After placement of the ports, the robot is brought toward the operative field in a similar manner to the left adrenalectomy approach. If the patient was rotated to the right to access the abdomen, they are now rotated back to the upright left lateral

**Fig. 25.7** Patient positioning and port placement for transabdominal robotic right adrenalectomy

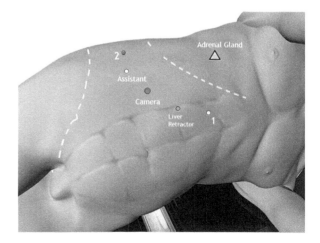

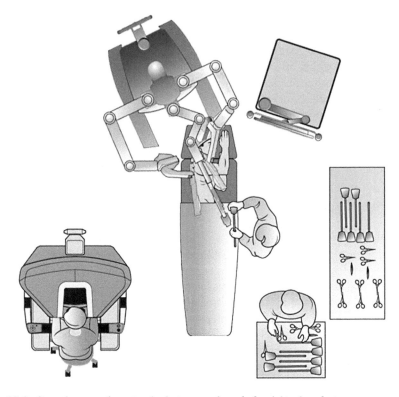

**Fig. 25.8** Operating room layout and robot approach angle for right adrenalectomy

decubitus position. While the bed remains flexed, the entire bed is then moved to a reverse Trendelenburg position to allow the bowel to retract downward with gravity. The robot is docked by driving the robot toward the surgical field along a line connecting the location of the adrenal gland and the camera port as shown by the angle of the robot in Fig. 25.8. This allows for the camera arm to align in the optimum working zone of the robot as well as minimize collisions with the working arms. The 30° robotic camera is then introduced to the abdomen in a downward looking orientation.

## Robotic Instrument Selection

To start the operation, a double fenestrated grasper is used through the lateral robotic port. An endowrist cautery hook or scissor cautery is placed through the medial working port. The Maryland bipolar or a curved bipolar forcep can be used through either port as needed to stop bleeding or seal small vessels. A robotic vessel sealer may also be used but is often not needed. Medium or large polymer clips and clip applier will be used for adrenal vein ligation along the inferior vena cava.

## Operative Technique

After insertion of the robotic instruments, a snake liver retractor is introduced through the medial 5 mm port by the assistant and positioned to provide gentle medial traction on the underside of the liver in order to provide exposure to the retroperitoneum (Fig. 25.9). The first step is mobilizing the right lobe of the liver. With medial retraction on the liver, the right triangular ligament is divided with the endowrist cautery hook or scissor cautery (Fig. 25.10). Freeing the liver from the diaphragm is continued medially to mobilize segments VI and VII of the liver. Care is taken not to proceed too far medially and injury the right hepatic vein. After mobilization of the right liver, the peritoneal layer covering the retroperitoneum is opened. Starting superiorly near the diaphragm, the endowrist cautery is used to divide the peritoneum approximately 3–5 mm from the underside of the liver. This is continued inferiorly in a hockey stick line following along the underside of the liver and then turning more southward just lateral and parallel to the vena cava as shown in Fig. 25.11 [6]. This can be continued out further laterally

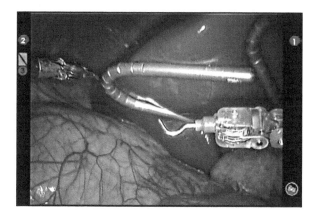

**Fig. 25.9** Initial placement of robotic instruments and liver retractor at the beginning of the operation

**Fig. 25.10** Taking down the triangular ligament of the right liver along the diaphragm to mobilize liver and expose right adrenal gland

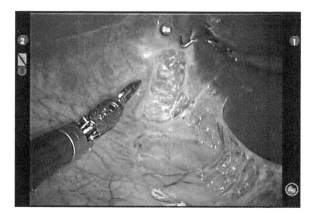

**Fig. 25.11** Opening of peritoneum along underside of liver and down the lateral border of the vena cava in a "hockey stick" line

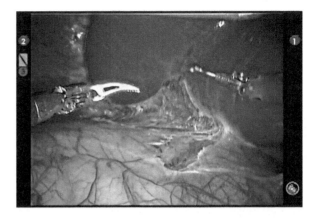

**Fig. 25.12** Dissection between lateral border of inferior vena cava and medial side of adrenal gland to expose right adrenal vein

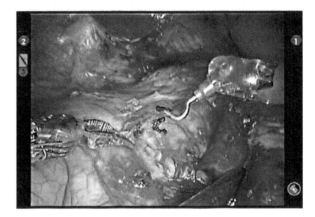

**Fig. 25.13** Isolating the right adrenal vein along the lateral border of the inferior vena cava. Image courtesy of Yusef Kudsi, MD

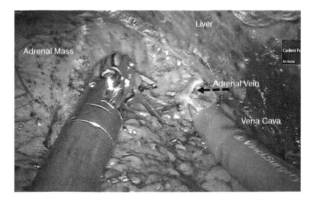

as well to follow the course of the right renal vein parallel to its superior aspect. Once the retroperitoneum is opened, blunt dissection along the lateral side of the inferior vena cava can expose the right adrenal vein (Figs. 25.12 and 25.13). Small vessels in this area can be divided with the robotic bipolar cautery. The location of the adrenal vein along the inferior vena cava can be variable and sometimes one will encounter multiple adrenal veins. Meticulous dissection in this area is critical as bleeding from the cava can be significant. Once the adrenal vein is identified and circumferentially dissected, a locking polymer clip is placed on the vena cava side and specimen side. If there is adequate length to the adrenal vein, a second clip can be placed on the vena cava side before dividing. Robotic shears are used to divide the adrenal vein.

After division of the adrenal vein, most of the remaining vessels can be divided with bipolar cautery. The peritoneal layer overlying the adrenal gland is then grasped and used as a handle to provide tension in the upward direction. Approaching from the inferior aspect of the adrenal gland, the bipolar cautery is then used to proceed in the relatively avascular plane beneath the adrenal gland. As noted previously, bleeding from small vessels in the retroperitoneal fat behind the adrenal gland can be sealed with the bipolar. Other than the adrenal vein medially, dissection through the plane along the vena cava and the underside of the liver is similarly avascular. Once the specimen is freed from its remaining attachments, it is placed into an endocatch bag for removal. The retroperitoneum is inspected for bleeding. Any visible bleeding can be stopped with cautery or hemostatic agents. The robotic instruments are then removed and the ports taken out under direct vision while the abdomen is desufflated. Often, the size of the adrenal tumor will necessitate enlargement one of the port incisions and further opening of the abdominal wall for specimen extraction. The robotic camera port, which would require fascial closure, is typically the incision chosen to enlarge. Once the specimen is removed, the abdominal wall is reapproximated in two layers.

## Post-operative Care

Patients are admitted for overnight observation and typically discharged on post-operative day (POD) 1. They are started on a clear diet on the operative day with the expectation that they will have regular food in the evening or by the next morning. A complete blood count (CBC) is checked in the morning of POD1. For pheochromocytomas, the decision to observe in the intensive care unit overnight is based on their immediate post-operative condition and hemodynamics with a low threshold for ICU admission. If their blood pressure has stabilized by post-operative day 1 they may also be discharged. In the cases of aldosteronoma, the patient's mineralocorticoid medications may be stopped immediately following the operation. Their other antihypertensive medications will likely have to be continued upon discharge and discontinued in a gradual fashion as it may take weeks for their blood pressure to decrease to a new baseline.

## Limitations

As with all robotic operations, the biggest limitation is lack of haptic feedback to the surgeon. This is particularly worrisome when retracting the spleen, liver or a fragile tumor with the robotic arm. In cases of pheochromocytoma, where manipulation of the tumor can have deleterious hemodynamic effects, one must be careful as well. Another limitation inherent in the system is collisions with the robot arms.

Robot-to-robot contact can easily mitigated by placing ports far enough apart to avoid interference but the problems we find are with the assistant navigating between the robot arms to work intra-abdominally. This is most pronounced with the snake liver retractor during the right adrenalectomy. The bulkiness of the robot arms and their position exterior to the patient makes it difficult for the assistant to thread between them and provide agile retraction of the liver. This difficulty may be obviated in a four robotic arm setup with the operating surgeon controlling the liver retraction robotically.

Some data suggest that robotic adrenalectomy may have benefits to the patient over laparoscopic surgery. A meta-analysis in 2014 comparing 277 robotic adrenalectomies to 323 laparoscopic adrenalectomies showed a statistically significant shorter length of stay and lower blood loss, though complication rate was the same and conversion to open was the same. The length of stay analysis, however, included data from institutions with a mean length of stay after laparoscopic adrenalectomy of 5 and 6 days. This would be well outside the norm in the United States where the majority of patients undergoing laparoscopic adrenalectomy are discharged on POD1 or 2. This study, as well as most others looking at robotic adrenalectomy, is limited by the quality of the source data and small numbers in the individual studies [3]. Better data are needed to show that robotic adrenalectomy has improved outcomes over laparoscopy.

## Conclusions

Like laparoscopy before it, robotic adrenalectomy provides another excellent surgical technique for approach to the adrenal gland. The transabdominal robotic approach is easily adapted by those who are familiar with laparoscopic adrenalectomy as the dissection is along familiar planes and the operations proceed in a similar manner. The greater flexibility of the wristed instruments and improved vision can make for more precise dissection. Because of the lack of haptic feedback, care needs to be taken especially in the case of pheochromocytoma due to the hemodynamic consequences of rough handling of the tumor. Overall, in properly selected patients, robotic surgery is a great tool for adrenalectomy and will continue to improve as technology advances.

## References

1. Lee J, El-Tamer M, Schifftner T, et al. Open and laparoscopic adrenalectomy: analysis of NSQIP. J Am Chem Soc. 2008;206:953–9.
2. Piazza L, Carigliano P, Scardili M, Sgroi AV, et al. Laparoscopic robot assisted right adrenalectomy and left ovariectomy. Chir Ital. 1999;51:465–6.
3. Branardo LF, Auturino R, Laydner H, et al. Robotic versus laparoscopic adrenalectomy: a systematic review and meta-analysis. Eur Urol. 2014;65(6):1154–61.
4. Ball MW, Hemal AK, Allaf MA. International Consultation on Urological diseases and European Association of Urology International Consultation on Minimally Invasive Surgery in Urology: laparoscopic and robotic adrenalectomy. BJU Int. 2016; doi:10.1111/bju.13592.
5. Ahmad G, Gent D, Henderson D, O'Flynn H, Phillips K, Watson A. Laparoscopic entry techniques. Cochrane Database Syst Rev. 2015;8:CD006583.
6. Smith CD, Weber CJ, Amerson JR. Laparoscopic adrenalectomy: new gold standard. World J Surg. 1999 Apr;23(4):389–96.

# Robotic-Assisted Transaxillary Thyroid and Parathyroid Surgery

Daniah Bu Ali, Sang-Wook Kang, and Emad Kandil

## Introduction

Over the last decade, there has been increased interest in improving quality of life as well as healthcare overall. Patients are more aware and active in the decision-making process, which has led to an increase in focusing on quality of life issues such as early return to normal activity and cosmetic appearance after a treatment. As a result, there has been an increased adoption of minimally invasive surgery in various surgical fields. In the area of head and neck surgery, minimally invasive and endoscopic surgical techniques were slow to be adopted due to some spatial and anatomical limitations, such as the lack of a pre-existing working space, the hypervascularities of target organs, and abundance of critical nerves and major vessels. However, using the features of the surgical robotic system, such as a three-dimensional magnified surgical view, hand-tremor filtration, fine-motion scaling, and precise and multiarticulated hand-like motions, scarless thyroid and parathyroid surgery using a remote site incision overcame many of the previous limitations.

**Electronic supplementary material:** The online version of this chapter (doi: 10.1007/978-3-319-51362-1_26) contains supplementary material, which is available to authorized users. Videos can also be accessed at http://link.springer.com/chapter/10.1007/978-3-319-51362-1_26.

D. Bu Ali, M.D.
Endocrine and Oncology Surgery Division, Department of Surgery, Tulane University School of Medicine, 1430 Tulane ave, New Orleans, LA 70112, USA
e-mail: dbuali@tulane.edu

S.-W. Kang, M.D.
Department of Surgery, Yonsei University College of Medicine, Seoul, South Korea
e-mail: oralvanco@yuhs.ac

E. Kandil, M.D., M.B.A., F.A.C.S., F.A.C.E. (✉)
Endocrine and Oncology Surgery Division, Department of Surgery, Tulane University School of Medicine, 1430 Tulane Ave, New Orleans, LA 70112, USA
e-mail: ekandil@tulane.edu

© Springer International Publishing AG 2018
A.D. Patel, D. Oleynikov (eds.), *The SAGES Manual of Robotic Surgery*,
The SAGES University Masters Program Series, DOI 10.1007/978-3-319-51362-1_26

Since the first introduction of robotic thyroidectomy using transaxillary approach in 2007, many studies have examined the technical aspects and surgical outcomes for robotic thyroid surgery and reported similar outcome. As a result, the robotic technique has become a promising remote access approach for the treatment of thyroid and parathyroid gland pathology in a select group of patients.

In this chapter, the robot-assisted transaxillary approach for thyroid and parathyroid surgery will be described.

## Indications and Patient Selection

### Thyroidectomy

Robotic approach can be considered in patients who have concerns of a visible neck scar, due to cosmetic impact or a previous history of healing with keloid or hypertrophic scar. The body build of the patient, volume of the thyroid gland, and the nodule size are factors that need to be assessed preoperatively as they can affect the decision to proceed with a robotic approach. Proper positioning is an essential part of the procedure, so certain conditions that can interfere with patients' positioning, such as limitation of neck or arm mobility, should also be considered preoperatively. Patient selection is based on the following criteria set by high volume centers, as there are no clearly established guidelines yet:

- Contraindications:
  - Absolute contraindication:
    History of radiation to the neck.
    Previous neck surgery.
    Substernal goiter.
    Thyroid cancer with invasion to adjacent structures.
    Metastatic thyroid cancer to the retropharyngeal or substernal lymph nodes.
    Poorly differentiated thyroid cancer.
  - Relative contraindication:
    Nodules more than 4 cm.
    Thyroid volumes more than 40 ml.
    Advanced thyroiditis.
    Conditions affecting neck or shoulder mobility, e.g., rotator cuff injury.
    Morbid obesity.

With experience, the surgeons might gradually extend their surgical indications for robotic thyroidectomy to include obese patients, cases of thyroiditis, Graves' disease [1], large thyroid nodules more than 4 cm, and lateral neck dissection [2]. However, it is advisable to be conservative at the beginning of the learning curve. The best candidates for the beginner surgeon are young female patients with small body build (BMI < 35) without any thyroiditis.

## Parathyroidectomy

Robotic parathyroidectomy is only indicated in patients with preoperatively well-localized primary hyperparathyroidism having a single gland disease. This procedure currently cannot be offered to patients with multi-gland disease or preoperatively poorly localized parathyroid glands, as it would require bilateral neck exploration, which is technically difficult to perform using a one side approach.

- Absolute contraindication:
  - Failure to localize the parathyroid gland preoperatively.
  - Preoperative biochemical or radiological evidence of multiglandular disease.
  - Previous neck surgery.
  - Previous radiation to the neck.
- Relative contraindication:
  - Parathyroid carcinoma.
  - Associated large goiter, or Graves' disease.

## Equipment and Instruments

A shoulder roll is required for neck extension and soft pillows are required for the arm positioning. For the flap creation, monopolar electro-cautery with long tip, long vascular Debakey forceps, two army-navy retractors, two lighted breast retractors (Fig. 26.1), and a vessel-sealing device are needed. An external retractor is required to maintain the working space during the procedure (Marina Medical, Sunrise, FL, USA) (Fig. 26.2).

For the robotic dissection portion of the procedure, the da Vinci S, Si, or Xi system (Intuitive, Inc., Sunnyvale, CA, USA) can be used along with a 30-degree down looking scope, 5 mm Maryland dissector (Intuitive, Inc.), and 8 mm Prograsp forceps (Intuitive, Inc.). A 5 mm harmonic curved shear (Intuitive, Inc.) is used as the robotic vessel-sealing device. Four trocars can be inserted through the single

**Fig. 26.1** Lighted breast retractor

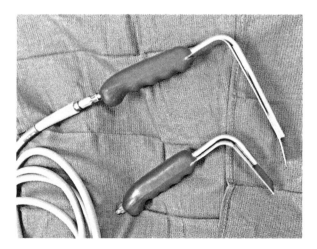

**Fig. 26.2** Modified
robotic thyroidectomy
retractor (Marina Medical,
Sunrise, FL, USA)

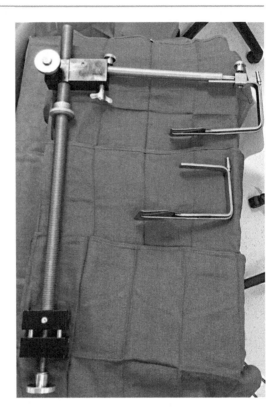

axillary incision: two 5 mm trocars, one 8 mm trocar, and one 12 mm trocar. During
the procedure a 5 mm laparoscopic suction and irrigation can be used by the assisting surgeon to retract structures such as sternocleidomastoid (SCM) muscle or trachea. Rolled gauze can be used for hemostasis during the procedure.

| Instruments and surgical equipment |
| --- |
| *Flap creation and maintenance of working space* |
| 2 Army-navy retractors |
| 2 Lighted breast retractors |
| Long Vascular Debakey forceps |
| Monopolar electrocautery (short and long tips) |
| Vessel sealing device |
| Special modified robotic thyroidectomy retractor (Marina Medical, Sunrise, FL, USA) |
| *Robotic instruments* |
| DaVinci Si or Xi robot system |
| Two 5-mm trocars |
| 8-mm trocar |
| 12-mm trocar |

| Instruments and surgical equipment |
| --- |
| 5-mm Maryland dissector |
| 8-mm Prograsp forceps |
| 5-mm Harmonic curved shear |
| 30 degree endoscope |
| Laparoscopic suction/irrigation |

## Surgical Technique

### Positioning

The patient is placed in the supine position and is intubated using one of the nerve integrity monitor endotracheal tubes to enable intraoperative monitoring of the recurrent laryngeal nerve. The neck is extended using a shoulder roll. The ipsilateral arm on the same side of the lesion is raised and flexed at the elbow with the forearm resting over the forehead, and secured in place with proper padding using soft pillows and foam (Fig. 26.3). By raising the arm, the distance between the incision and anterior neck will be shortened. The contralateral arm is tucked in on the side of the patient. Caution has to be taken not to overextend the shoulder in order to avoid traction injury of the brachial plexus. Nerve monitoring of the radial, median, and ulnar nerves using somatosensory evoked potential (SSEP) (Biotronic, Ann Arbor, MI) can be used to help avoid stretching of any of these nerves.

Intraoperative ultrasound is usually performed at the beginning of the procedure to assess the relation of the thyroid to the internal jugular vein and carotid artery. In cases of robotic-assisted parathyroidectomy, the location of the pathological parathyroid gland can be confirmed by performing intraoperative ultrasound.

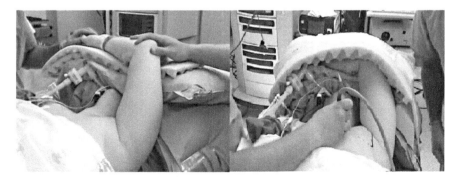

**Fig. 26.3** Patient positioning in transaxillary approach; the arm is raised and flexed at the elbow resting comfortably over the patients face. Preoperative ultrasound is performed to assess the relation of the internal jugular vein and carotid to the thyroid

## Incision and Flap Creation

### Incision

- The neck, anterior chest, and the ipsilateral axilla are prepped and draped.
- The incision location landmarks are the thyroid prominence, sternal notch, and the anterior axillary line. A 60° oblique line is drawn from the thyroid prominence to the axilla and a transverse line is drawn from the sternal notch to the axilla. Afterward, a 5–6 cm skin incision can be made between the two lines at the anterior axillary line along the lateral border of pectoralis major muscle. This will create a completely hidden incision in the axillary folds (Fig. 26.4).

### Flap Creation

1. Using electrocautery, the subcutaneous flap is created superficial to the pectoralis major muscle fascia up to the clavicle. The army-navy and lighted breast retractors are used to facilitate this step (Fig. 26.5).
2. Subplatysmal dissection is performed after crossing the clavicle until the two heads of (SCM) are identified. The flap dissection is continued medially to the medial border of the SCM.

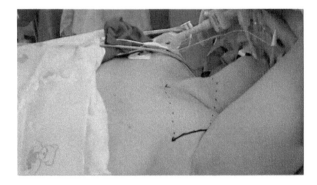

**Fig. 26.4** The skin incision landmarks, it is placed at the anterior axillary line between two lines, an oblique line from the thyroid prominence and a transverse line from the sternal notch

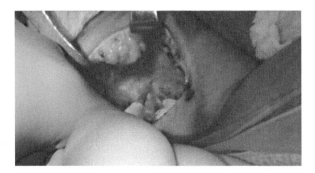

**Fig. 26.5** Flap creation superficial to the pectoralis major muscle fascia

3. The avascular plane between the clavicular and sternal heads of the SCM is created. The omohyoid muscle is considered a great landmark of the superior pole of the thyroid gland. Great care should be taken to avoid injury to the internal and external jugular vein during this dissection (Fig. 26.6, 26.7, and 26.8).
4. The superior belly of omohyoid muscle is retracted or divided and then the thyroid is separated from the overlying strap muscles using the electrocautery or a vessel-sealing device until the contra lateral side of the thyroid gland is fully exposed.
5. The blade of the special thyroid modified self-retaining retractor is placed through the axillary incision retracting the flap, the sternal head of SCM, and the strap muscles. It is mounted to the bed from the contralateral side of the operating table. Appropriate maintenance of the working space is an important aspect during the procedure. A suction tube should be attached to the suction channel of the retractor to remove the smoke during the procedure (Fig. 26.9).

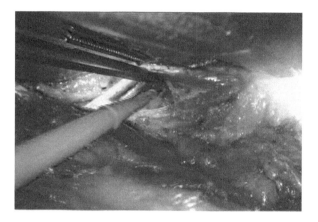

**Fig. 26.6** Opening of the avascular plane between the two heads of SCM

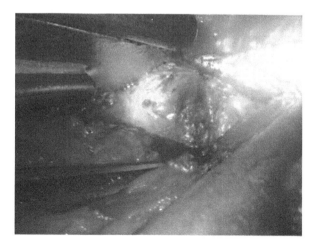

**Fig. 26.7** The omohyoid muscle, which is a landmark of the upper pole, is identified after opening the plane between the two heads of SCM

**Fig. 26.8** After dividing the omohyoid muscle the strap muscles, thyroid, and internal jugular vein are exposed

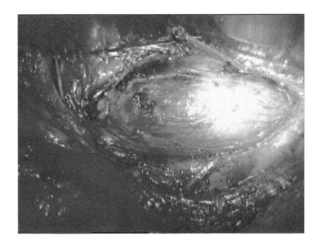

**Fig. 26.9** The external modified robotic thyroidectomy retractor is placed and connected to suction to eliminate the smoke during the procedure

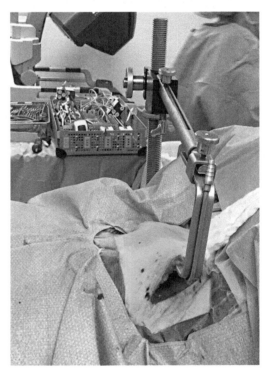

## Robot Docking

The robot is docked from the contralateral side of the table. A 30-degree down view endoscope and three robotic instruments are secured to the robotic arms and inserted through the single axillary incision. The 12 mm trocar is placed in the middle of the

**Fig. 26.10** Placement of the endoscope, the trocar is placed at the center of the lower edge and the scope is inserted in an upward direction

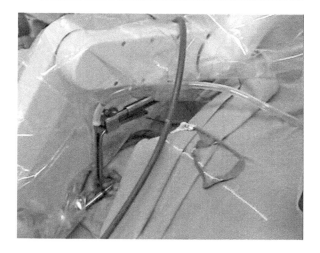

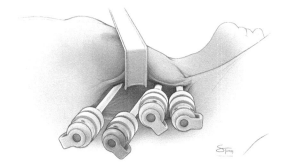

**Fig. 26.11** Placement of trocars in a left side approach; the scope is placed at the middle of the lower edge of the incision, the prograsp placed taround the upper middle area of incision, the Maryland to the right lateral end of the incision and harmonic curved shear at the left lateral end

axillary incision on the lower edge and the camera is inserted in an upward direction (Fig. 26.10). The 8 mm trocar is placed at the upper edge of the incision, and the Prograsp forceps is inserted in downward direction. The two 5 or 8 mm trocars are placed as far apart as possible at the lateral ends of the incision, and the Maryland dissector is inserted at the non-dominant side of the surgeon in an upward direction and the Harmonic curved shear is inserted so it can be used by the dominant hand of the surgeon. Proper placement of the instruments and maintaining appropriate space between the arms is a crucial step of the procedure to avoid collision of the robotic arms (Fig. 26.11, 26.12, 26.13, and 26.14).

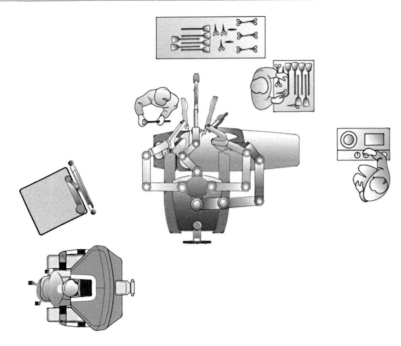

**Fig. 26.12** Room setup for Si robot, left side approach

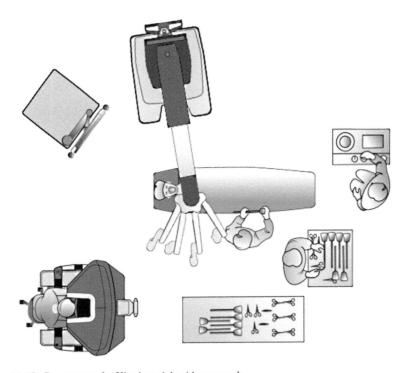

**Fig. 26.13** Room setup for Xi robot, right side approach

**Left Side Approach**
Yellow: Harmonic
Green : Prograsp
Pink : Maryland

**Right side approach**
Yellow : Prograsp
Pink : Harmonic
Green : Maryland

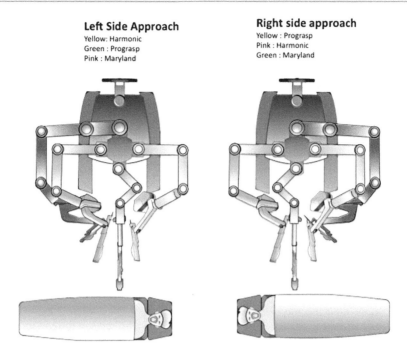

**Fig. 26.14**   Robotic arms configuration for Si robot

## Thyroidectomy

1. The vagus nerve is stimulated initially using the nerve monitor probe, which is introduced into the field by the assistant.
2. The laparoscopic suction/irrigation is introduced by the assistant through the axillary incision, and used to downward retract the internal jugular vein and clavicular head of the SCM.
3. The upper pole of thyroid is retracted medially and inferiorly using the Prograsp forceps. The superior thyroid vessels are dissected and divided using the Harmonic curved shear. Care has to be taken to divide them closer to the thyroid to avoid injury of the external branch of the superior laryngeal nerve. Further dissection of the upper pole is continued until it is dissected from the cricothyroid muscle. This will allow identification and preservation of the superior parathyroid gland.
4. The Prograsp forceps is repositioned and the thyroid is retracted medially, then the thyroid middle vein is dissected and divided using the Harmonic curved shears.
5. Meticulous dissection at the tracheoesophageal groove is performed until the recurrent laryngeal nerve (RLN) is identified and its functional integrity is confirmed using the nerve monitor probe. Dissection of the RLN is carried until its insertion into the cricothyroid muscle.
6. The inferior pedicle is dissected and divided using the Maryland and Harmonic curved shear after careful dissection of the RLN.

7. The thyroid is dissected carefully medial to the RLN. It is shaved from the trachea until reaching the contralateral side. Caution has to be taken at Berry's ligament region to avoid direct and indirect thermal injury to the RLN by the Harmonic curved shear active blade.

8. The thyroid lobe and isthmus are divided from the remaining thyroid lobe and the specimen is extracted through the axillary incision (Video 26.1).

9. In cases of total thyroidectomy, after performing ipsilateral lobectomy, subcapsular dissection of the contralateral lobe is performed. The RLN and parathyroid glands are identified. The superior pedicle is then dissected and divided followed by dissection of the inferior pedicle. Then, the remaining thyroid is separated from the trachea and extracted through the axillary incision. In some cases, such as in a prominent trachea or male patient, tilting the operating table 10–15° can help to achieve better exposure of the contralateral tracheoesophageal groove.

10. The vagus nerve and RLN are re-stimulated using the nerve monitor probe at the end of the procedure. Hemostasis is secured and confirmed prior to completion of the procedure.

11. The external retractor is removed followed by careful inspection for hemostasis at the flap. A drain is inserted through a separate incision below the axillary incision, then the incision is closed in two layers: interrupted subcutaneous closure followed by a continuous subcuticular closure.

## Parathyroidectomy

1. The vagus nerve is initially stimulated using the nerve stimulator probe.

2. The thyroid is retracted medially using the Prograsp forceps; the pathological parathyroid gland is identified with careful dissection.

3. Meticulous dissection in the tracheoesophageal groove is performed until the recurrent laryngeal nerve is identified and its functional integrity is confirmed by nerve stimulation using the nerve monitor probe.

4. Circumferential dissection of the parathyroid gland is performed via the utilization of Harmonic curved shears and Maryland dissectors until the pedicle of the inferior thyroid artery branches is identified and divided.

5. The specimen is extracted using an endo-catch bag through the axillary incision and sent for frozen section for confirmation.

6. Serial blood samples are drawn for intra-operative parathyroid hormone (IOPTH) levels at scheduled interval; one baseline at the beginning of the procedure, one pre-excision followed by scheduled 10 and 15 min levels post-excision. A drop of 50% or more of the IOPTH level from the baseline or pre-excision level indicates a curative surgery by successful removal of the culprit parathyroid gland.

7. Hemostasis is secured and the vagus nerve is re-stimulated at the end of the procedure, followed by undocking of the robot.

8. The retractor is removed and a drain is inserted through a separate incision below the axillary incision. The incision is closed in two layers: interrupted subcutaneous and continuous subcuticular.

## Postoperative Care

The drain is usually kept in place until the output is less than 30 ml/day. Most patients will have their drains removed in 2 or 3 days. Discharging the patient depends on the surgeons' experience and preference; however, in our experience, most patients are discharged on the same day of surgery.

## Precautions During the Procedure

### Positioning

Neuropraxia of the brachial plexus is a rare possible risk that can happen during improper positioning, likely caused by overextension of the shoulder leading to traction of the brachial plexus. It usually causes temporary paralysis of the arm that recovers within a few weeks. This can be prevented by avoiding overextension and over medial-rotation of the shoulder while positioning the arm. In addition, the use of the nerve monitor of the radial, median, and ulnar nerves using SSEP can be very helpful, which can alert you if there was loss of signal of the nerve during the procedure allowing adjustment of the arm positioning when needed.

### Flap Creation

During flap creation, injury to the skin flap by button-hole perforation or thermal injury should be avoided by following the proper surgical plane along the subplatysmal layer and using the lighted breast retractor. One should avoid injury to the internal jugular vein or carotid while opening the avascular plane between the two heads of SCM. The best way to avoid this complication is careful dissection following the anatomical plane and direct identification of these structures.

## Robotic Dissection

One should avoid the rare risk of thermal tracheal or esophageal injuries by making sure all arms are in view during energy application.

## Advantages of Robotic Thyroid and Parathyroid Surgery

Several studies have reported on the safety and feasibility of robotic thyroid and parathyroid surgery, with surgical outcomes comparable to conventional open and endoscopic approaches. In one meta-analysis study, we found no difference in the incidence of recurrent laryngeal nerve injury, permanent hypocalcaemia, hematoma, seroma, chyle leak, and tracheal injury in robotic approaches compared to open and endoscopic approaches [3].

Robotic surgery has several advantages compared to the conventional open approach. The main advantage is the cosmetic effect of a hidden scar in the axilla, which might be an important factor for young females where a visible neck scar might have significant cosmetic impact on them. Several studies reported greater cosmetic satisfaction in robotic approach compared to the open approach [4–7]. Technically, the robotic approach has several advantages compared to the endoscopic approaches. First, it provides a stable three-dimensional view that makes it easier to identify and preserve the recurrent laryngeal nerve and parathyroid gland. Additionally, the downscaling and tremor elimination features enable the surgeon to perform precise movements. The multiarticulated arms and endowrist instruments facilitate the work in deep and narrow places and enable wide range of movement. During robotic surgery, the surgeon is in control of the entire procedure, and is not depending on an assistant compared to the endoscopic approach [7–10].

The ergonomics provided by the robot reduces the musculoskeletal discomfort to the surgeon [9, 11]. A multicenter study by Lee et al. showed that surgeons' neck and back pain were lower in robotic thyroidectomy compared to open and endoscopic thyroidectomy. This can be attributed to the position of the surgeon, as he or she sits at a console and performs the surgery with the aid of stereoscopic vision and robotically controlled instruments with the monitor placed at his eye level, which minimize the postural changes to the neck and shoulders [10].

Interestingly, there is a reported rapid learning curve in robotic-assisted thyroidectomy in comparison to endoscopic approaches. One should perform 35–45 robotic cases compared to 55–70 in the endoscopic approach to reach the peak of their learning curve [12].

The high cost of robotic thyroid surgery compared to the open and endoscopic approaches is the main disadvantage, and this is due to the longer operative time and equipment cost [13]. However, there is less risk of complications, shorter hospitalizations, and lower cost when thyroid surgery is performed by high volume surgeons compared to low volume surgeons.

## Conclusion

Robotic thyroid and parathyroid surgeries provide great functional and cosmetic benefits with acceptable surgical outcomes when compared to the conventional open procedure. We anticipate that with future improvements of the robotic technology the indications of robotic thyroid and parathyroid surgery will expand along with improved surgical outcomes.

## References

1. Kandil E, Noureldine S, Abdel Khalek M, Alrasheedi S, Aslam R, Friedlander P, et al. Initial experience using robot- assisted transaxillary thyroidectomy for Graves' disease. J Visc Surg. 2011;148(6):e447–51.

2. Kang SW, Lee SH, Ryu HR, Lee KY, Jeong JJ, Nam KH, et al. Initial experience with robot-assisted modified radical neck dissection for the management of thyroid carcinoma with lateral neck node metastasis. Surgery. 2010;148(6):1214–21.
3. Kandil E, Hammad AY, Walvekar RR, Hu T, Masoodi H, Mohamed SE, et al. Robotic thyroidectomy versus nonrobotic approaches: a meta-analysis examining surgical outcomes. Surg Innov. 2016;23(3):317–25.
4. Lee J, Nah KY, Kim RM, Ahn YH, Soh E, Chung WY. Differences in postoperative outcomes, function, and cosmesis: open versus robotic thyroidectomy. Surg Endosc. 2010;24(12):3186–94.
5. Tae K, Ji YB, Jeong JH, Lee SH, Jeong MA, Park CW. Robotic thyroidectomy by a gasless unilateral axillo-breast or axillary approach: our early experiences. Surg Endosc. 2011;25(1):221–8.
6. Tae K, Ji YB, Cho SH, Lee SH, Kim DS, Kim TW. Early surgical outcomes of robotic thyroidectomy by a gasless unilateral axillo-breast or axillary approach for papillary thyroid carcinoma: 2 years' experience. Head Neck. 2012;34(5):617–25.
7. Kang SW, Jeong JJ, Nam KH, Chang HS, Chung WY, Park CS. Robot-assisted endoscopic thyroidectomy for thyroid malignancies using a gasless transaxillary approach. J Am Coll Surg. 2009;209(2):e1–7.
8. Kandil EH, Noureldine SI, Yao L, Slakey DP. Robotic transaxillary thyroidectomy: an examination of the first one hundred cases. J Am Coll Surg. 2012;214(4):558–64.
9. Kang SW, Lee SC, Lee SH, Lee KY, Jeong JJ, Lee YS, et al. Robotic thyroid surgery using a gasless, transaxillary approach and the da Vinci S system: the operative outcomes of 338 consecutive patients. Surgery. 2009;146(6):1048–55.
10. Lee J, Kang SW, Jung JJ, Choi UJ, Yun JH, Nam KH, et al. Multicenter study of robotic thyroidectomy: short-term postoperative outcomes and surgeon ergonomic considerations. Ann Surg Oncol. 2011;18(9):2538–47.
11. Lee YM, Yi O, Sung TY, Chung KW, Yoon JH, Hong SJ. Surgical outcomes of robotic thyroid surgery using a double incision gasless transaxillary approach: analysis of 400 cases treated by the same surgeon. Head Neck. 2014;36(10):1413–9.
12. Lee J, Yun JH, Choi UJ, Kang SW, Jeong JJ, Chung WY. Robotic versus endoscopic thyroidectomy for thyroid cancers: a multi-institutional analysis of early postoperative outcomes and surgical learning curves. J Oncol. 2012;2012:734541.
13. Cabot JC, Lee CR, Brunaud L, Kleiman DA, Chung WY, Fahey 3rd TJ, et al. Robotic and endoscopic transaxillary thyroidectomies may be cost prohibitive when compared to standard cervical thyroidectomy: a cost analysis. Surgery. 2012;152(6):1016–24.

# Robotic Lobectomy

**27**

Benjamin Wei and Robert Cerfolio

## Introduction

Minimally invasive lobectomy has traditionally been performed using video-assisted thoracoscopic surgery (VATS) techniques. The first robotic lobectomies were reported in 2003 by Morgan et al. and Ashton et al. [1, 2]. Since then, the use of robotic technology for lobectomy has become increasingly common.

## Patient Selection and Preoperative Considerations

The evaluation of candidates for robotic lobectomy includes the standard preoperative studies for patients undergoing pulmonary resection. For patients with suspected or biopsy-proven lung cancer, whole-body PET-CT scan is currently the standard of care. Pulmonary function testing including measurement of diffusion capacity (DLCO) and spirometry is routine. Mediastinal staging can consist of either endobronchial ultrasound-guided fine-needle aspiration biopsy (EBUS-FNA) or mediastinoscopy, depending on expertise. Certain patients may warrant additional testing, including stress test, brain MRI if concern exists for metastatic disease, and/or dedicated computed tomography scan with intravenous contrast or MRI if concern exists for vascular or vertebral/nerve invasion, respectively.

B. Wei, M.D.
Cardiothoracic Surgery, Department of Surgery, University of Alabama
Birmingham—Medical Center, 1720 2nd Avenue South, Birmingham, AL 35294, USA
e-mail: bwei@uab.edu

R. Cerfolio, M.D., M.B.A. (✉)
Thoracic Surgery, Department of Surgery, University of Alabama Birmingham—Medical
Center, 1720 2nd Avenue South, Birmingham, AL 35294, USA
e-mail: rcerfolio@uabmc.edu

© Springer International Publishing AG 2018
A.D. Patel, D. Oleynikov (eds.), *The SAGES Manual of Robotic Surgery*,
The SAGES University Masters Program Series, DOI 10.1007/978-3-319-51362-1_27

Investigators have shown that thoracoscopic lobectomy is safe in patients with a predicted postoperative forced expiratory volume (FEV1) or DLCO <40% of predicted [3]. We consider robotic lobectomy feasible in these patients as well.

At present, we view vascular invasion, locally invasive T4 lesions, Pancoast tumors, and massive tumor (>10 cm) as contraindications for a robotic approach to lobectomy. The need for reconstruction of the airway, chest wall invasion, presence of induction chemotherapy and/or radiation, prior thoracic surgery, and hilar nodal disease are not contraindications for robotic-assisted lobectomy for experienced surgeons.

## Conduct of Operation

### Preparation

A well-trained team that communicates effectively is a priority for successful performance of robotic lobectomy. Criteria for a well-trained team include: documented scores of 70% or higher on simulator exercises, certificate of robotic safety training and cockpit awareness, weekly access to the robot, familiarity with the robotic and the instruments, and a mastery of the pulmonary artery from both an anterior and posterior approach. Currently, the da Vinci surgical system console (Intuitive Surgical; Sunnyvale, CA) is the only FDA-approved device available for robotic lobectomy. Proper location of the robot should be established prior to the operation. The third robotic arm will need to be located so that it will approach the patient from the posterior. The approach of the robot to the patient depends on whether or not an Si or Xi system is used. For the Si system, the robot is driven from over to patient shoulder at a 15° angle off the longitudinal access of the patient (Fig. 27.1). The patient will need to be turned so that the axis of the patient is 90° away from the typical position (i.e. head near the anesthesia workstation) to facilitate this. The use of long ventilator tubing and wrapping up this and other monitoring lines with a towel secured to the side of the bed is helpful to minimize interference with the surgeon/assistant. For the Xi system, the robot can approach from the patient's side and the patient's head can remain oriented towards the anesthesiologist's work station (Fig. 27.2). Precise placement of the double lumen endotracheal tube and the ability to tolerate single lung ventilation should be established prior to draping the patient, as repositioning the tube will be virtually impossible once the robot is docked.

### Patient Positioning/Port Placement

The patient is positioned in lateral decubitus position and the operating table flexed to open up the intercostal spaces. The patient should be moved posteriorly as much as possible so that the patient's arms can fit on the bed in front of the patient's head. Axillary rolls and arm boards are unnecessary (Fig. 27.3). The robotic ports are inserted in the seventh intercostal space for upper/middle lobectomy and in the

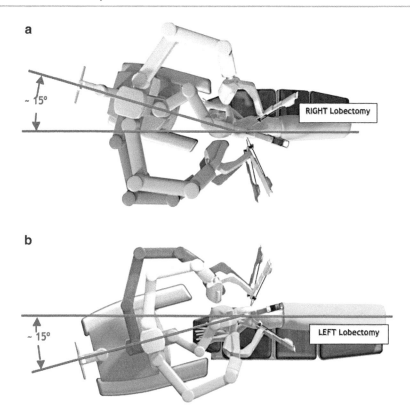

**Fig. 27.1** Angle of approach of robot docking for lobectomy (da Vinci Si system) (**a**) right lobectomy, (**b**) left lobectomy

eighth intercostal space for lower lobectomy. Typical port placement is shown in Fig. 27.4 for a right robotic lobectomy. The ports are marked as follows: robotic arm 3 (5 or 8 mm port) is located 1–2 cm lateral from the spinous process of the vertebral body, robotic arm 2 (8 mm) is 10 cm medial to robotic arm 3, the camera port (we prefer the 12 mm camera) is 9 cm medial to robotic arm 2, and robotic arm 1 (12 mm) is placed right above the diaphragm anteriorly. The assistant port is triangulated behind the camera port and the most anterior robotic port, and as inferior as possible without disrupting the diaphragm. We use a zero-degree camera for this operation. Insufflation of the camera or assistant port with carbon dioxide is used to depress the diaphragm, decrease bleeding, and compress the lung.

## Mediastinal Lymph Node Dissection

After examining the pleura to confirm the absence of metastases, the next step during our performance of robotic lobectomy is removal of the mediastinal lymph nodes, for staging, and also to help expose the structures of the hilum.

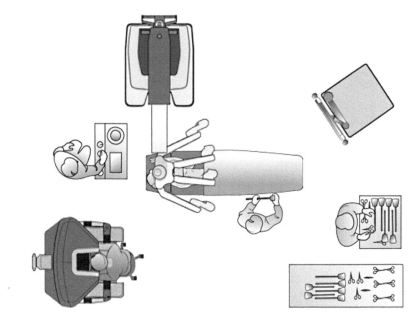

**Fig. 27.2** Angle of approach of robot docking for lobectomy (da Vinci Xi system) and possible room layout

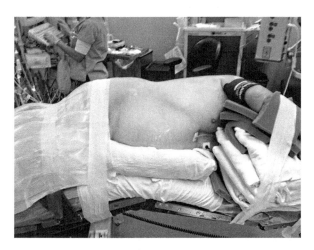

**Fig. 27.3** Patient position for robotic lobectomy, viewed from anterior

- *Right side*—The inferior pulmonary ligament is divided. Lymph nodes at stations 8 and 9 are removed. Robotic arm 3 is used to retract the lower lobe medially and anteriorly in order to remove lymph nodes from station 7. Robotic arm 3 is used to retract the upper lobe inferiorly during dissection of stations 2R and 4R, clearing the space between the SVC anteriorly, the esophagus posteriorly, and the azygos

**Fig. 27.4** Port placement for right robotic lobectomy. *C* camera port, *1* robotic arm 1, *2* robotic arm 2, *3* robotic arm 3, *A* assistant port, *MAL* mid-axillary line

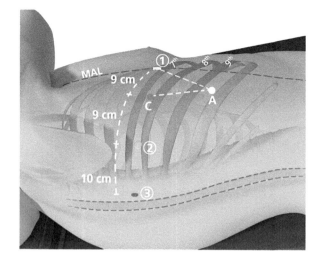

vein inferiorly. Avoiding dissection too far superiorly can prevent injury to the right recurrent laryngeal nerve that wraps around the subclavian artery.

- *Left side*—The inferior pulmonary ligament is divided to facilitate the removal of lymph node station 9. The nodes in station 8 are then removed. Station 7 is accessed in the space between the inferior pulmonary vein and lower lobe bronchus, lateral to the esophagus. The lower lobe is retracted medially/anteriorly with robotic arm 3 during this process. Absence of the lower lobe facilitates dissection of level 7 from the left. Finally, robotic arm three is used to wrap around the left upper lobe and pressed it inferior to allow dissection of stations 5 and 6. Care should be taken while working in the aorto-pulmonary window to avoid injury to the left recurrent laryngeal nerve. Station 2 L. cannot typically be accessed during left-sided mediastinal lymph node dissection due to the presence of the aortic arch, but the 4 L. node is commonly removed.

## Wedge Resection

Wedge resection of a nodule may be necessary to confirm the presence of cancer prior to proceeding with lobectomy. Because the current iteration of the robot does not offer tactile feedback, special techniques may be necessary to identify a nodule that is not obvious on visual inspection. An empty ring forceps may be used via the assistant port to palpate the nodule. Alternatively, preoperative marking of the nodule with a dye marker injected via navigational bronchoscopy can help facilitate location of the nodule. Preoperative confirmation of a cancer diagnosis with tissue biopsy is helpful to avoid being unable to locate the nodule intraoperatively. In the future, the use of injected indocyanine green (ICG) may also allow surgeons to visualize nodules intraoperatively [4].

## The Five Lobectomies

A certain degree of adaptability is necessary for performance of robotic lobectomy. Structures may be isolated and divided in the order that the patient's individual anatomy permits. What follows is a description of an outline of the typical conduct of each lobectomy.

### Right Upper Lobectomy

- The right upper lobe is then reflected anteriorly to expose the bifurcation of the right main stem bronchus. There is usually a lymph node here that should be dissected out to expose the bifurcation. The right upper lobe bronchus is then encircled and divided. Care must be taken to apply only minimal retraction on the specimen in order to avoid tearing the remaining pulmonary artery branches.
- Retraction of the right upper lobe laterally and posteriorly with robot arm 3 helps expose the hilum.
- The bifurcation between the right upper and middle lobar veins is developed by dissecting it off the underlying pulmonary artery.
- The 10R lymph node between the truncus branch and the superior pulmonary vein should be removed or swept up towards the lung, which exposes the truncus branch.
- The superior pulmonary vein is encircled with the vessel loop and then divided. The truncus branch is then divided.
- Finally, the posterior segmental artery to the right upper lobe is exposed, the surrounding N1 nodes removed, and the artery encircled and divided.
- The upper lobe is reflected again posteriorly, and the anterior aspect of the pulmonary artery is inspected to make sure that there are no arterial branches remaining. If not, then the fissure between the upper and middle lobes, and the upper and lower lobes, is then divided. This is typically done from anterior to posterior, but may be done in the reverse direction if the space between the pulmonary artery and right middle lobe is already developed. During completion of the fissure, the right upper lobe should be lifted up to ensure that the specimen bronchus is included in the specimen.

### Right Middle Lobectomy

- Retraction of the right middle lobe laterally and posteriorly with robot arm 1 helps expose the hilum.
- The bifurcation between the right upper and middle lobar veins is developed by dissecting it off the underlying pulmonary artery. The right middle lobe vein is encircled and divided.

- The fissure between the right middle and lower lobes, if not complete, is divided from anterior to posterior. Care should be taken to avoid transecting segmental arteries to the right lower lobe.
- The right middle lobe bronchus is then isolated. It will be running from left to right in the fissure. Level 11 lymph nodes are dissected from around it. It is encircled and divided, taking care to avoid injuring the right middle lobar artery that is located directly behind it.
- Dissection of the fissure should continue posteriorly until the branches to the superior segment are identified. Then the one or two right middle lobar segmental arteries are isolated and divided.
- Stapling of middle lobar structures may be facilitated by passing the stapler from posterior to anterior, to have a greater working distance.
- The fissure between right middle and upper lobes is then divided.

## Right Lower Lobectomy

- The inferior pulmonary ligament should be divided to the level of the inferior pulmonary vein.
- The bifurcation of the right superior and inferior pulmonary veins should be dissected out. The location of the right middle lobar vein should be positively identified to avoid inadvertent transection.
- A subadventitial plane on the ongoing pulmonary artery should be established. If the major fissure is not complete, then it should be divided. The superior segmental artery and the right middle lobe arterial branches are identified. The superior segmental artery is isolated and divided. The common trunk to right lower lobe basilar segments may be taken as long as this does not compromise the middle lobar segmental artery/arteries; otherwise, dissection may have to extend further distally to ensure safe division.
- The inferior pulmonary vein is divided.
- The right lower lobe bronchus is isolated, taking care to visualize the right middle lobar bronchus crossing from left to right. The surrounding lymph nodes, as usual, are dissected and the bronchus divided. If there is any question of compromising the right middle lobe bronchus, the surgeon can ask the anesthesiologist to hand-ventilate the right lung to confirm that the middle lobe expands.

## Left Upper Lobectomy

- Retraction of the left upper lobe laterally and posteriorly with robot arm 3 helps expose the hilum.
- The presence of both superior and inferior pulmonary veins is confirmed, and the bifurcation dissected.
- The lung is then reflected anteriorly with robotic arm 3 and interlobar dissection is started, going from posterior to anterior.

- If the fissure is not complete then it will need to be divided. Reflecting the lung posteriorly again and establishing a subadventitial plane will be helpful. The branches to the lingula are encountered and divided in the fissure during this process. The posterior segmental artery is also isolated and divided. Division of the lingular artery or arteries can be done before or after division of the posterior segmental artery.
- The superior pulmonary vein is isolated then divided. Because the superior pulmonary vein can be fairly wide, it may require that the lingular and upper division branches be transected separately.
- Often the next structure that can be divided readily will be the left upper lobar bronchus, as opposed to the anterior and apical arterial branches to the left upper lobe. The upper lobe bronchus should be encircled and divided, often passing the stapler from robotic arm 1 in order to avoid injuring the main pulmonary artery.
- Finally, the remaining arterial branches are encircled and divided.

## Left Lower Lobectomy

- The inferior pulmonary ligament should be divided to the level of the inferior pulmonary vein. The lower lobe is then reflected posteriorly by robotic arm 3.
- The bifurcation of the left superior and inferior pulmonary veins should be dissected out.
- The lung is reflected anteriorly by robotic arm 3. The superior segmental artery is identified. The posterior ascending arteries to the left upper lobe are frequently visible from this view also. The superior segmental artery is isolated and divided. The common trunk to left lower lobe basilar segments may be taken as long as this does not compromise the middle lobar segmental artery/arteries; otherwise, dissection may have to extend further distally to ensure safe division. If the fissure is not complete, this will need to be divided to expose the ongoing pulmonary artery to the lower lobe.
- After division of the arterial branches, the lung is reflected again posteriorly. The inferior pulmonary vein is divided.
- The left lower lobe bronchus is isolated. The surrounding lymph nodes, as usual, are dissected and the bronchus divided.
- For left lower lobectomy, it may be simpler to wait until after resection is performed before targeting the subcarinal space for removal of level 7 lymph nodes.

## Review of Literature

Reported series of robotic lobectomy to date have been notable for a fairly low conversion rate, low mortality rate, and comparable morbidity to VATS approaches (Table 27.1). We will soon publish our results with over 500 consecutive robotic lobectomies, the largest series ever reported. Between September 2010 and September 2015, there were 1304 consecutive operations scheduled for robotic resection by one

**Table 27.1** Results reported in series of robotic-assisted lobectomies

| | Year | n | Conversion rate | Morbidity | Perioperative mortality | Median LOS | Other notes |
|---|---|---|---|---|---|---|---|
| Cerfolio et al. [5] | 2011 | 168 | 7.7% | 27% | 0% | 2 days | Decreased morbidity, improved QOL, shorter LOS than open lobectomy |
| Park et al. [6] | 2006 | 30 | 12% | 26% | 0% | 4.5 days | |
| Veronesi et al. [7] | 2009 | 54 | 13% | 20% | 0% | 4.5 days | Shorter LOS than open lobectomy |
| Gharagozloo et al. [8] | 2009 | 100 | | 21% | 3% | 4 days | |

*LOS* length of stay, *QOL* quality of life

thoracic surgeon. They included 502 planned robotic lobectomies (37 were converted to thoracotomy, 11 of which were for bleeding from a major vascular injury, additionally 2 major vascular injuries were repaired robotically) and 130 planned segmentectomies (2 were converted to thoracotomy, both for bleeding from a major vascular injury). Overall, there were 16 patients with major vascular injuries (1.2%). Thirteen occurred during lobectomy (13/502 = 2.6%), two during segmentectomy (2/130 = 1.5%), and one during a mediastinal tumor resection. Of the 13 that occurred during lobectomy, five occurred during left upper lobectomy, four during right upper lobectomy, two during right lower lobectomy, and two during left lower lobectomy. All injuries were immediately packed with pressure from a rolled-up sponge that was already in the operative field at the time of injury. A minimum of 7 min of pressure was held. In the first eight patients, an elective thoracotomy was performed after packing. In the last eight patients, the injury was unpacked and examined; two injuries were able to be repaired using robotic minimally invasive techniques, while the remaining six patients required thoracotomy.

With increasing experience, operating times for robotic lobectomy have been shown to decrease; at our institution, robotic lobectomies with complete mediastinal lymph node dissection can routinely be done in 1.5–2 h from incision to skin closure. The single comparison with VATS lobectomy published to date, by Louie et al., demonstrates similar blood loss, operative time, ICU stay, and length of stay between robotic and VATS, but did show benefits of robotic lobectomy in terms of duration of narcotic use and time to return to usual activities [9]. Park et al. have reported 5-year survival rates for 310 patients with stage I non-small cell lung cancer of ~90% following robotic lobectomy, which is comparable to both VATS and open lobectomy [10]. Our experience has been that robotic lobectomy facilitates a thorough mediastinal lymph node dissection, which we believe is associated with a greater accuracy of staging and therefore more optimal adjuvant treatment.

## Tips and Tricks/Troubleshooting

- The dissection and removal of lymph nodes between lobar and segmental structures (bronchi, arteries, veins) helps facilitate their isolation.
- Although the temptation when performing dissection is to avoid encountering these structures, approaching them carefully but emphatically will result in a more accurate and faster dissection.
- Appropriate retraction is essential for the steps outlined above. The assistant can be used to help with retraction.
- The passing of vascular staplers around fragile structure such as the pulmonary artery and/or vein deserves special attention. Carefully orchestrated moves and clear communication is needed between the bedside assistant and the surgeon. We have developed our own communication system between the bedside assistant and the surgeon to prevent iatrogenic injuries. This uses the anvil of the stapler as the hour hand of a clock and the degree of articulation is also quantified and communicated.
- Robotic instruments should be initially inserted under *direct vision* during thoracic surgery for their initial placement. Once safely positioned, instruments then can be quickly and safely inserted or changed for other instruments by properly using the memory feature of the robot that automatically inserts any new instruments to a position that is exactly 3 mm proximal to its latest position. However, if this feature is used, it is incumbent on the surgeon to ensure that no vital structure has moved into the path of that newly placed instrument. The most common structure would be the lung.
- A rolled-up sponge should always be immediately accessible when working around vascular structures. If an injury occurs, the first step should be to tamponade the structure with the sponge. A minor injury may respond to this packing alone. If bleeding is massive or persists, a thoracotomy will be necessary. Lap pads should be inserted via the assistant port and packed around the injury to control bleeding. The robot is then de-docked and a thoracotomy made.
- The "drop zone" for the specimen should be well away from the pulmonary artery, which can be injured during this process if care is not taken.
- The robotic arms are removed under direct vision with insufflation discontinued in order to confirm the absence of bleeding.

Table 27.2 shows how to trouble shoot common problems encountered during robotic lobectomy.

## Conclusion

Robotic lobectomy can be done with very low morbidity and mortality, as we and other investigators have demonstrated, and is clearly advantageous when compared to open lobectomy with regard to short-term outcomes, both in community and academic settings [10, 11]. Early and 5-year survival rates appear to be similar

**Table 27.2**  Troubleshooting of common problems during robotic lobectomy

| Problems | Solutions |
|---|---|
| Robotic arms are not responding to hand movement | 1.  Ensure trocar's remote center is in chest |
| | 2.  Ensure trocar's docked properly to robotic arms |
| | 3.  Ensure sterile plastic gown covering robotic arms is not interfering with wheeled mechanism of robot |
| | 4.  Ensure surgeons' hand not maximized at console |
| The camera is fogging | 1.  Place humidified $CO_2$ insufflation through non-robotic access port (and not through the camera port) |
| | 2.  Pre-heat the camera |
| | 3.  Evacuate smoke from intra-operative field |
| There are conflicts between robotic arms 3 & 1 or 2 | 1.  Ensure at least 10 cm between robotic arm 3 and closest robotic arm (robotic arm 1 or 2) |
| | 2.  Use 5 mm thoracic lung grasper as the instrument of choice through the most posterior robotic arm |
| | 3.  After docking, ensure the link 2 s of robotic arms are aligned parallel to one another |
| | 4.  When surgeon toggles between robotic arm 3 and 2 or 1, ensure the non-active instrument is placed anteriorly towards chest wall |
| The bipolar cautery or thoracic dissector is not working | Ensure bipolar… |
| | 1.  …source is connected to robot |
| | 2.  … energy source is functioning |
| | 3.  … cord is not damaged |
| There is a sudden loss of working space | 1.  Ensure DLET is properly positioned |
| | 2.  Inflate more air in bronchial cuff |
| | 3.  Ensure no leaks out of ports if using a completely portal technique |
| | 4.  Ensure all valves are closed on ports |
| | 5.  Do not place sucker in chest on suction unless immersed under water or blood |
| You are unable to achieve proper angle of stapler to come across vessels or fissures | 1.  Try placing stapler through robotic access port or robotic arm 1 or 2 to achieve best angle |
| | 2.  Use a stapler which maximizes the degrees of rotation and articulation |
| | 3.  Do not force the stapler; tie vessels with suture or |
| | 4.  Use 8 mm robotic clips on vessel |
| There is difficulty in bagging specimen | 1.  Use a bag that provides easy opening and closing by bed-side assistant |
| | 2.  Place bag under trocar prior to deployment |
| | 3.  Place bag in the most anterior-superior aspect of chest to maximize use of gravity, space, and keep bag away from stapled hilar structures |
| | 4.  Use robotic arm 3 to place specimen into bag and then hold back of the bag in place while stuffing specimen into bag with robotic arms 1 & 2 |

*DLET* double lumen endotracheal tube

between robotic, VATS, and open lobectomy [12, 13]. With proper training and experience, robotic lobectomy can become part of the fundamental armamentarium of the modern thoracic surgeon.

## References

1. Morgan JA, Ginsburg ME, Sonett JR, et al. Advanced thoracoscopic procedures are facilitated by computer-aided robotic technology. Eur J Cardiothorac Surg. 2003;23:883–7.
2. Ashton RC, Connery CP, Swistel DG, DeRose JJ. Robot-assisted lobectomy. J Thorac Cardiovasc Surg. 2003;126:292–3.
3. Burt BM, Kosinski AS, Shrager JB, et al. Thoracoscopic lobectomy is associated with acceptable morbidity and mortality in patients with predicted postoperative forced expiratory volume in 1 second or diffusing capacity for carbon monoxide less than 40% of normal. J Thorac Cardiovasc Surg. 2014;148:19–28.
4. Daskalaki D, Aguilera F, Patton K, Giulianotti PC. Fluorescence in robotic surgery. J Surg Oncol. 2015;112:250–6.
5. Cerfolio RJ, Bryant AS, Skylizard L, Minnich DJ. Initial consecutive experience of completely portal robotic pulmonary resection with 4 arms. J Thorac Cardiovasc Surg. 2011;142:740–6.
6. Park BJ, Flores RM, Rusch VW. Robotic assistance for video-assisted thoracic surgical lobectomy: technique and initial results. J Thorac Cardiovasc Surg. 2006;131:54–9.
7. Veronesis G, Galetta D, Maisonneuve P, et al. Four-arm robotic lobectomy for the treatment of early-stage lung cancer. J Thorac Cardiovasc Surg. 2010;140:19–25.
8. Gharagozloo F, Margolis M, Tempesta B, et al. Robot-assisted lobectomy for early-stage lung cancer: report of 100 consecutive cases. Ann Thorac Surg. 2009;88:380–4.
9. Farivar AS, Cerfolio RJ, Vaillieres E, et al. Comparing robotic lung resection with thoracotomy and video-assisted thoracoscopic surgery cases entered in the Society of Thoracic Surgeons database. Innovations. 2014;9:10–5.
10. Kent M, Wang T, Whyte R, et al. Open, video-assisted thoracic surgery, and robotic lobectomy: review of a national database. Ann Thorac Surg. 2014;97:236–42.
11. Adams RD, Bolton WD, Stephenson JE, et al. Initial multicenter community robotic lobectomy experience: comparisons to a national database. Ann Thorac Surg. 2014;97:1893–8.
12. Park BJ, Melfi F, Mussi A, et al. Robotic lobectomy for non-small cell lung cancer (NSCLC): long-term oncologic results. J Thorac Cardiovasc Surg. 2012;143:383–9.
13. Yang HX, Woo KM, Sima CS, et al. Long-term survival based on the surgical approach to lobectomy for clinical stage I nonsmall lung cancer: comparison of robotic, video-assisted thoracic surgery, and thoracotomy lobectomy. Ann Surg. 2016.

# 28

Ray K. Chihara and Manu S. Sancheti

## Introduction

Mediastinal pathology historically required maximum exposure through incisions such as median sternotomy, lateral thoracotomy, and anterolateral thoracotomy with or without transverse sternotomy (clamshell), leading to long hospital stay and recovery. The development of video-assisted thoracoscopic surgery (VATS) for mediastinal procedures allowed smaller incisions, shorter hospital stay, and faster recovery time [1]. VATS has been utilized for various mediastinal pathologies including the thymus, germ cell, cysts, neurogenic tumors, and malignant or meta-static lesions such as thymoma, liposarcoma, and adenocarcinoma [2]. Advances in robotic surgery have given surgeons an additional tool to visualize, navigate, and dissect the mediastinum. The benefits of robotics as compared to VATS include articulating instruments, three-dimensional visualization, scaling down of operative movements, and lack of tremor. Such improvements are particularly paramount in areas like the mediastinum due to its small space and many vital structures. Disadvantages are the lack of tactile sensation, higher costs, initial learning curve, and lack of standardized approaches to robotic mediastinal procedures. In this chapter, approaches to robotic mediastinal procedures are detailed, specifically catego-rized into three anatomical sections: the anterior, middle, and posterior mediastinum. The anterior mediastinum is the space in the chest between the anterior border of the pericardium and the sternum. The middle mediastinum is the space in the chest between the anterior border of the pericardium and the posterior border of the peri-cardium. The posterior mediastinum is the space in the chest between the posterior border of the pericardium and the vertebrae. The mediastinal pleura is the lateral boundaries for this space.

R.K. Chihara, M.D., Ph.D. (✉) • M.S. Sancheti, M.D.
Cardiothoracic Surgery, Emory University Hospital/Emory University, The Emory Clinic,
1365 Clifton Road NE, Atlanta, GA 30322, USA
e-mail: rchihar@emory.edu; manu.suraj.sancheti@emory.edu

© Springer International Publishing AG 2018
A.D. Patel, D. Oleynikov (eds.), *The SAGES Manual of Robotic Surgery*,
The SAGES University Masters Program Series, DOI 10.1007/978-3-319-51362-1_28

## General Operative Evaluation for Robotic Mediastinal Procedures

Preoperative evaluation for robotic mediastinal procedures is generally the same as open cases with several caveats. Computed tomography (CT) with contrast is essential in evaluation of mediastinal pathology and important mediastinal structures to determine if the lesion can be resected safely. The association of the lesion with rib spaces is vital for planning port placement. History of prior chest procedures may indicate higher risk for conversion to open procedure due to adhesive disease in the chest and may change surgical approach. Pulmonary function testing is recommended for robotic mediastinal procedures, as poor pulmonary function may not allow for single lung ventilation necessary for mediastinal robotic surgery. Lung isolation is achieved with the combination of carbon dioxide insufflation at 8–10 mmHg as well as selective ventilation via a double lumen endotracheal tube or bronchial blocker.

## Reasons for Conversion to Open

The most common reasons for conversion are chest wall adhesions and inability to discern the appropriate anatomy for dissection. Causes include prior instrumentation of the pleural cavity via thoracotomy or thoracoscopy, pleural space infections, malignant involvement of the pleural space, and decreased working space from inability to insufflate the pleural space with carbon dioxide. Other reasons for conversion to open include the mass is in close proximity of vital mediastinal structures and inability to tolerate single lung ventilation. The later causes for conversion are largely avoided with appropriate preoperative work up of the patient.

## General Rules for Port Placement and Robotic Positioning in Mediastinal Masses

Port placement and robotic positioning is a key aspect of successful mediastinal robotic operations. Port sites are ideally placed in a triangular pattern at least 10 cm away from the target lesion. The camera should be in the center with robotic arms at least 10 cm away from the camera port to decrease conflict between the robotic arms. Access port placement for the assistant should ideally be 10 cm away from robotic ports posterior to the engaged robotic arms to minimize assistant to robot arm collisions. The imaging studies are key in determining appropriate port sites especially for masses in the middle mediastinum and posterior mediastinum where variability in tumor location is more common. The position of the robot should generally be placed at an angle allowing the instruments to be pointing at the dissection area and in a manner where the robotic arms are extended out approximately half way to maximum extension using the range indicator on the robot. Such robot positioning allows for the maximum mobility and increases angles of dissection.

## Approach to Anterior Mediastinal Pathology

### Introduction to Anterior Mediastinal Procedures

Anterior mediastinal pathology for which robotic surgery has been utilized include: thymus for myasthenia gravis, thymoma, lymphoma/lymph node excisional biopsy, germ cell tumors, parathyroid, and thyroid tissues. Specific preoperative consideration may be necessary for anterior mediastinal pathology. Myasthenia gravis patients have increased risks for general anesthesia requiring preoperative preparation with pyridostigmine, IVIG, or plasmapheresis. IVIG should be given 2 weeks prior to planned resection. Potential anesthetic related issues include resistance to depolarizing paralytic agents, cholinergic crisis for neuromuscular blocking reversal agents, increased risks of aspiration, increased risks of respiratory failure, and continued requirements for intubation and ventilator use postoperatively. If the differential for the anterior mediastinal mass includes thymoma, screening for symptoms related to myasthenia gravis should be completed to direct further laboratory investigation for definitive diagnosis of myasthenia gravis to avoid potential anesthesia-related complications.

### Indications for Robotic Anterior Mediastinal Mass Resection

Cross-sectional imaging, CT and/or MRI, is required to evaluate the association of the anterior mediastinal mass to surrounding mediastinal structures to discern resectability of the lesion. In the case of a thymoma, complete resection is required for adequate treatment due to risk of recurrence. Therefore, Masaoka stage I tumors, enclosed within the thymic capsule, have been deemed acceptable for minimally invasive techniques [3]. Some data suggest possible equivalent efficacy of minimally invasive resections for Masaoka stage II tumors, but requires further validation for robotic-assisted resections [4]. Robotic resections for anterior mediastinal germ cell tumors are indicated for mature teratomas and dermoid cysts. Seminomas and non-seminomas are treated primarily with radiation and chemotherapy, respectively. If a mass remains after initial treatment of seminomas or non-seminomas, further medical treatment may be indicated or surgical resection if tumor markers AFP and beta-HCG are negative and remaining mass does not involve mediastinal structures. Excision of enlarged anterior mediastinal lymph nodes may also be appropriate for diagnosis of lymphoma or staging for other malignancies.

### Anterior Mediastinal Mass Case Scenario

The patient was a 67 year-old man who was undergoing work up for unintentional weight loss. The work up included a CT scan, revealing an incidental anterior mediastinal mass surrounded by thymus and thymic fat (Fig. 28.1). He had no history of myasthenia gravis. Differential diagnosis included thymic hyperplasia, thymic carcinoma, thymoma, and lymphoma. The patient elected to undergo resection of the anterior mediastinal mass.

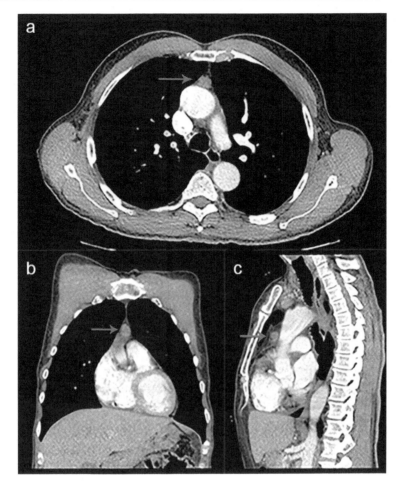

**Fig. 28.1** CT scan for an anterior mediastinal mass. *Red arrows* point to the anterior mediastinal mass. (**a**) Axial, (**b**) coronal, (**c**) sagittal. Anterior mediastinal mass does not appear to involve surrounding mediastinal structures and appears to be encapsulated by thymus and surrounding thymic fat.

## Surgical Equipment Used

- da Vinci 0-degree camera
- EndoWrist® (Bipolar) Maryland forceps or EndoWrist® One™ Vessel sealer
- EndoWrist® Grasper—Cadiere Forceps × 2
- EndoWrist® Clip Applier—small and large
- Kittner roll gauze sponges
- 5 mm Optiview trocar
- 12 mm Optiview trocar
- 8 mm instrument cannula × 2
- 5 mm thoracoscope
- Endo Catch bag

## Patient Positioning

Anterior mediastinal masses may be approached from the right or the left side of the chest. In our example, a right-sided approach was used. The patient is placed in supine position with a jellyroll or rolled sheet along the posterior mid-clavicular line to elevate the operative side. The arms are tucked with the arm on the operative side allowed to sit slightly below the OR table to allow more space for the robotic arms.

Port sites were determined by preoperative imaging studies (Fig. 28.1). The port sites are positioned along the mid-anterior axillary line for the robotic port 1 and camera port. Robotic port 2 was positioned in the anterior axillary line as shown in Fig. 28.2. In the example case, port 1 was placed in the third intercostal space, camera port in the fifth intercostal space, and port 2 in the seventh intercostal space. When the anterior mediastinal mass sits high in the chest, port placement in the second, fourth, and sixth intercostal spaces may be advantageous. The rib spaces and port sites are marked, then the patient is prepped and draped in usual fashion (Fig. 28.3).

## Port Insertion and Positioning of the Robot

After making a 5 mm incision at the camera port, the chest is entered using the 5 mm Optiview trocar and the 5 mm laparoscope. Stabilize the trocar with your non-dominant hand, while passing the scope and trocar into the chest seeing the layers of the chest wall until lung is visualized (Fig. 28.4). The pleural space is insufflated with carbon dioxide set at 10 mmHg pressure and inspected for adhesions and evaluated for malignant involvement. Decision can be made at this time to convert to an open procedure or continue with placement of the robotic ports 1 and 2. Using the 5 mm laparoscope for visualization, the 8 mm robotic cannulas are placed into port sites 1 and 2. The thick black line on the 8 mm port is positioned just within the intercostal muscle. The 5 mm port is removed and the incision is then extended to fit a 12 mm

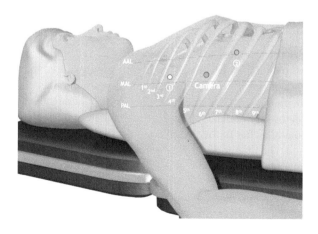

**Fig. 28.2**  Port placement for robotic anterior mediastinal mass resection. *AAL* anterior axillary line, *MAL* mid-axillary line, *PAL* posterior axillary line. Port sites are labeled *blue* for camera port, *yellow* for robotic port 1, *green* for robotic port 2

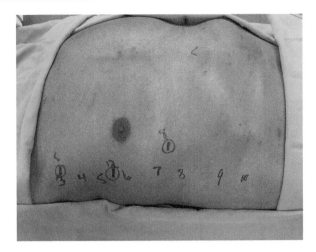

**Fig. 28.3**  Positioned and marked for anterior mediastinal mass resection

Optiview port with depth just past the chest wall confirmed with the 5 mm laparo-scope in one of the 8 mm port sites. The robot is then driven into the operative field from the contralateral side and perpendicular to the patient centered on the camera trocar as depicted in Fig. 28.5. The ports are then secured into the robotic arms. The 0-degree da Vinci camera is passed into the center camera port. The Cadiere forceps are placed into port site 1 followed by the Maryland bipolar forceps (or robotic vessel sealer) into port site 2 under robotic camera visualization. Bipolar is set at 70 W.

## Anterior Mediastinal Mass Excision Operative Steps

The phrenic nerve is first identified along the pericardium, as this nerve must be pre-served and defines the posterior border of the dissection. We use the Maryland bipo-lar forceps to initiate the dissection of the mediastinal pleura just anterior to the phrenic nerve running along the superior vena cava (Fig. 28.6). The Kittner roll gauzes are inserted into the thoracic cavity through the access port to assist with absorbing minor bleeding and assist with retraction. The dissection of the mediasti-nal pleura is extended caudad to the inferior pole of the thymic tissue above the dia-phragm denoting the right-sided inferior border of dissection. The mediastinal pleural incision is then extended cephalad to the innominate vein (Fig. 28.7). Care must be taken as the dissection nears the innominate vein, as clips may be necessary to divide vein branches to the thymus. Thymic tissue underneath the innominate is dissected free. The thymic tissues are dissected off the pericardium posteriorly to the medias-tinal pleura on the left side which is incised at the same level as on the right side. Occasionally, the phrenic nerve may not be visible on the left side. If there is con-cern, a 5 mm thoracoscope can be placed into the left pleural space to visualize the left phrenic nerve. The anterior dissection is started just medial to the internal mam-mary vessels (Fig. 28.8). Arterial branches may need to be clipped and divided

**Fig. 28.4** Thoracic cavity entry using 5 mm Optiview trocar with 5 mm laparoscope. (**a**) Subcutaneous fat layer, (**b**) muscle layer, (**c**) lung parenchyma visualized

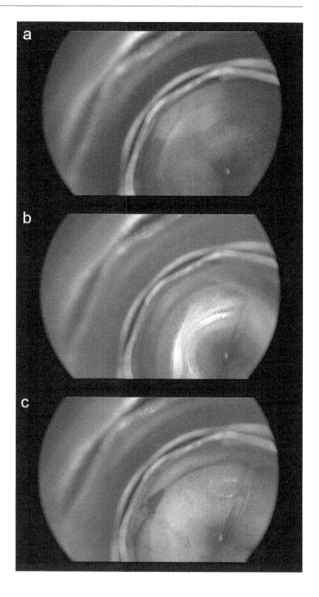

supplying the thymus. The right-sided superior pole of the thymus is then dissected free using caudad and posterior traction (Fig. 28.9). A clip is usually necessary at the superior aspect of the pole to control bleeding. The dissection is then carried over to the left superior pole, which is similarly dissected away from the inferior neck (Fig. 28.10). The dissection is then carried over to the mediastinal pleura on the anterior aspect of the dissection along the sternum. The left pleural space is entered anteriorly taking care not to injure the left internal mammary artery. The thymus is retracted over to the right side and the left lobe of the thymus is dissected free (Fig. 28.11). The robotic instruments are retracted and robot disengaged from the ports. The 5 mm laparoscope is placed into port site 1 and the Endo Catch bag is then

**Fig. 28.5** Robot position in respect to the patient for anterior mediastinal mass resection

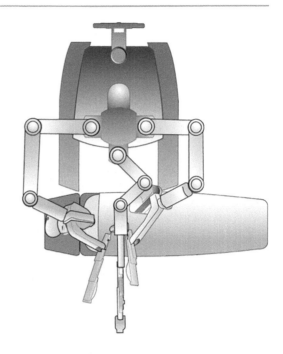

**Fig. 28.6** Initial dissection plane for anterior mediastinal mass resection

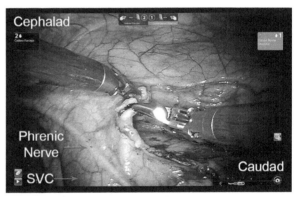

**Fig. 28.7** Identification of the Innominate vein

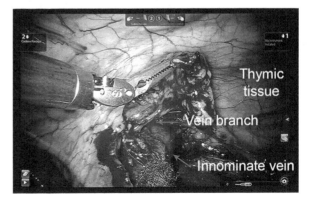

**Fig. 28.8** Identification of the internal mammary vessels. Defines the superior and anterior dissection plane

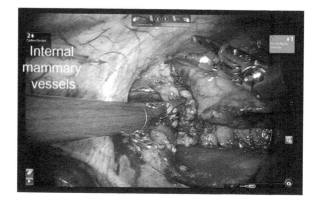

**Fig. 28.9** Identification of the right superior thymic pole

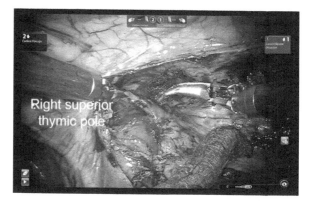

**Fig. 28.10** Identification of the left superior thymic pole

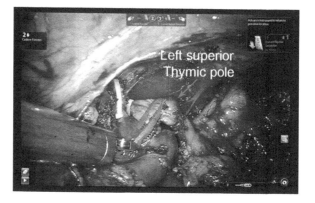

used in the 12 mm camera port. A blunt grasper is used to place the specimen into the bag and removed from the pleural cavity. The incision may need to be widened to accommodate the removal of the specimen. The port sites are then closed with 2-0 vicryl suture followed by 4-0 monocryl subcuticular skin closure. The anterior mediastinal mass was found to be a thymoma, Masaoka stage I on pathology.

**Fig. 28.11** Completion of
the anterior mediastinal
mass resection

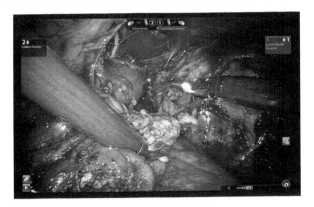

## Approach to Middle Mediastinal Pathology

Middle mediastinal masses include most commonly lymph nodes and congenital bronchogenic cysts and pericardial cysts. Lymph nodes in the middle mediastinum are addressed mainly with mediastinoscopy, which is a minimally invasive technique to sample paratracheal and subcarinal lymph nodes of interest. Bronchogenic cysts, most common, and pericardial cysts, second most common, are rare congenital entities found in the middle mediastinum [5]. Bronchogenic cysts and pericardial cysts have been addressed with robotic assistance in several case reports [6–8].

### Indications for Resection

Bronchogenic cysts can be symptomatic due to extrinsic compression, have infection risks if they rupture, and rare transformation to malignant lesions [9]. Resection is indicated for both lesions that are symptomatic and asymptomatic and are amenable to straightforward resection to avoid future complications. Surveillance of the lesion may be more appropriate for asymptomatic lesions in high-risk patients or asymptomatic lesions located in a precarious area. Resection for diagnostic purposes is also indicated if the type of mediastinal cyst is in question. Pericardial cysts are benign lesions where resection is indicated for rare symptomatic lesions or for diagnostic purposes.

### Middle Mediastinal Mass Example Case Scenario

The patient is a 66 year-old woman with history of mantle cell lymphoma who underwent computed tomography scan, revealing an incidental middle mediastinal cyst in the aortopulmonary window that abutted the esophagus, trachea, pulmonary artery, and aorta (Fig. 28.12). Differential diagnosis included bronchogenic cyst, pericardial cyst, and less likely a foregut cyst. The patient was given

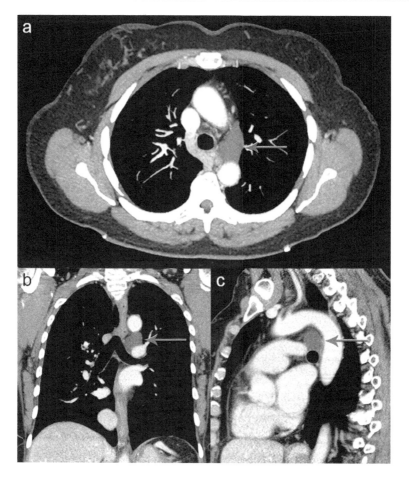

**Fig. 28.12**  CT scan for middle mediastinal cyst. *Red arrow* points to the cyst. The cyst abuts the aorta, pulmonary artery, esophagus, trachea, and left main stem bronchus. (**a**) Axial, (**b**) coronal, (**c**) sagittal

recommendations for observation versus resection, which included risks of injury to vital structures such as aorta, pulmonary artery, trachea esophagus, left vagus, and recurrent laryngeal nerve resulting in voice hoarseness. The patient elected for resection due to her concerns with prior malignancy.

## Surgical Equipment Used

- da Vinci 30-degree camera
- EndoWrist® (Bipolar) Maryland forceps or EndoWrist® One™ Vessel sealer
- EndoWrist Grasper—Cadiere Forceps × 2
- 12 mm Optiview trocar × 2
- 8 mm instrument cannula × 3

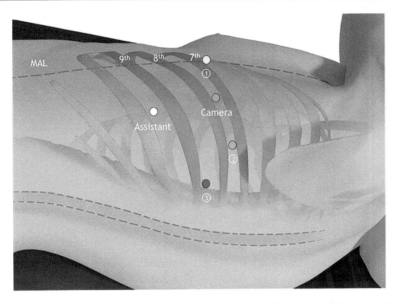

**Fig. 28.13** Port placement for middle mediastinal cyst excision. Camera port is *blue*, robotic port 1 is *yellow*, robotic port 2 is *green*, robotic port 3 is *red*. Assistant port is *white*

## Patient Positioning

For middle mediastinal masses, patient positioning will depend on the location of the tumor. In most cases, a right or left lateral decubitus position will be appropriate for resection. A right lateral decubitus position, left side up, on a reversed OR table was used for the example case due to the laterality of the lesion and to allow space for docking the robot.

A three-armed robot was chosen for this procedure along with an access port. Port sites were determined by preoperative imaging studies (Fig. 28.12). The camera port was positioned in the seventh intercostal space mid-axillary line. Robotic port 1 was positioned in the sixth intercostal space just outside the anterior axillary line. Robotic port 2 was positioned in the seventh intercostal space along the posterior axillary line. Robotic port 3 was positioned in the eighth intercostal space just anterior to the paraspinal muscles. The access port was positioned in the ninth intercostal space triangulated between robotic port sites 1 and 2 (Fig. 28.13).

## Port Insertion and Positioning of the Robot

The robotic camera and a 12 mm Optiview trocar can be used as an alternative to using the 5 mm laparoscope with the Optiview trocar as demonstrated for the anterior mediastinal mass case. A 12 mm incision is made at the planned camera port site followed by guiding the robotic camera and 12 mm Optiview trocar into the thoracic cavity visualizing the layers of the chest wall until lung parenchyma is seen (Fig. 28.14).

**Fig. 28.14**  Thoracic
cavity entry using 12 mm
Optiview trocar with
robotic camera.
(**a**) Subcutaneous fat layer,
(**b**) muscle layer, (**c**) lung
parenchyma visualized

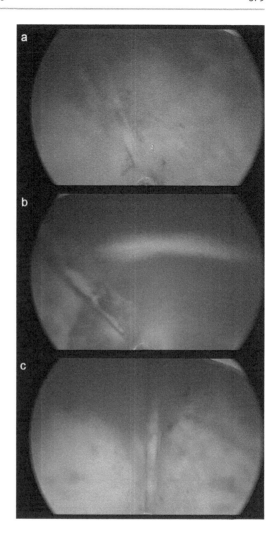

The carbon dioxide insufflation tube is connected to the 12 mm port to insufflate the pleural space for inspection of the thoracic cavity. Using the robotic camera for visualization, the 8 mm instrument cannulas are placed into robotic port sites 1, 2, and 3. Another 12 mm trocar is placed for assistance. Special care must be taken for posteriorly positioned ports to ensure the placement is anterior and lateral to the paraspinal muscles to avoid oozing. The OR table was turned 90° and the robot was then driven into operative field from cephalad direction perpendicular to the patient centered on the camera trocar as depicted in Fig. 28.15. The ports are then secured into the robotic arms. The 30-degree da Vinci camera is passed into the center camera port. The bipolar Maryland forceps was placed into the port site 1 followed by the Cadiere forceps into port sites 2 and 3. Energy for the bipolar Maryland forceps was set at 70 W for dissection due to proximity of the left vagus nerve and recurrent laryngeal nerve.

**Fig. 28.15** Robot position in respect to the patient for middle mediastinal cyst resection

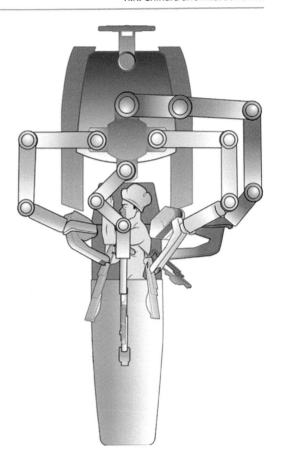

## Middle Mediastinal Cyst Excision Operative Steps

The lung is pushed away anteriorly using the Robotic arm 3 with the Cadiere forceps instrument to expose the aortopulmonary window (Fig. 28.16). The mediastinal pleura was entered using robotic arms 1 and 2 centered around the camera port to begin the dissection of the cyst away from vital structures starting with the aorta (Fig. 28.17). The assistance port is used for suctioning and retraction. As the dissection is carried medially towards the trachea, the left vagus and recurrent laryngeal nerve is visualized and preserved (Fig. 28.18). The cyst is then released from the trachea and esophagus. Blunt dissection is carried anteriorly, while retracting the cyst anteriorly and laterally away from the pulmonary artery (Fig. 28.19). Once the cyst is fully released, a sterile cut glove finger was placed into the apex of the thoracic cavity via the access port and the specimen was then removed (Fig. 28.20). The middle mediastinal cyst was lined with mesothelial cells on pathology consistent with a pericardial cyst.

**Fig. 28.16** Exposure of the aortopulmonary window

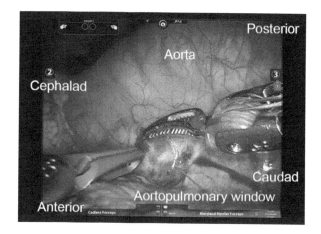

**Fig. 28.17** Dissection of the middle mediastinal cyst away from the aorta

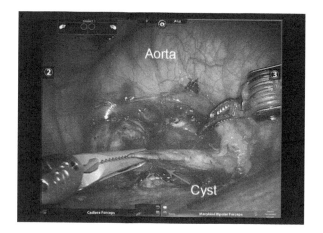

**Fig. 28.18** Identification of the left recurrent laryngeal nerve for preservation

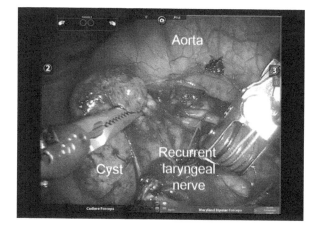

**Fig. 28.19** Dissection of the cyst away from the pulmonary artery

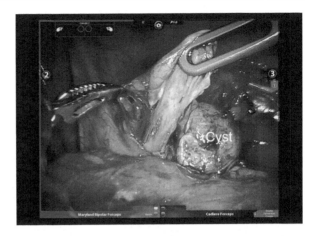

**Fig. 28.20** Removal of the specimen using a cut sterile glove finger

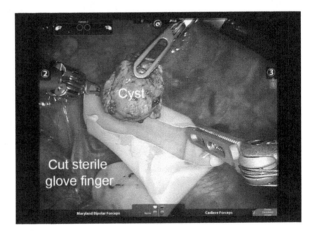

## Approach to Posterior Mediastinal Pathology

Posterior mediastinal pathology for which robotic surgery has been utilized include: neurofibroma, schwannoma, neuroganglioma, ganglioneuroblastoma, paraganglioma, and foregut duplication cysts. Mediastinal foregut duplications cysts are rare entities with case reports found in literature regarding the use of robotics in the pediatric population. Foregut duplication cysts can be approached in similar fashion to middle mediastinal cysts with the exception of not resecting the medial common mucosal wall aspect of the cyst. The most common adult posterior mediastinal masses are neurogenic in origin.

## Indications for Robotic Posterior Mediastinal Mass Resection

Most adult neurogenic tumors are benign; however, resection is usually indicated in adults due to rare risk of possible malignancy [5]. There are preoperative considerations for posterior mediastinal solid tumors of neurogenic origin. Patients with suspicious history of hypertension are evaluated for a functional paraganglioma with serum and urine catecholamine levels, as hypertensive crisis is a possible fatal intraoperative complication without the appropriate preoperative medical treatment [5]. Patients with neurogenic posterior mediastinal masses are screened for compressive spinal cord symptoms because such symptoms may indicate an intraspinal involvement of the tumor. Magnetic resonance imaging is the diagnostic study of choice in patients with neurogenic tumors, as this imaging modality is sensitive for identifying dumbbell- or hourglass-shaped involvement of the intravertebral foramen [5]. If intraspinal involvement is detected, a combined Robotic and posterior neurosurgical approach may be necessary to treat the tumor.

## Posterior Mediastinal Mass Case Scenario

A 59 year-old man presents to clinic with previously discovered posterior mediastinal mass that has grown in size on comparison computed tomography scan (Fig. 28.21). Past medical history was significant for previous lymphoma that had been in remission for over 5 years and well-controlled hypertension. The patient denied headaches, palpitations, or night sweats. He was referred for CT-guided biopsy of this mass with pathology consistent with Schwannoma. Magnetic resonance imaging was obtained, which did not identify involvement of the intravertebral foramen. After discussion about continued surveillance versus resection, the patient elected for surgical management.

## Surgical Equipment Used

- da Vinci 0-degree camera
- EndoWrist® (Monopolar) Permanent cautery spatula
- EndoWrist® (Bipolar) Maryland forceps or EndoWrist® One™ Vessel sealer
- EndoWrist® Grasper - Cadiere Forceps × 2
- EndoWrist® Clip Applier — small and large
- Kittner roll gauze sponges
- 12 mm Optiview trocar × 2
- 8 mm instrument cannula × 2
- Endo Catch bag

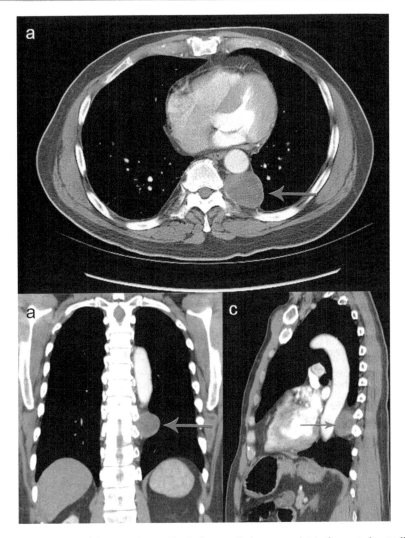

**Fig. 28.21** CT scan of the posterior mediastinal mass. *Red arrows* point to the posterior medias-tinal mass. The mass abuts the aorta. (**a**) Axial, (**b**) coronal, (**c**) sagittal

## Patient Positioning

Posterior mediastinal mass resections are approached from either right or left lateral decubitus position depending on the location of the mass. For the case example, the patient was placed in the right lateral decubitus position. The OR table is placed in reverse direction for the positioning of the patient to accom-modate the robot.

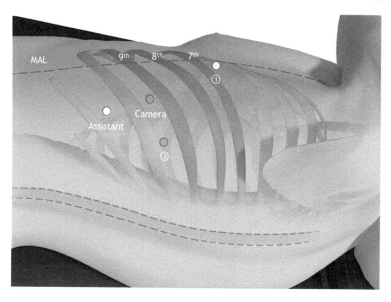

**Fig. 28.22** Port placement for the posterior mediastinal mass resection. Camera port is *blue*. Robotic port 1 is *yellow*. Robotic port 2 is *green*. Assistant port is *white*

A 3-arm robot was chosen for the case along with an access port. Port sites were determined by preoperative imaging studies (Fig. 28.21). In our example, a posterior mediastinal mass was found in the left pleural cavity at the level of the T9 vertebral body. The camera port was positioned along the mid-axillary line ninth intercostal space. Robotic port 1 was positioned in the anterior axillary line seventh intercostal space. Robotic port 2 was marked for the posterior axillary line in the ninth intercostal space. The accessory port was marked for the tenth intercostal space triangulated between robotic ports 1 and 2 (Fig. 28.22).

## Port Insertion and Positioning of the Robot

Entry into the thoracic cavity is accomplished using the Optiview trocar technique as described in the anterior and middle mediastinal sections of this chapter. The pleural cavity is insufflated with carbon dioxide and assessed. The 8 mm instrument cannulas were placed into the robotic port sites previously marked robotic port sites 1 and 2. The OR table was turned 90° and the robot was then driven into operative field from anterior-cephalad direction to the patient centered on the camera trocar as depicted in Fig. 28.23. The ports are then secured into the robotic arms. The 0-degree da Vinci camera is passed into the center camera port. The monopolar cautery spatula was placed into the port site 2 followed by the Cadiere forceps into port site 1. The monopolar cautery was set at 30 W and bipolar Maryland forceps set at 70 W.

**Fig. 28.23** Robot
positioning in respect to
patient for posterior
mediastinal mass resection

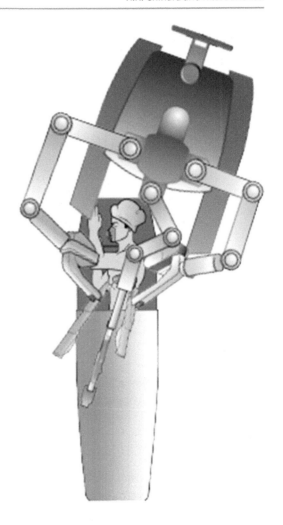

## Posterior Mediastinal Mass Excision Operative Steps

The assistant retracted the lung anteriorly through the access port using a blunt grasper holding a Kittner roll gauze sponge to expose the posterior mediastinal mass. Robotic arm 1 was used to retract the mass superiorly to initiate dissection of the mass along inferiorly using the monopolar cautery spatula (Fig. 28.24). Feeding vessels are identified during the dissection (Fig. 28.25). An intercostal artery branch was found feeding the tumor inferiorly requiring clips (Fig. 28.26). Bipolar Maryland forceps were used once dissection became close to the vertebral foramina to decrease risk of nerve stimulation. The dissection is carried over medially with continued retraction using robotic arm 1 medially and anteriorly (Fig. 28.27). The anteromedial dissection is accomplished with retraction of the aorta using robotic arm 1 and the assistant retracting the mass posteriorly (Fig. 28.28). A plane of dissection can be created easily along a rib when identified (Fig. 28.29).

**Fig. 28.24** Identification of intrathoracic mass and inferior dissection plane. Courtesy of Dr. Allan Pickens, Emory University, Atlanta, GA

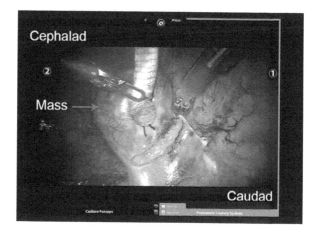

**Fig. 28.25** Identification of a tumor feeding blood vessel. Courtesy of Dr. Allan Pickens, Emory University, Atlanta, GA

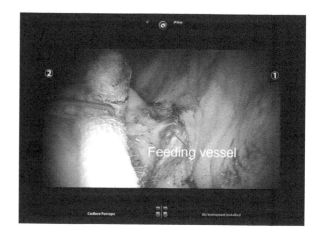

**Fig. 28.26** Identification, dissection, and clipping of an intercostal artery feeding the tumor. Courtesy of Dr. Allan Pickens, Emory University, Atlanta, GA

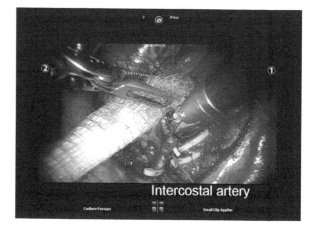

**Fig. 28.27** Posterior and lateral dissection of the mass. The robotic arm retracts the mass anteriorly. Courtesy of Dr. Allan Pickens, Emory University, Atlanta, GA

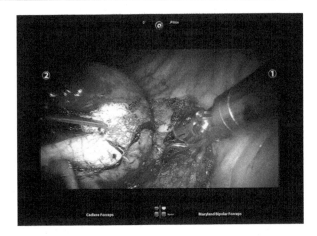

**Fig. 28.28** Anterior and medial dissection of the mass. The robotic arm retracts the aorta anteriorly. The suction irrigator retracts the tumor posteriorly. Courtesy of Dr. Allan Pickens, Emory University, Atlanta, GA

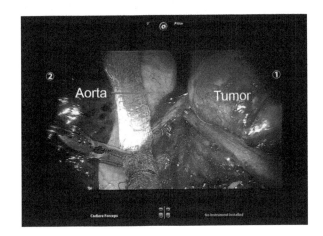

**Fig. 28.29** Identification of a rib as a marker for the posterior dissection plane. Courtesy of Dr. Allan Pickens, Emory University, Atlanta, GA

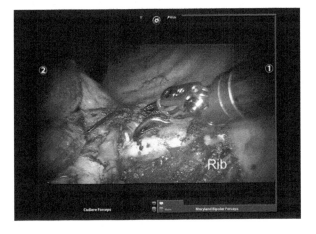

**Fig. 28.30** Removal
of the specimen using
the Endo Catch bag
through the access port.
Courtesy of Dr. Allan
Pickens, Emory University,
Atlanta, GA

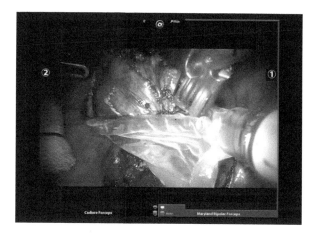

After the last tumor attachments are ligated in the superior and medial aspect of the dissection, the Endo Catch bag was placed into the assistant port with subsequent removal of the specimen after the trocar incision was enlarged (Fig. 28.30). Pathology revealed a schwannoma.

## Summary

Robotic assistance is useful for navigating and dissecting the mediastinal space. Vision is enhanced by using the binocular 3D robotic camera and dexterity is improved by having surgical instruments with superior articulation in respect to thoracoscopic equipment. Future advances in equipment and technology such as haptic feedback would further increase the value of robotic assistance in delicate mediastinal operations. The most common indicated procedures were presented in detail for the anterior, middle, and posterior mediastinal lesions. The principles learned from these examples may be applied to a wide variety of lesions in the mediastinum. Continued research and development in robotic surgical techniques will be necessary as advances are made to current robotic technology.

## References

1. Straughan DM, Fontaine JP, Toloza EM. Robotic-assisted videothoracoscopic mediastinal surgery. Cancer Control. 2015;22(3):326–30.
2. Demmy TL, et al. Multicenter VATS experience with mediastinal tumors. Ann Thorac Surg. 1998;66(1):187–92.
3. Ye B, et al. Video-assisted thoracoscopic surgery versus robotic-assisted thoracoscopic surgery in the surgical treatment of Masaoka stage I thymoma. World J Surg Oncol. 2013;11:157.
4. Yuan ZY, et al. Comparative study of video-assisted thoracic surgery versus open thymectomy for thymoma in one single center. J Thorac Dis. 2014;6(6):726–33.

5. Juanpere S, et al. A diagnostic approach to the mediastinal masses. Insights Imaging. 2013;4(1):29–52.
6. Asaf BB, Kumar A, Vijay CL. Robotic excision of paraesophageal bronchogenic cyst in a 9-year-old child. J Indian Assoc Pediatr Surg. 2015;20(4):191–3.
7. Toker A, et al. Resection of a bronchogenic cyst in the first decade of life with robotic surgery. Interact Cardiovasc Thorac Surg. 2014;19(2):321–3.
8. Bacchetta MD, et al. Resection of a symptomatic pericardial cyst using the computer-enhanced da Vinci Surgical System. Ann Thorac Surg. 2003;75(6):1953–5.
9. Ribet ME, Copin MC, Gosselin B. Bronchogenic cysts of the mediastinum. J Thorac Cardiovasc Surg. 1995;109(5):1003–10.

# Robotic-Assisted Cardiac Surgery

Emmanuel Moss and Michael E. Halkos

## Introduction

The first robotic-assisted cardiac surgery using the da Vinci robot was reported by Carpentier in 1998 [1]. Due to the complexity of cardiac surgical operations, broader adoption of robotic technology has been slower than other specialties; however, with recent technological advances and concurrent growing demand for less invasive procedures, it is now becoming a significant part of the armamentarium for the treatment of cardiac valvular and coronary artery disease. In addition to smaller incisions and improved cosmesis, the theoretical advantages of minimally invasive cardiac surgery include shorter intensive care unit and hospital stays, decreased perioperative complications, and an earlier return to the patient's preoperative functional level. The da Vinci Surgical system (Intuitive Surgical, Sunnyvale, CA, USA) is currently the only robotic surgical system approved by the United States Food and Drug Association (FDA) for cardiac surgery. When used in conjunction with advanced perfusion systems, myocardial protection strategies, and operative techniques that have been developed to facilitate minimal access surgery, the advantages of robotic technology over video-assisted thoracoscopic surgery are clear. The robot's high definition 3-dimensional video capabilities and articulating wrists with six degrees of freedom allow for greater freedom of movement in an enclosed space compared to traditional long-shafted instruments. Robotic-assisted cardiac surgical procedures have been shown safe and feasible, with a growing body of literature

E. Moss, M.D., M.Sc., F.R.C.S.C.
Division of Cardiac Surgery, Jewish General Hospital/McGill University 3755 Cote Ste Catherine Ave, Suite A-520, Montreal, H3T 1E2 Quebec, Canada
e-mail: emmanuel.moss@mcgill.ca

M.E. Halkos, M.D., M.Sc. (✉)
Cardiothoracic Surgery, Emory University School of Medicine,
Medial Office Tower, 6th Floor, 550 Peachtree Street NE, Atlanta, GA 30308, USA
e-mail: mhalkos@emory.edu

© Springer International Publishing AG 2018
A.D. Patel, D. Oleynikov (eds.), *The SAGES Manual of Robotic Surgery*,
The SAGES University Masters Program Series, DOI 10.1007/978-3-319-51362-1_29

showing equivalent or improved perioperative outcomes. In addition to describing robotic-assisted coronary bypass surgery, this chapter will outline robotic technology's application to other cardiac surgical procedures.

## Robotic-Assisted Coronary Artery Bypass

Minimally invasive coronary bypass has evolved significantly over the last decade. While most techniques have in common a sternal sparing approach, technological advances have allowed surgeons to progress from left internal mammary harvest (LIMA) under direct vision (minimally invasive direct coronary artery bypass, MIDCAB), to endoscopic harvest (endoscopic atraumatic coronary artery bypass, ENDOACAB), to robotic harvest (robotic-assisted coronary artery bypass), and finally to totally endoscopic robotic CABG (TECAB). With the exception of TECAB, these other procedures include a LIMA-LAD anastomosis performed through a left mini-thoracotomy incision of varying sizes. Robotic-assisted Coronary Artery Bypass Graft (CABG) is our preferred technique, giving the operator superior visualization and control during LIMA harvest compared to other techniques, while avoiding the complexity of TECAB. The anastomosis is performed through a small 4–5 cm non-rib-spreading anterior minithoracotomy, located precisely over the Left Anterior Descending (LAD) target.

## Patient Selection

As with many minimally invasive procedures, patient selection is key to a successful operation. Surgeons must ensure that coronary anatomy is suitable by evaluating the caliber and quality of the LAD, anticipating the planned anastomotic site as it relates to LIMA length, and recognizing an intramyocardial LAD path. A patient's body habitus is important as well, with ideal candidates being non-obese and having large thoracic cavities and generous intercostal spaces. In obese patients, landmarks can be obscured making port placement difficult, and intrathoracic adipose tissue can obscure the LIMA and LAD leading to a difficult harvest and anastomosis, respectively.

While robotic-assisted CABG is limited to bypassing only 1 or 2 vessels (LAD and/or a Diagonal branch), the technique can be applied more broadly to patients that may benefit from a hybrid coronary revascularization (HCR) strategy. The criteria include an LAD target that is appropriate for a mini-thoracotomy approach, and non-LAD targets that are appropriate for percutaneous coronary intervention (PCI).

## Indications/Contraindications

Indications for robotic-assisted CABG are similar to traditional CABG. There are two typical patient subgroups that are often referred for this procedure. (1) Relatively low-risk patients with LAD disease that wish to avoid sternotomy, but seek the durability of CABG. (2) Sicker patients, considered high risk for sternotomy, with

LAD disease that is not suitable for PCI or medical therapy. These patients may or may not have non-LAD targets that require PCI. These subgroups can present with either isolated LAD disease or with multivessel CAD that have anatomy amenable to a hybrid revascularization approach.

Contraindications include left chest adhesions (e.g. previous thoracotomy, empyema, etc.), morbid obesity, untreated left subclavian stenosis, and severe lung disease. Coronary anatomical contraindications include an LAD that is intramyocardial, small, heavily calcified, or diffusely diseased. Some of the above are relative contraindications, dependent on surgeon experience and patient comorbidities.

## Operating Room Setup and Overview of Operative Technique

The patient is placed in supine position with the left chest lifted 15°. The left shoulder hangs over the edge of the bed, with the left arm hanging slightly below the table to maximize mobility of the right (superior) robotic arm (Fig. 29.1). The chest, abdomen, and legs of the patient are prepared as for traditional CABG, with the sterile field extended to the left midaxillary line to allow for placement of the robotic arms. Three incisions are made in the left chest to accommodate the robotic camera and two robotic arms (Figs. 29.2 and 29.3). These are placed in approximately the third, fifth, and seventh intercostal spaces, although it may vary slightly depending on individual patient anatomy.

Figure 29.4 shows a sketch of a typical operating room setup. The robot is advanced from the patient's right side to allow docking onto the left-sided ports. The assistant and scrub nurse must have an unhindered view of the vision cart, which should be placed toward the patient's feet. A monopolar spatula instrument is placed in the right arm and a microbipolar forceps in the left. The chest is insufflated with carbon dioxide at 12 mmHg to push the mediastinal structures medial and inferior, facilitating visualization. This pressure can be adjusted depending on the patient's response to the controlled pneumothorax. Most commonly, anesthesia

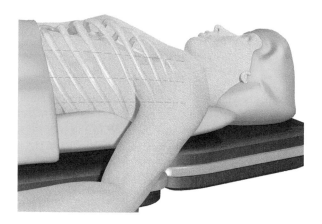

**Fig. 29.1** Arm positioning during robotic-assisted CABG. The patient's left shoulder lies flush with the edge of the operating room table, while the arm is allowed to hang below the plane of the table. This allows the superior (*right*) robotic arm to move freely

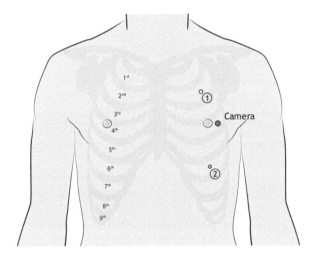

**Fig. 29.2** Port placement. Superior port (*green*) is placed in the second or third intercostal space. The camera port (*blue*) is placed at the midsternal level, at a 45° angle to the chest wall. The inferior port (*green*) in placed in the sixth or seventh intercostal space at the level of the distal third of the clavicle

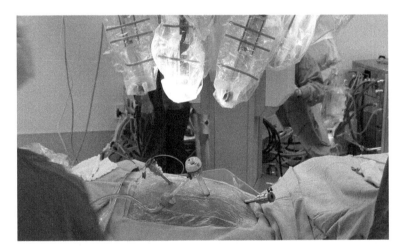

**Fig. 29.3** View of the left hemithorax following port placement

adjustments with preload and minor vasopressors allow for hemodynamic stability during the entire LIMA harvest. Figure 29.5 shows a thoracoscopic view of the LIMA and surrounding structures. With the robot docked, the surgeon can then proceed to the robotic console and complete the LIMA harvest, pericardiotomy, and identification of the LAD. Following administrating heparin, the LIMA is divided between clips and hemostasis along the entire mammary bed is verified.

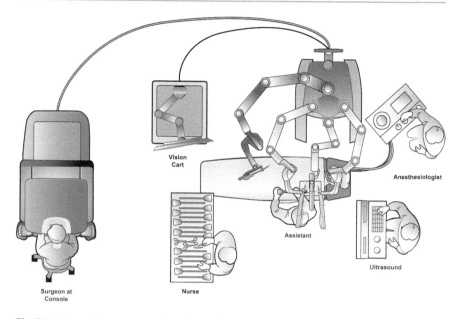

**Fig. 29.4** Operating room setup for robot-assisted CABG

**Fig. 29.5** Thoracoscopic
view of proximal LIMA
and surrounding structures

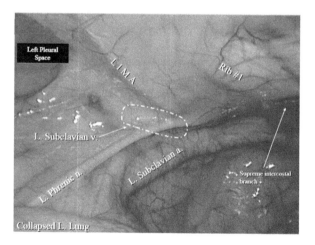

The robot is then undocked and the minithoracotomy site is planned. Under thoracoscopic guidance, a long spinal needle is passed through the anterior chest wall, allowing precise localization of both the ideal LAD anastomotic site and the intercostal space most appropriate to approach it. This allows for a precise 3–4 cm anterolateral thoracotomy. Once the thoracotomy is performed, a soft-tissue retractor (Medtronic, Minneapolis, MN) is placed between the ribs to provide optimal visualization without requiring the use of a rib-spreader. After retrieving the LIMA into the field, an endoscopic coronary stabilizer (Octopus Nuvo, Medtronic

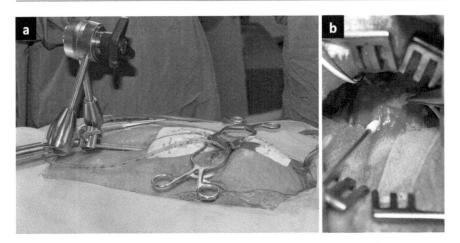

**Fig. 29.6** (a) Soft tissue and self-retaining retractors are shown, with the Medtronic Nuvo stabilizer inserted through the lower robotic port site. (b) LIMA-LAD anastomosis being completed with the aid of an intracoronary shunt

Corporation, Minneapolis, Minn) is advanced through the left robotic arm incision and the hand-sewn off-pump LIMA-LAD anastomosis is performed (Fig. 29.6). Use of an intracoronary shunt is recommended to avoid any concerns for hemodynamic or electrical instability during the anastomosis. Subsequently, hemostasis is verified, the stabilizer is removed, the lung reinflated over the LIMA pedicle, and the incisions are closed, leaving a left pleural chest tube that is placed through the left arm port. Unlike traditional cardiac surgery, patients can often be extubated in the operating room, which facilitates "fast track" transfer out of the intensive care unit and discharge home on postoperative day 2 or 3. Figure 29.7 shows a photograph at 1 month following surgery.

## Outcomes

Compared to other techniques for minimally invasive CABG, we believe that the technique described above provides the optimal combination of practicality, patient benefit, and operating room efficiency, as well as potential broad adoption for the cardiac surgical community [2]. In 2014, we published our institution's series of 307 patients who underwent robotic-assisted CABG surgery, with low mortality (1.3%), a low incidence of perioperative stroke (0.3%), and a 97% graft patency [3]. Nesher and colleagues published a series of 146 consecutive robotic-assisted CABGs with a 96.3% patency rate and no in-hospital deaths [4]. More recently, Harskamp and colleagues performed a meta-analysis including 941 patients who had undergone either minimally invasive CABG or PCI with drug eluting stents and found a lower incidence of repeat revascularization with CABG and otherwise

**Fig. 29.7** Photograph taken 1 month following surgery

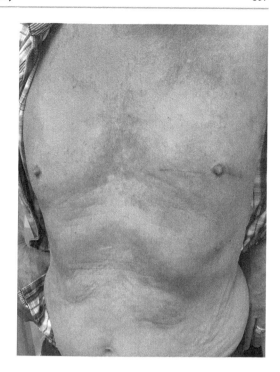

similar clinical outcomes [5]. Compared to traditional CABG, patients benefit from a shorter length of hospital stay, faster recovery, decreased need for perioperative blood transfusions, and similar cardiovascular outcomes at 3 years [6].

## Robotic-Assisted TECAB

While robotic-assisted LIMA harvest is an excellent alternative to traditional CABG, some surgeons have transitioned to robot-assisted totally endoscopic coronary artery bypass (TECAB). The benefits of TECAB are even less tissue trauma because the need for a minithoracotomy is obviated, and the potential to perform multivessel bypass, including to the circumflex and right coronary territories. The first significant series, reported by Mohr and colleagues in 2001, described 27 patients who underwent LIMA harvest and endoscopic LIMA to LAD anastomosis using the da Vinci telemanipulation system [7]. In 2006, a multicenter FDA-sanctioned trial demonstrated the safety and efficacy of TECAB using the da Vinci system in 85 patients [8]. Since that time, select centers have begun to routinely perform multivessel TECAB with excellent results [9]. Unfortunately, the complexity of the operation and significant learning curve result in prolonged operative times and possibly increased complication rates early in a surgeon's experience [10, 11]. Despite overall good short-term results with TECAB, the aforementioned shortcomings have limited its widespread adoption.

## Hybrid Coronary Revascularization (HCR)

With good outcomes for minimally invasive CABG surgery established, increasing demand for minimally invasive procedures, mediocre outcomes with saphenous vein grafts, and improved results with PCI using drug-eluting stent (DES), hybrid coronary revascularization (HCR) has garnered attention from surgeons, cardiologists, and patients. While many minimally invasive CABG techniques have been described, we feel that robotic-assisted CABG is ideally suited for this revascularization strategy in appropriate coronary anatomy. The robotic-assisted LIMA harvest is a relatively simple and short procedure and allows for versatility when combining with non-LAD PCI, which can be performed either before, after, or concomitantly with the surgical procedure. HCR has been repeatedly shown to be safe and effective compared to traditional CABG and PCI [5, 12–16]. When compared to CABG, several reports have found excellent results with shorter ICU and hospital lengths of stay, decreased perioperative blood loss and transfusion requirements, shorter intubation time, and improved patient satisfaction. These advantages are likely particularly true in sicker or potentially frail patients. Although long-term outcomes with HCR are lacking, this strategy is quickly becoming an important option in the revascularization algorithm.

## Robotic-Assisted Mitral Valve Surgery

Technological advances with the cardiopulmonary bypass machine and perfusion options have fueled a growing trend toward less invasive "sternal sparing" mitral valve surgery. Compared to sternotomy, these techniques are associated with shorter hospital lengths of stay, improved cosmesis, and earlier return to preoperative functional level. Non-sternotomy mitral valve surgery began with larger right anterior minithoracotomy approaches and subsequently evolved to smaller incision minithoracotomy incisions with videoscopic assistance. While these techniques are still commonly used today with excellent reported results in high volume centers, they are hindered by technical challenges such as limited visualization, the mandatory use of long-shafted instruments, and considerations for patient anatomy (e.g. small chests, obesity, etc.). Robotic-assisted surgery addresses these limitations with unparalleled visualization and improved dexterity that enables application to a broader range of patients. Since the first report of robotic-assisted mitral valve surgery in 1999 [17], the technique has evolved considerably and can now be performed in minimally traumatic fashion with five 1–2 cm incisions in the right thorax, in addition to a 3 cm femoral cutdown for venous and arterial cannulation [18]. Several high volume academic centers have since published excellent results using robotic-assisted techniques for mitral valve surgery [19–21].

As technology and surgical techniques have improved, surgeons have been able to safely perform concomitant procedures such as atrial septal defect repair, tricuspid valve repair or replacement, and the Cox-Maze procedure for atrial fibrillation. These procedures are generally well-tolerated, adding little increase in morbidity.

## Other Robotic-Assisted Intracardiac Procedures

The versatility and improved dexterity that is delivered by robotic technology has led to its use in a variety of other cardiac surgical procedures.

*Isolated atrial fibrillation surgery*—This therapy can be delivered using either transcatheter or surgical techniques. Robotic technology alleviates some of the technical challenges of the thoracoscopic Maze procedure while minimizing morbidity. In 2009, Rodriguez and colleagues reported their series of stand-alone robotic atrial fibrillation surgery, with an 88% freedom from AF at 6-month in 71 patients [22].

*Atrial septal defect closure*—Robotic-assisted repair of isolated atrial septal defects is now performed routinely in adults. A series reported by Bonaros and colleagues described 17 patients, ranging from 16 to 35 years of age, with excellent safety and efficacy outcomes [23].

*Epicardial pacemaker lead placement*—When transcatheter left ventricular pacemaker lead placement is not feasible, the surgical procedure is traditionally performed via a left anterior minithoracotomy. Performing the procedure with robotic-assistance has been proposed by some surgeons as an option to decrease procedure-related morbidity in a patient population that often suffers from multiple comorbidities [24].

*Intracardiac mass resection*—There are limited numbers of reports describing resection of left and right atrial tumors; however, the procedure is being performed frequently in actual practice. One of the first series was reported in 2005 by Murphy and colleagues [25]. We recently reported the largest series to date of left atrial tumor resection and showed it to be safe with improved perioperative outcomes [26].

*Pediatric cardiac surgery*—Although robotic technology is better suited for use in adult cardiac surgery, robotic-assisted procedures have been described in children as well. In 2005, Suematsu and colleagues reported six successful vascular ring repairs and nine patent ductus arteriosis closures [27].

## Conclusion

It is up to cardiac surgeons to adapt to the growing demand for less invasive procedures without compromising short- or long-term patient outcomes. Robotic technology allows surgeons to perform gold standard interventions through smaller incisions with minimal morbidity. Despite the slow early adoption in cardiac surgery, robotic cardiac surgical procedures are now routinely performed in many centers across North America and around the world. This has been due to pioneering work by innovative surgeons and their numerous publications over the last decade demonstrating safety and efficacy in the application of robotic technology to cardiac surgery.

# References

1. Carpentier A, Loulmet D, Aupècle B, Kieffer JP, Tournay D, Guibourt P, et al. [Computer assisted open heart surgery. First case operated on with success]. C R Acad Sci III. 1998;321(5):437–42.
2. Halkos ME, Vassiliades TA, Myung RJ, Kilgo P, Thourani VH, Cooper WA, et al. Sternotomy versus nonsternotomy LIMA-LAD grafting for single-vessel disease. Ann Thorac Surg. 2012;94(5):1469–77.
3. Halkos ME, Liberman HA, Devireddy C, Walker P, Finn AV, Jaber W, et al. Early clinical and angiographic outcomes after robotic-assisted coronary artery bypass surgery. J Thorac Cardiovasc Surg. 2014;147(1):179–85.
4. Nesher N, Bakir I, Casselman F, Degrieck I, De Geest R, Wellens F, et al. Robotically enhanced minimally invasive direct coronary artery bypass surgery: a winning strategy? J Cardiovasc Surg (Torino). 2007;48(3):333–8.
5. Harskamp RE, Williams JB, Halkos ME, Lopes RD, Tijssen JGP, Ferguson TB, et al. Meta-analysis of minimally invasive coronary artery bypass versus drug-eluting stents for isolated left anterior descending coronary artery disease. J Thorac Cardiovasc Surg. 2014;148(5):1837–42.
6. Harskamp RE, Bagai A, Halkos ME, Rao SV, Bachinsky WB, Patel MR, et al. Clinical outcomes after hybrid coronary revascularization versus coronary artery bypass surgery: a meta-analysis of 1,190 patients. Am Heart J. 2014;167(4):585–92.
7. Mohr FW, Falk V, Diegeler A, Walther T, Gummert JF, Bucerius J, et al. Computer-enhanced "robotic" cardiac surgery: experience in 148 patients. J Thorac Cardiovasc Surg. 2001;121(5):842–53.
8. Argenziano M, Katz M, Bonatti J, Srivastava S, Murphy D, Poirier R, et al. Results of the prospective multicenter trial of robotically assisted totally endoscopic coronary artery bypass grafting. Ann Thorac Surg. 2006;81(5):1666–75.
9. Bonaros N, Schachner T, Lehr E, Kofler M, Wiedemann D, Hong P, et al. Five hundred cases of robotic totally endoscopic coronary artery bypass grafting: predictors of success and safety. Ann Thorac Surg. 2013;95(3):803–12.
10. Bonatti J, Schachner T, Bonaros N, Öhlinger A, Danzmayr M, Jonetzko P, et al. Technical challenges in totally endoscopic robotic coronary artery bypass grafting. J Thorac Cardiovasc Surg. 2006;131(1):146–53.
11. Bonaros N, Schachner T, Wiedemann D, Oehlinger A, Ruetzler E, Feuchtner G, et al. Quality of life improvement after robotically assisted coronary artery bypass grafting. Cardiology. 2009;114(1):59–66.
12. Kiaii B, McClure RS, Stewart P, Rayman R, Swinamer SA, Suematsu Y, et al. Simultaneous integrated coronary artery revascularization with long-term angiographic follow-up. J Thorac Cardiovasc Surg. 2008;136(3):702–8.
13. Gao C, Yang M, Wu Y, Wang G, Xiao C, Liu H, et al. Hybrid coronary revascularization by endoscopic robotic coronary artery bypass grafting on beating heart and stent placement. Ann Thorac Surg. 2009;87(3):737–41.
14. Reicher B, Poston RS, Mehra MR, Joshi A, Odonkor P, Kon Z, et al. Simultaneous "hybrid" percutaneous coronary intervention and minimally invasive surgical bypass grafting: feasibility, safety, and clinical outcomes. Am Heart J. 2008;155(4):661–7.
15. Kon ZN, Brown EN, Tran R, Joshi A, Reicher B, Grant MC, et al. Simultaneous hybrid coronary revascularization reduces postoperative morbidity compared with results from conventional off-pump coronary artery bypass. J Thorac Cardiovasc Surg. 2008;135(2):367–75.
16. Halkos ME, Vassiliades TA, Douglas JS, Morris DC, Rab ST, Liberman HA, et al. Hybrid coronary revascularization versus off-pump coronary artery bypass grafting for the treatment of multivessel coronary artery disease. Ann Thorac Surg. 2011;92(5):1695–701;discussion 1701–2.
17. Falk V, Autschbach R, Krakor R, Walther T, Diegeler A, Onnasch JF, et al. Computer-enhanced mitral valve surgery: toward a total endoscopic procedure. Semin Thorac Cardiovasc Surg. 1999;11(3):244–9.

18. Murphy DA, Miller JS, Langford DA, Snyder AB. Endoscopic robotic mitral valve surgery. J Thorac Cardiovasc Surg. 2006;132(4):776–81.

19. Nifong LW, Rodriguez E, Chitwood WR. 540 consecutive robotic mitral valve repairs including concomitant atrial fibrillation cryoablation. Ann Thorac Surg. 2012;94(1):38–42;discussion 43.

20. Suri RM, Burkhart HM, Daly RC, Dearani JA, Park SJ, Sundt TM, et al. Robotic mitral valve repair for all prolapse subsets using techniques identical to open valvuloplasty: establishing the benchmark against which percutaneous interventions should be judged. J Thorac Cardiovasc Surg. 2011;142(5):970–9.

21. Mihaljevic T, Pattakos G, Gillinov AM, Bajwa G, Planinc M, Williams SJ, et al. Robotic posterior mitral leaflet repair: neochordal versus resectional techniques. Ann Thorac Surg. 2013;95(3):787–94.

22. Rodriguez E, Cook RC, Chu MWA, Chitwood Jr WR. Minimally invasive bi-atrial cryomaze operation for atrial fibrillation. Oper Tech Thorac Cardiovasc Surg. 2009;14(3):208–23.

23. Bonaros N, Schachner T, Oehlinger A, Ruetzler E, Kolbitsch C, Dichtl W, et al. Robotically assisted totally endoscopic atrial septal defect repair: insights from operative times, learning curves, and clinical outcome. Ann Thorac Surg. 2006;82(2):687–93.

24. Kamath GS, Balaram S, Choi A, Kuteyeva O, Garikipati NV, Steinberg JS, et al. Long-term outcome of leads and patients following robotic epicardial left ventricular lead placement for cardiac resynchronization therapy. Pacing Clin Electrophysiol. 2011;34(2):235–40.

25. Murphy DA, Miller JS, Langford DA. Robot-assisted endoscopic excision of left atrial myxomas. J Thorac Cardiovasc Surg. 2005;130(2):596–7.

26. Moss E, Halkos ME, Miller JS, Murphy DA. Comparison of endoscopic robotic versus sternotomy approach for the resection of left atrial tumors. Innovations (Phila). 2016;11(4):274–7.

27. Suematsu Y, Mora BN, Mihaljevic T, del Nido PJ. Totally endoscopic robotic-assisted repair of patent ductus arteriosus and vascular ring in children. Ann Thorac Surg. 2005;80(6):2309–13.

# Index